Dysphagia Assessment and Treatment Planning

A TEAM APPROACH

Third Edition

Dysphagia Assessment and Treatment Planning

A TEAM APPROACH

Third Edition

Rebecca Leonard, PhD
Katherine A. Kendall, MD

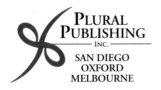

PLURAL
PUBLISHING
INC.

SAN DIEGO
OXFORD
MELBOURNE

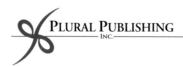

5521 Ruffin Road
San Diego, CA 92123

e-mail: info@pluralpublishing.com
Web site: http://www.pluralpublishing.com

49 Bath Street
Abingdon, Oxfordshire OX14 1EA
United Kingdom

Library of Congress Cataloging-in-Publication Data

Dysphagia assessment and treatment planning : a team approach / [edited] by
Rebecca Leonard and Kathy Kendall.—Third edition.
     p. ; cm.
 Includes bibliographical references and index.
 ISBN-13: 978-1-59756-525-7 (alk. paper)
 ISBN-10: 1-59756-525-3 (alk. paper)
 I. Leonard, Rebecca, editor of compilation. II. Kendall, Katherine (Staff physician),
editor of compilation.
 [DNLM: 1. Deglutition Disorders—diagnosis. 2. Deglutition Disorders—therapy.
3. Patient Care Planning. 4. Patient Care Team. WI 250]

 616.3'23—dc23
                              2012049160

Contents

Introduction

The second edition of this book, published in 2008, remains relatively current even four years later. But, of course, areas that were just emerging at that time have since been expanded, and new ideas, both in assessment and treatment, have been elaborated, as well. Our goal is to update topic areas previously addressed, and to expand on some that we felt received too little attention in the earlier edition(s). We hope that the text will be of interest to all medical and other professionals involved in dysphagia. Particular target audiences may be new to the area, for example, graduate students in speech-language pathology, new clinicians, medical specialists who have just been recruited to participate in a dysphagia team, or are hoping to develop a team.

Information not covered extensively in the second edition, including the bedside swallow evaluation, noninvasive instruments sometimes used in these evaluations, and surveys and rating scales commonly used in dysphagia practice, are addressed in this version of the text (Chapter 8). Throughout the text, pros and cons are considered with respect to both assessment and treatment techniques in an attempt to encourage clinicians to think critically about the tools or strategies they implement in their own clinical practices. The chapter on neurogenic dysphagia (Chapter 4) has undergone extensive revision, with a great deal

more emphasis on CVA, and more definitive discussions of other causes of dysphagia in the general area of "neurogenic" disorders. Similarly, the chapter on dysphagia related to head and neck pathology (Chapter 3) has been revised to address current treatment approaches and the growing information base regarding their implications, for example, radiation, chemotherapy, as well as new surgical approaches, for swallowing function. New information regarding eosinophillic esophagitis and its importance in pediatric populations is addressed in Chapter 9. Chapter 12, concerned with radiological evaluation, addresses the extremely important issue of radiation exposure to patients undergoing fluoroscopic evaluation, and stresses the need for maximizing the study's potential. In addition, the anterior-posterior screen, and the value it brings to the usual dynamic swallow study (DSS), is emphasized. The unique value of endoscopy, and differences between endoscopic and fluoroscopic observations of the same events, for example, aspiration, penetration, are reviewed in Chapter 11. In Chapter 18, substantial effort has been expended to provide updates on existing treatments, including behavioral, medical, and surgical, and to introduce new information that has become available since the previous edition. Chapters by our nursing (Chapter 7), dietetic (Chapter 10) and physician specialists (Chapters 1 to 6,

12, and 13) explain critical features of their practices, but also underscore the huge value of these individuals in a team approach to dysphagia. New media clips provide good and representative examples of both normal and disordered swallowing, and instrumental approaches to swallowing assessment.

The use of objective measures from fluoroscopy studies has greatly influenced our team's approach to dysphagia, and is again a particular focus of the text (Chapters 14 through 17). New tools that are inexpensive and easy to use have greatly streamlined the measurement process, and these are considered in depth. In addition, the applications of objective measurements and other data in assessing individual patient's risk and potential for oral feeding are elaborated. A media clip illustrating the making of measures is included. In our experience, making measures of the mechanical events that comprise a swallow is one of the very best ways to learn about swallowing; we strongly encourage readers to give them a try!

We are particularly excited about the inclusion of a workbook with the text that will provide structured exercises accompanying each chapter. The idea for the workbook, authored primarily by Dr. Barkmeier-Kramer, reflects our interest in providing thoughtful practice assignments to readers and, in particular, students new to this specialty area, that may help further their understanding of dysphagia. Readers have suggested that a clarification of terms not likely to be familiar to this audience would be constructive, and we agree. Consequently, for each chapter, we attempt to define new concepts and terminology as they are introduced. This should reduce confusion and lead to improved comprehension. A text that contains excellent information, piques readers' interest and enthusiasm, and, at the same time, is readily comprehensible, is our goal.

The unique value of this book, reflected in each edition to date, is the multidisciplinary approach presented. Too often, speech-language pathologists function clinically with insufficient interaction with, or understanding of, the roles of other professionals involved, or potentially involved, with their patients. Dysphagia, perhaps of all the disorders SLPs deal with, is best approached by a team. It is no one specialist's domain; rather, clinicians from a number of specialties offer resources that are both novel and necessary to optimal patient management. This text incorporates the information, tools, and views of a multidisciplinary dysphagia team that works together on a daily basis. Knowledge bases and skill sets unique to each member are relied on and valued in our joint effort to manage patients. The same commitment and talent these specialists offer to their colleagues and patients is evident in the text, reflecting both a responsibility for, and pleasure in, educating others. For the last 25 years, a "team approach" has characterized our approach to dysphagic patients, and we feel strongly that this represents current "best practice." Our own team has been smaller or larger, represented at one time by only 2 SLPs and a radiologist and, more recently, by the many specialists who have contributed to this text. But, in every case, what we learned, and were able to offer to patients benefited directly from our interaction and collaboration. We hope readers will learn from, and enjoy, this new edition.

Acknowledgments

The authors gratefully acknowledge the significant contributions of the members of the U.C. Davis Dysphagia Team, current and past, to this project. Their enthusiasm, skill, knowledge, and insights, were key in their function as members of our Team, and in this text. We are extremely fortunate to have developed and maintained a strong interdisciplinary and collegial approach to the management of our patients, and we firmly believe that it represents an excellent model for professionals involved in the management of dysphagia. We also thank those patients and volunteer subjects who have shared their time and efforts willingly and generously to our collection of normative and other data.

Contributors

Jacqui Allen, MD, FRACS
Otolaryngologist, Senior Lecturer
University of Auckland
North Shore Hospital
Takapuna, Auckland
New Zealand
Chapters 4 and 12

Peter C. Belafsky, MD, MPH, PhD
Professor & Director, Center for Voice
    & Swallowing
Department of Otolaryngology
University of California, Davis
Sacramento, California
Chapters 5, 6, and 13

Margie Crandall, RN, PhD
Family Health Nursing
Pediatric Clinical Nurse Specialist
Chapter 9

Susan J. Goodrich, MS
Senior Speech Pathologist
Voice Speech Swallow Center
Department of Otolaryngology
University of California, Davis
Sacramento, California
Chapters 5, 6, and 13

Katherine A. Kendall, MD, FACS
Associate Professor
Division of Otolaryngology
University of Utah
Salt Lake City, Utah
Chapters 1, 2, 3, 17, and 18

Rebecca Leonard, PhD
Professor, Department of
    Otolaryngology/Head and Neck
    Surgery

Director, Voice-Speech-Swallowing
    Center
University of California, Davis
Sacramento, California
Chapters 11, 14, 16, 17, and 18

Beverly Lorens, MS, RD
Senior Clinical Dietition, retired
Food and Nutition Services
University of California Davis Medical
    Center
Sacramento, California
Academy of Nutrition and Dietics
Chapter 10

Susan McKenzie, MS
Senior Speech Pathologist
Voice and Swallowing Center
University of California Davis
Sacramento, California
Chapters 14, 15, 17, and 18

Janet Pitcher, RN, MSN, PNP
Child Neurology Nurse Practioner
University of California Davis Medical
    Center
Sacramento, California
Chapter 9

Catherine J. Rees Lintzenich, MD
Associate Professor Otolaryngology
    Head and Neck Surgery
Center for Voice and Swallowing
    Disorders
Wake Forest University School of
    Medicine
Winston-Salem, North Carolina
Chapters 5, 6, and 13

Ann E. F. Sievers
ENT Nurse Expert
Department of Patient Care Services
 and Otolaryngology
University of California, Davis
Sacramento, California
Chapter 7

Alice I. Walker, MS
Senior Speech Language Pathologist
Department of Otolaryngology
University of California, Davis
Sacramento, California
Chapter 8

1

Anatomy and Physiology of Deglutition

Katherine A. Kendall

Familiarity with the anatomy and physiology of normal deglutition enables a more focused approach to the evaluation of patients with disordered swallowing. This chapter discusses those head and neck structures involved in swallowing and reviews the sequence of events resulting in a successful swallow.

The oral cavity, oropharynx, and esophagus can be thought of as a series of expanding and contracting chambers, divided by muscular sphincters. Propulsion of a bolus through this part of the alimentary tract is the result of forces or positive pressure developed behind the bolus, as well as a vacuum or negative pressure developed in front of the bolus. The creation of propulsion pressures depends on the sequential contraction and expansion of the chambers of the upper aerodigestive tract and the competency of the sphincters dividing the chambers. Any disturbance in the functional elements or coordination of this system is likely to result in less efficient transfer of a bolus from the oral cavity to the stomach, resulting in dysphagia. Swallowing involves coordination of the sequence of activation and inhibition for more than 25 pairs of muscles in the mouth, pharynx, larynx, and esophagus. An understanding of how the structures of the head and neck interact and coordinate to bring about the propulsion pressures required for normal swallowing is vital for the clinician involved in the evaluation and treatment of patients with swallowing complaints.

For simplicity, the act of deglutition is traditionally divided into four parts: the preparatory phase, the oral phase, the pharyngeal phase, and the esophageal phase (Dodds, Stewart, & Logemann, 1990; Miller, 1982).

PREPARATORY PHASE

The preparatory phase of swallowing includes mastication of the bolus, mixing it with saliva, and dividing the food for transport through the pharynx and esophagus. The preparatory phase takes place in the oral cavity, the first chamber in the swallowing system. This oral preparatory phase of swallowing is almost entirely voluntary and can be interrupted at any time.

During bolus preparation, facial muscles play a role in maintaining the bolus on the tongue and between the teeth for chewing. Specifically, the obicularis oris muscle, the circular muscle of the lips, maintains oral competence and can be considered as the first sphincter of the swallowing system. The buccinator muscle of the cheek contracts to keep the bolus from pooling in the pockets formed by the gingival buccal sulcii. These muscles receive neural input from the facial nerve or cranial nerve VII (Figures 1–1A, 1–1B, and 1–1C).

Most of the movement and positioning of the bolus is carried out by the tongue muscles. In addition to four intrinsic muscles, the tongue has four extrinsic muscles: the genioglossus, palatoglossus, styloglossus, and hyoglossus muscles (Figure 1–2). Along with the genioglossus muscle, the intrinsic muscles act primarily to alter the shape and tone of the tongue while the other three extrinsic muscles aid in

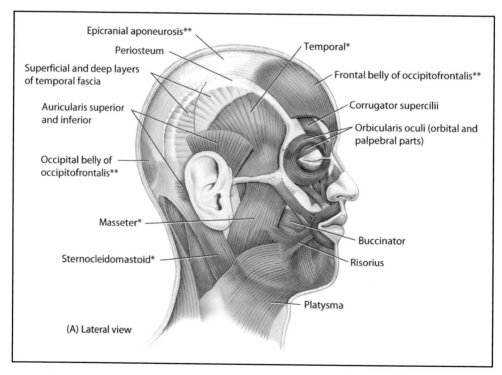

Figure 1–1. A. Facial musculature shown in relationship to muscles of head and neck. (Reprinted with permisison from Moore & Dalley, 2006, *Clinically Oriented Anatomy*, 5th ed., Williams and Wilkins, Balitmore, p. 934, figure 7-4a.) *(continues)*

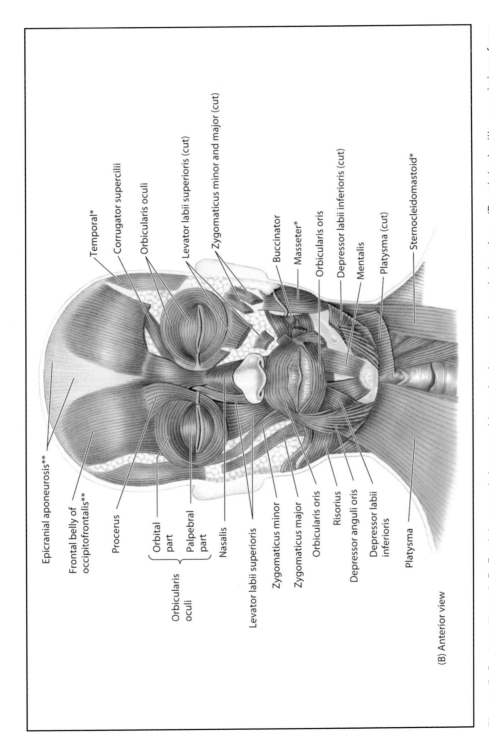

Epicranial aponeurosis**

Frontal belly of
occipitofrontalis**

Procerus

Orbicularis
oculi
{ Orbital
part
Palpebral
part

Nasalis

Levator labii superioris

Zygomaticus minor

Zygomaticus major

Orbicularis oris

Risorius

Depressor anguli oris

Depressor labii
inferioris

Platysma

Temporal*

Corrugator supercilii

Orbicularis oculi

Levator labii superioris (cut)

Zygomaticus minor and major (cut)

Buccinator

Masseter*

Orbicularis oris

Depressor labii inferioris (cut)

Mentalis

Platysma (cut)

Sternocleidomastoid*

(B) Anterior view

Figure 1-1. (continued) **B.** Facial musculature and buccinator muscle, anterior view. (Reprinted with permisssion from Moore & Dalley, 2006, *Clinically Oriented Anatomy,* 5th ed., Williams and Wilkins, Baltimore, p. 935, figure 7-4b.) (continues)

3

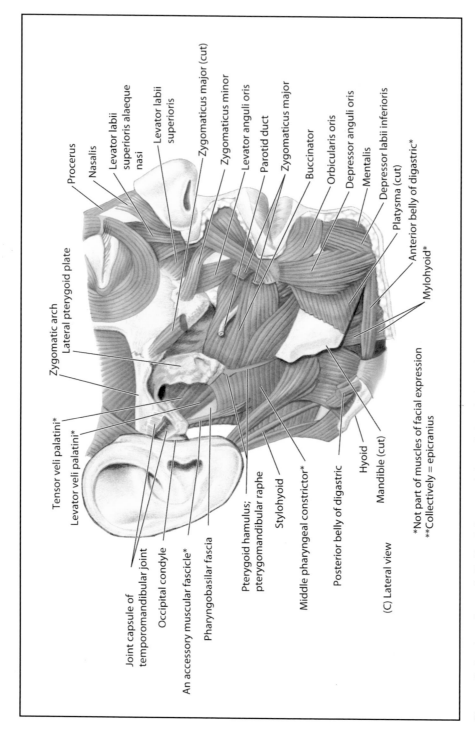

Figure 1-1. *(Continued)* **C.** Facial musculature, lateral view. (Reprinted with permissison from Moore & Dalley, 2006, *Clinically Oriented Anatomy,* 5th ed., Williams and Wilkins, Baltimore, p. 935, figure 7-4c.)

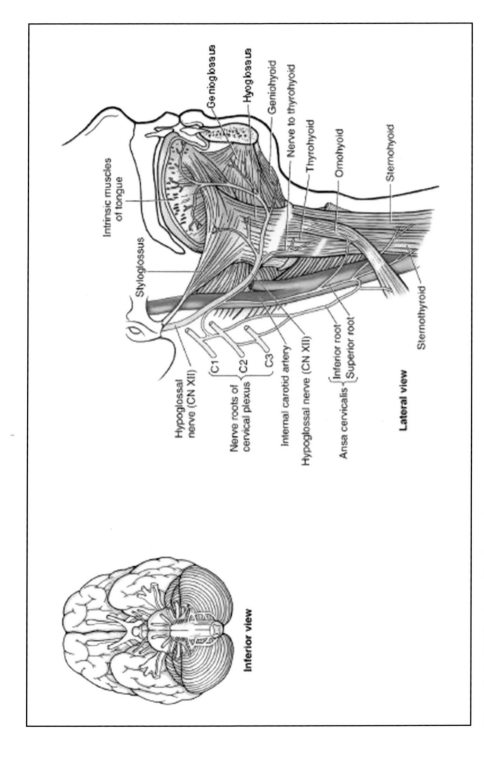

Figure 1–2. Distribution of the hypoglossal nerve. (Reprinted with permission from Moore & Dalley, 2006. *Clinically Oriented Anatomy*, 5th ed., Williams and Wilkins, Baltimore, p. 1154, figure 9-15.)

the positioning of the tongue relative to other oral cavity and pharyngeal structures. Cranial nerve XII, the hypoglossal nerve, carries the motor nerve fibers that innervate both the intrinsic and extrinsic tongue muscles, except for the palatoglossus muscle (see Figure 1–2). A branch of the pharyngeal plexus from the vagus nerve (X) sends motor fibers to innervate the palatoglossus muscle. A high density of mechanoreceptors within and on the surface of the tongue indicates that the tongue is an important sensory region for determining the size of the bolus. Sensory information from the anterior two-thirds of the tongue is carried back to central swallowing control centers via the lingual nerve, a branch of the trigeminal nerve or cranial nerve V. Sensory information from the posterior one-third of the tongue is carried centrally by the glossopharyngeal nerve, or cranial nerve IX (Figures 1–3A and 1–3B). During the bolus preparatory phase of deglutition, the posterior part of the tongue elevates against the soft palate, which pushes downward to keep the bolus from escaping prematurely into the pharynx. The palate is the second sphincter in the swallowing system. Contraction of the palatoglossus muscles approximates the palate and posterior tongue, effectively closing the back of the oral cavity (Figures 1–4 and 1–5).

Mastication of the bolus involves the masseter muscles, the temporalis muscles, and the medial and lateral pterygoid muscles. This muscle group is known collectively as the muscles of mastication. Motor fibers controlling the contraction of these muscles are carried in branches of the trigeminal nerve (V) (Figure 1–6).

Salivation

Successful transfer of a food bolus from the oral cavity into the esophagus requires the mixing of the bolus with saliva. Saliva lubricates and dilutes the bolus to a consistency proper for swallowing. Saliva contains two major types of protein secretion: an enzyme for digesting starches, and mucous for lubricating purposes. Normal salivary secretion ranges from 1.0 to 1.5 liters per day. Saliva also plays an important role in maintaining healthy oral tissues. It is bacteriostatic and controls the pathogenic bacteria normally present in the oral cavity that are largely responsible for dental caries. The secretion of saliva is controlled by the salivatory nucleus in the brainstem. The nerve fibers of the parasympathetic nervous system carry signals from the salivatory nucleus to the salivary glands (Guyton, 1981).

ORAL PHASE

The bolus is propelled from the oral cavity to the pharynx during the oral phase of swallowing. The top of the tongue is placed on the superior alveolar ridge behind the maxillary central incisors. Voluntary opening of the pharynx then begins with elevation of the soft palate and depression of the posterior tongue (see video clip of straw drinking in the materials folder for Chapter 1). In this way, there is expansion of the posterior oral cavity and a chute forms down which the bolus moves into the pharynx. Elevation of the palate occurs as a result of contraction of the levator veli palatini muscle. The levator veli palatini muscle receives motor innervation from the

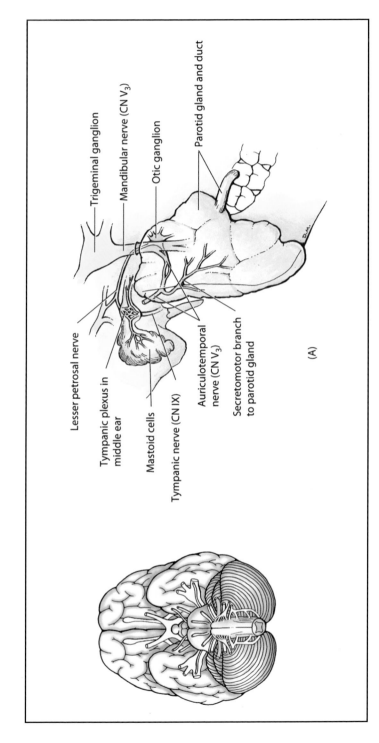

Figure 1–3. Distribution of the glossopharyngeal nerve (*A, B*). (Reprinted with permissison from Moore & Dalley, 2006, *Clinically Oriented Anatomy,* 5th ed., Williams and Wilkins, Baltimore, p. 1148, figure 9-10B.) *(continues)*

Trigeminal ganglion

Mandibular nerve (CN V$_3$)

Otic ganglion

Parotid gland and duct

Lesser petrosal nerve

Tympanic plexus in middle ear

Mastoid cells

Tympanic nerve (CN IX)

Auriculotemporal nerve (CN V$_3$)

Secretomotor branch to parotid gland

(A)

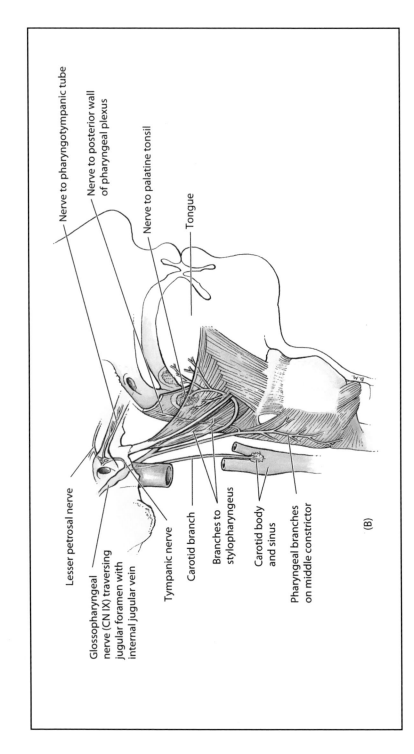

Nerve to pharyngotympanic tube

Nerve to posterior wall of pharyngeal plexus

Nerve to palatine tonsil

Tongue

Lesser petrosal nerve

Glossopharyngeal nerve (CN IX) traversing jugular foramen with internal jugular vein

Tympanic nerve

Carotid branch

Branches to stylopharyngeus

Carotid body and sinus

Pharyngeal branches on middle constrictor

(B)

Figure 1–3. *(continued)*

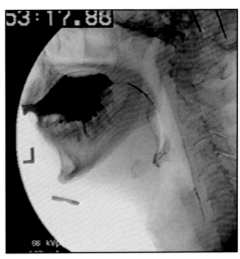

Figure 1–4. Lateral view from videofluorscopic swallowing study: oral phase. Note bolus in the oral cavity on the superior surface of the tongue. Palate closes against tongue base to close posterior oral cavity from oropharynx.

vagus nerve (X) via the pharyngeal plexus. The hyoglossus muscle (XII), and to a lesser extent the styloglossus muscle (XII), are active in posterior tongue depression. The anterior half of the tongue is then pressed against the maxillary alveolar ridge and the anterior half of the hard palate in rapid sequence, moving the bolus posteriorly on the dorsum of the tongue. Contraction of the obicularis oris and buccinator muscles prevents pressure escape forward, out of the mouth, or laterally.

Soft palate elevation allows the bolus to pass through the tonsillar pillars. Once the soft palate is fully elevated, it contacts the adjacent pharyngeal walls in a valving action that acts to prevent penetration of the bolus or escape of air pressure into the nasopharynx. The side walls of the nasopharynx, consisting of the superior pharyngeal constrictor muscle, also appose one another to make a more forceful closure of the nasopharynx (Figure 1–7). Motor nerve fibers from the vagus nerve (X) via the pharyngeal plexus innervate the superior pharyngeal constrictor and palatal musculature. The hyoid bone is then

moderately elevated in preparation for the pharyngeal phase of swallowing. Early hyoid bone elevation occurs primarily as a result of mylohyoid muscle contraction. Motor innervation of the mylohyoid muscle comes from a branch of the trigeminal nerve (V).

The muscles involved in the oral phase of swallowing represent three anatomical regions: the suprahyoid suspensory muscles (which affect the position of the posterior tongue and thus, the hyoid bone), the muscles surrounding the tonsillar pillars, and the muscles involved in the closure of the nasopharynx. Muscles that discharge during the oral phase of swallowing include the muscles of the face, (specifically, those within the lips and cheeks), the tongue muscles, the superior pharyngeal constrictor, the styloglossus, stylohyoid, geniohyoid, and mylohyoid muscles with the palatoglossus and palatopharyngeus muscles demonstrating their maximal activity later. The anterior and posterior bellies of the digastric muscle participate in the subsequent elevation of the hyoid and larynx (see Figures 1–1A, 1–1B, and 1–6E).

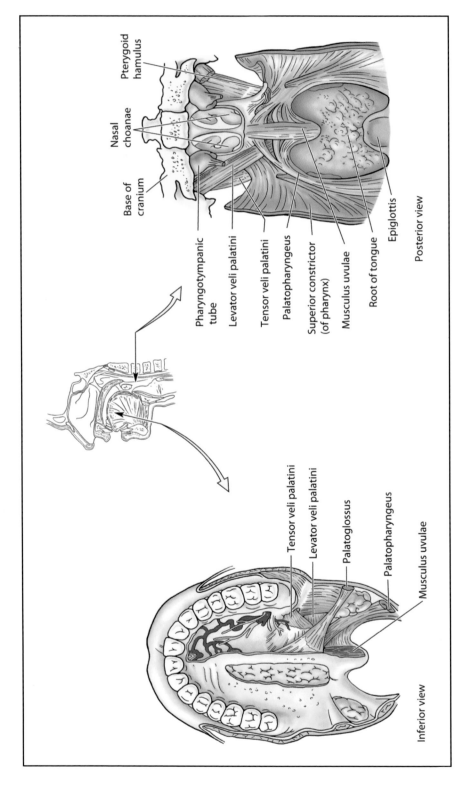

Figure 1-5. Palate and oral cavity (posterior view) showing tensor veli palatini and levator veli palatini muscles. (Reprinted with permission from Moore & Dalley, 2006, *Clinically Oriented Anatomy*, 5th ed., Williams and Wilkins, Baltimore, p. 829, figure 8-45.)

Pterygoid hamulus

Nasal choanae

Base of cranium

Pharyngotympanic tube

Levator veli palatini

Tensor veli palatini

Palatopharyngeus

Superior constrictor (of pharynx)

Musculus uvulae

Root of tongue

Epiglottis

Posterior view

Tensor veli palatini

Levator veli palatini

Palatoglossus

Palatopharyngeus

Musculus uvulae

Inferior view

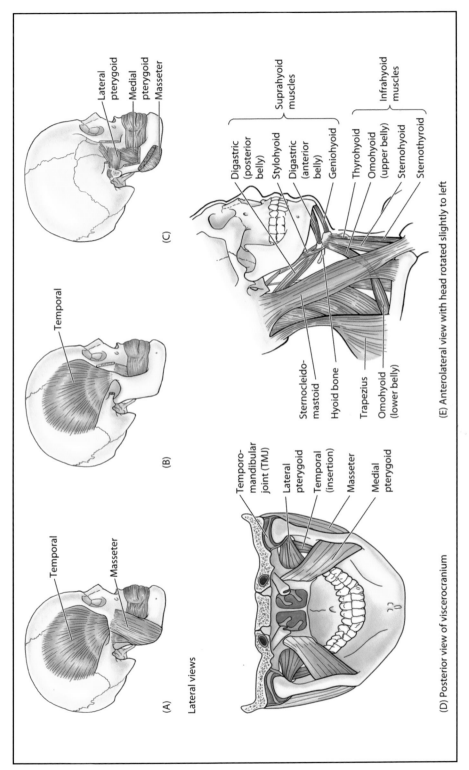

Figure 1-6. Muscles of mastication (**A–E**). (Reprinted with permission from Moore & Dalley, 2006. *Clinically Oriented Anatomy*, 5th ed., Williams and Wilkins, Baltimore, p. 988, figure 7-12.)

(A)

Temporal

Masseter

Lateral views

(B)

Temporal

(C)

Lateral pterygoid

Medial pterygoid

Masseter

(D) Posterior view of viscerocranium

Temporomandibular joint (TMJ)

Lateral pterygoid

Temporal (insertion)

Masseter

Medial pterygoid

(E) Anterolateral view with head rotated slightly to left

Digastric (posterior belly)

Stylohyoid

Digastric (anterior belly)

Geniohyoid

Suprahyoid muscles

Thyrohyoid

Omohyoid (upper belly)

Sternohyoid

Sternothyroid

Infrahyoid muscles

Sternocleidomastoid

Hyoid bone

Trapezius

Omohyoid (lower belly)

11

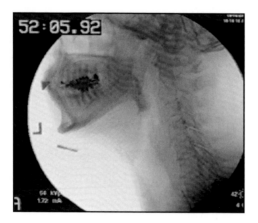

Figure 1-7. Lateral view from videofluoroscopic swallowing study: oropharyngeal phase. Note elevation of palate and contact with posterior pharyngeal wall.

PHARYNGEAL PHASE

Passage of food through the pharynx and into the esophagus occurs during the pharyngeal phase of swallowing. Respiration and swallowing must be coordinated during this portion of the swallow, since both functions occur through the common portal of the pharynx, but not simultaneously. Because respiration must cease during the pharyngeal phase of deglutition, the central control of pharyngeal swallowing must involve an efficient, automatic mechanism. The pharyngeal phase of swallowing is also involuntary and, once initiated, the pharyngeal phase is an irreversible motor event.

At the onset of the pharyngeal phase of swallowing, the tongue carries the bolus into the oropharynx as the entire posterior mass of the tongue is rolled backward on the hyoid bone, while maintaining the bolus on the tongue surface. The mandibular muscles (medial and lateral pterygoid muscles, masseter and temporalis muscles [V])

contribute to stabilization of the tongue base during the development of the tongue's pistonlike movements, and this stabilization of the tongue is more critical with boluses of thicker consistency. The mandible is held in a closed position during swallowing.

As the bolus is propelled posteriorly by the pistonlike movement of the tongue, the pharynx, as a whole, elevates and then contracts to create a descending peristaltic wave. Elevation of the pharynx occurs when the paired palatopharyngeus muscles contract (X). The walls of the pharyngeal chamber stiffen because of the sequential contraction of its three constrictors (X) (Figures 1–8, 1–9A, and 1–9B). As the oropharynx is a closed cavity at the time of bolus passage, the pressure generated by the tongue and pharyngeal walls provides a force that drives the bolus inferiorly. Simultaneously, the hyoid and larynx rise and are pulled forward under the root of the tongue by the contraction of the suprahyoid muscles. The larynx moves with the hyoid bone because it is attached to the hyoid bone by the thyrohyoid membrane and paired thyrohyoid muscles. This anterior movement of the larynx simultaneously protects the larynx from penetration by the bolus and expands the hypopharyngeal chamber causing a decrease of pressure in the pharyngoesophageal (PE) segment. This decrease in pressure in front of the bolus, along with the piston action of the tongue base against the pharyngeal constrictors, drives the bolus through the pharynx and into the upper esophagus (Figure 1–10).

As the bolus is driven inferiorly and the larynx begins to move forward, the epiglottis folds down over the laryn-

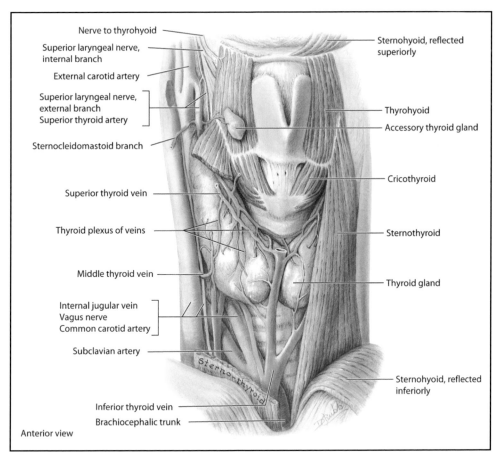

Nerve to thyrohyoid
Superior laryngeal nerve, internal branch
External carotid artery
Superior laryngeal nerve, external branch
Superior thyroid artery
Sternocleidomastoid branch
Superior thyroid vein
Thyroid plexus of veins
Middle thyroid vein
Internal jugular vein
Vagus nerve
Common carotid artery
Subclavian artery
Inferior thyroid vein
Brachiocephalic trunk
Anterior view

Sternohyoid, reflected superiorly
Thyrohyoid
Accessory thyroid gland
Cricothyroid
Sternothyroid
Thyroid gland
Sternohyoid, reflected inferiorly

Figure 1–8. Anterior view of larynx and neck. (Reprinted with permissison from Moore & Dalley, 2006, *Clinically Oriented Anatomy*, 3rd ed., Williams and Wilkins, Baltimore, p. 1085, figure 8-23.)

geal opening. The epiglottis moves from an upright to a horizontal position and then tips downward. This positional change of the epiglottis is caused mainly by elevation of the hyoid and larynx as well as by contraction of the paired thyrohyoid muscles followed by contraction of the intrinsic laryngeal muscles to close the vocal folds. The abductors of the vocal folds, the posterior cricoarytenoid muscles, are inhibited during this phase, ensuring closure of the vocal folds. The true and ventricular vocal folds play a major role in protecting the laryngeal vestibule by constricting the laryngeal aperture. The larynx closes anatomically from below upward: first, the vocal folds, then the vestibular folds, then the lower vestibule (approximation and forward movement of the arytenoids), and then the upper vestibule (horizontal position of the epiglottis that contacts the closed arytenoids). Opening of the larynx proceeds from above downward. Many of the mechanisms that contribute to airway protection also contribute to bolus transportation as closure of the larynx

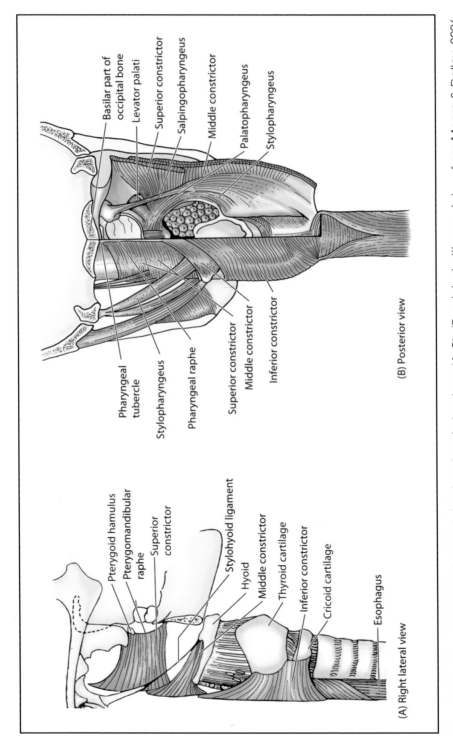

Figure 1-9. Muscles of the pharynx: lateral and posterior views (**A, B**). (Reprinted with permisisson from Moore & Dalley, 2006. *Clinically Oriented Anatomy*, 3rd ed., Williams and Wilkins, Baltimore, p. 1107, figure 8-6.)

Basilar part of occipital bone
Levator palati
Superior constrictor
Salpingopharyngeus
Middle constrictor
Palatopharyngeus
Stylopharyngeus

Pharyngeal tubercle
Stylopharyngeus
Pharyngeal raphe

Superior constrictor
Middle constrictor
Inferior constrictor

(B) Posterior view

Pterygoid hamulus
Pterygomandibular raphe
Superior constrictor
Stylohyoid ligament
Hyoid
Middle constrictor
Thyroid cartilage
Inferior constrictor
Cricoid cartilage
Esophagus

(A) Right lateral view

14

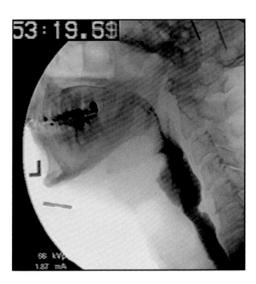

Figure 1-10. Lateral view from videofluoroscopic swallowing study: pharyngeal phase. Note anterior displacement of hyoid and larynx with expansion of the hypopharynx. The tongue base contacts the posterior pharyngeal wall. Subject has a cricopharyngeal bar at cervical vertebra 5.

creates pressures that promote movement of the bolus away from the larynx and into the upper esophagus (Figures 1–10 and 1–11) (Doty & Bosma, 1956; Kidder, 1995).

The upper esophageal sphincter, also known as the pharyngoesophageal (PE) segment, is the third and final sphincter involved in the oropharyngeal phase of deglutition. At rest, the sphincter is closed by the tonic contraction of the cricopharyngeus muscle. Inhibition of the tonic contraction, which results in relaxation and allows for opening of the sphincter, starts at the onset of the oropharyngeal phase of swallowing and lasts until the cricopharyngeus muscle becomes active and propels the bolus into the esophagus. Both laryngeal elevation (which pulls the cricoid lamina away from the posterior pharyngeal

wall) and cricopharyngeal relaxation are essential for normal opening of the pharyngoesophageal segment for bolus passage (see Figures 1–8, 1–10, and 1–11). Manometric studies have shown that a successful swallow depends on the tongue driving pressure and the negative pressure developed in the PE segment more than the peristaltic-like pressure of the constrictors (McConnel, 1988a, 1988b).

Once the bolus passes into the pharyngoesophageal segment, the force of the pharyngeal contraction eliminates the bolus from the level of the glottic opening. If pharyngeal contractions do not fully clear the bolus from the pharynx while the laryngeal aperture is closed, then a portion of the residual bolus will be aspirated upon reopening the airway and inhalation. The pharyngeal phase of swallowing is completed when the soft palate returns to its original position and the larynx is reopened for respiration.

The oropharyngeal phase of swallowing is a complex sequence of not only excitatory but also inhibitory events that take place generally in less than one second. It involves a set of striated muscles that always participate in the fundamental motor pattern. Electromyographic studies of the muscles involved in the pharyngeal phase of swallowing have delineated that the onset of swallowing begins with a contraction of the mylohyoid muscle. At the same time or very shortly thereafter, the anterior digastric and the pterygoid muscles begin to contract (innervation from the trigeminal nerve V) followed by the geniohyoid (XII), stylohyoid (VII), styloglossus (XII), posterior tongue, superior constrictor (X), palatoglossus (X), and palatopharyngeus

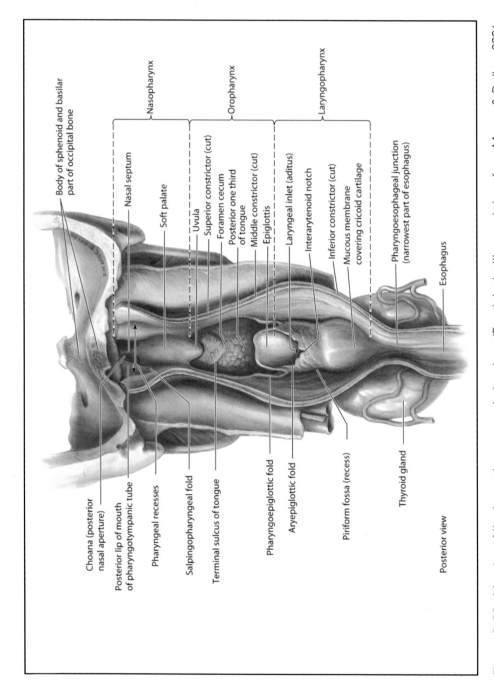

Figure 1-11. Muscles of the hypopharynx, posterior view. (Reprinted with permission from Moore & Dalley, 2006, *Clinically Oriented Anatomy*, 5th ed., Williams and Wilkins, Baltimore, p. 1102, figure 8-36.)

Body of sphenoid and basilar part of occipital bone

Nasal septum

Soft palate

Uvula

Superior constrictor (cut)

Foramen cecum

Posterior one third of tongue

Middle constrictor (cut)

Epiglottis

Laryngeal inlet (aditus)

Interarytenoid notch

Inferior constrictor (cut)

Mucous membrane covering cricoid cartilage

Pharyngoesophageal junction (narrowest part of esophagus)

Esophagus

Nasopharynx

Oropharynx

Laryngopharynx

Choana (posterior nasal aperture)

Posterior lip of mouth of pharyngotympanic tube

Pharyngeal recesses

Salpingopharyngeal fold

Terminal sulcus of tongue

Pharyngoepiglottic fold

Aryepiglottic fold

Piriform fossa (recess)

Thyroid gland

Posterior view

muscles (innervation from pharyngeal plexus: X). This group of muscles is called the "leading complex." The middle and inferior constrictor muscles then contract in an overlapping sequence. The oropharyngeal sequence ends when the wave of contraction reaches the upper esophageal sphincter. Electrophysiologic studies have shown that any background electrical activity in the swallowing muscles is inhibited with the onset of electrical activity in the leading complex and that inhibition is also found in the muscles of the leading complex just before they contract during swallowing (Doty, 1968; Doty & Bosma, 1956; Hrycyshyn & Basmajian, 1972; Miller, 1982).

Neural Control of the Pharyngeal Phase of Swallowing

The complex oropharyngeal muscle contraction and relaxation sequence that results in a successful swallow is triggered and controlled by a group of neurons within the reticular formation of the brainstem. These neurons are collectively referred to as a central pattern generator because they drive a sequence of complex but repetitive movements. The neurons of the central pattern generator directly stimulate several pools of motoneurons located in various brainstem cranial motor nuclei responsible for excitatory and inhibitory signals to the muscles of the oropharynx involved in swallowing. Peripheral feedback from sensory receptors in the muscles and mucosa of the pharynx is thought to modify the swallow sequence via direct input to the neurons of the central pattern gen-

erator. The central pattern generator can therefore be subdivided into three systems: an afferent input system from peripheral sensory mechanisms to the center, an efferent system corresponding to the motor outputs from the center to the muscles of the pharynx, and an organizing system corresponding to the interneuronal network within the brainstem that programs the motor pattern. Within the central pattern generator, some neurons may participate in activities other than swallowing such as respiration, mastication, and vocalization. Respiration is also likely controlled via a central pattern generator that coordinates with the swallowing pattern generator to integrate swallowing and respiratory functions (Altschuler, Bao, Bieger, Hopkins, & Miselis, 1989; Broussard & Altschuler, 2000; Doty & Bosma, 1956; Jean, 1990; Jean, Car, & Roman, 1975).

Afferent Input to the Central Pattern Generator

Branches from three cranial nerves: the trigeminal (V), the glossopharyngeal (IX), and the vagus (X) provide peripheral sensory feedback to the central pattern generator. The most sensitive oropharyngeal mucosal receptor regions for the stimulation of the swallowing sequence are innervated by fibers of the glossopharyngeal nerve via the pharyngeal plexus and by the superior laryngeal nerve (SLN) via the vagus nerve. Stimulation of the superior laryngeal nerve induces pure swallowing with a short latency, and this finding has led to the belief that the fibers of the SLN constitute the main afferent pathway involved in the initiation of swallowing.

Stimulation of the glossopharyngeal nerve facilitates swallowing, but alone, does not trigger the pure motor pattern of oropharyngeal swallowing (Doty& Bosma, 1956; Jean, 1990, 2001; Kessler & Jean, 1985; Miller, 1982; Ootani, Umezaki, Shin, & Murata, 1995).

Both the glossopharyngeal and the superior laryngeal nerve send fibers to the nucleus tractus solitarius (NTS) in the brainstem. The nucleus tractus solitarius is the principal sensory nucleus of the pharynx and esophagus and all the afferent fibers involved in initiating or facilitating swallowing converge in the nucleus tractus solitarius, mainly in the interstitial subdivision. Almost all of the nucleus tractus solitarius neurons that are involved in swallowing are activated with stimulation of the SLN. Most of the same NTS neurons can be activated by stimulation of the glossopharyngeal nerve. During swallowing, stimulation of sensory receptors in the pharynx by the posterior movement of the bolus is thought to initiate the involuntary pharyngeal phase of swallowing coordinated by the central pattern generator via the superior laryngeal nerve (Altschuler, 2001; Jean, 2001).

Although the oropharyngeal swallowing motor sequence is centrally organized, it can change in response to peripheral afferent information. The same irreversible muscle sequence is exhibited during swallowing of food, liquids or saliva but sensory information received from peripheral receptors can modulate the central network activity to adapt the swallowing motor sequence according to bolus consistency and size. Oropharyngeal muscle contraction timing, duration, and likely intensity, change with changes in bolus size and consistency. Sensory feedback

likely modifies the central program, by adjusting the motor outputs depending on the contents of the oropharyngeal tract. In other words, continuous sensory feedback from the pharynx may influence the neurons of the central pattern generator and thus modulate the central program. Considerable variability in the sequence of events that occurs during the pharyngeal phase of swallowing can be appreciated on videofluoroscopic studies of swallowing in normal individuals. Ablation of sensory feedback does not, however, disrupt sequential discharge of the cranial motor nerve fibers that occurs during swallowing (Hamdy et al., 1997; Hamdy, Mikulis, et al., 1999; Hamdy, Rothwell, et al., 1999; Jean, 2001; Kendall, 2002; Kendall, McKenzie, Leonard, Gonçalves, & Walker, 2000; Kendall, Leonard, & McKenzie, 2003).

Higher Cortical Input to the Central Pattern Generator

Higher cortical input is also thought to influence the coordination of swallowing by the central pattern generator. Many of the neurological disorders that result in dysphagia do not involve the brainstem but rather affect a wide range of supramedullary central neural regions. In addition, the fact that swallowing can be initiated voluntarily without stimulation of the pharynx by a bolus, such as in a "dry" swallow, indicates that input from cerebral cortex can trigger swallowing.

The mechanism by which higher cortical centers impact swallowing function is poorly understood, but it appears that a widespread network of brain regions participate in the control of swallowing. It is hypothesized that speech movements and perhaps the oral phase of swallowing rely on the lateral regions of the primary motor cortex and the premotor areas that are mapped somatotopically to the anterior vocal tract. There are a number of subcortical sites, including the corticofugal swallowing pathway, which can trigger or modify swallowing, in particular the internal capsule, subthalamus, amygdala, hypothalamus, substantia nigra, mesencephalic reticular formation and monoaminergic brain stem nuclei. Many studies of central swallowing control emphasize the importance of the inferior precentral gyrus. The anterior insula/claustrum and the cerebellum are also likely active in the initiation of voluntary swallowing (Barlow & Burton, 1990; Hamdy, Rothwell, Brooks, Bailey, Aziz, & Thompson, 1999; Kendall, Leonard, & McKenzie, 2003; Mosier & Bereznaya, 2001; Zald & Pardo, 1999).

Motor Output from the Central Pattern Generator

The main motor nuclei of the brainstem involved in deglutition are the hypoglossal (XII) motor nucleus and the nucleus ambiguus (X) (Figure 1–12). The cell bodies of the hypoglossal nucleus are organized myotopically, related to the different tongue muscles innervated by the hypoglossal motoneurons. The nucleus ambiguus is organized in a rostrocaudal pattern with respect to the motoneurons innervating the esophagus, pharynx and larynx. The esophageal motoneurons are localized in the rostral compact formation of the nucleus, the pharyngeal and soft palate motoneurons are in the intermediate semicompact formation and most of the laryngeal motoneurons are in the caudal loose formation of the nucleus. The organization scheme results in sequential firing of the motoneurons within the nucleus ambiguus during swallowing. Because the neurons in the nucleus fire sequentially during swallowing, each group of neurons in this chain may control more and more distal regions of the swallowing chain and be responsible for the successive firing behavior. In addition to excitatory drive, these motoneurons may also receive inhibitory inputs or have complex intrinsic properties that are activated by the swallowing sequence.

The motoneurons also exhibit extensive dendritic extensions into the adjacent reticular formation with a distinct pattern for each muscle group. Because the reticular formation is the location of the neuronal network that is the central pattern generator, these dendrites provide an anatomical basis for the interaction of the swallowing motoneurons and the neurons of the central pattern generator (Bieger & Hopkins, 1987; Doty, & Bosma, 1956; Gestreau, Dutschmann, Obled, & Bianchi, 2005; Lawn, 1966, 1988; Tomomune & Takata, 1988; Zoungrana, Amri, Car, & Roman, 1997).

It has been reported that when the motoneurons responsible for the beginning of the swallowing sequence fire, the neurons controlling the more distal parts of the tract are inhibited and their activity is delayed. In some cases, the activity of distal neurons is inhibited before the motor activity of proximal muscle groups is initiated. These inhibitory mechanisms may contribute directly to the sequential excitation of the motoneurons. Via mechanisms

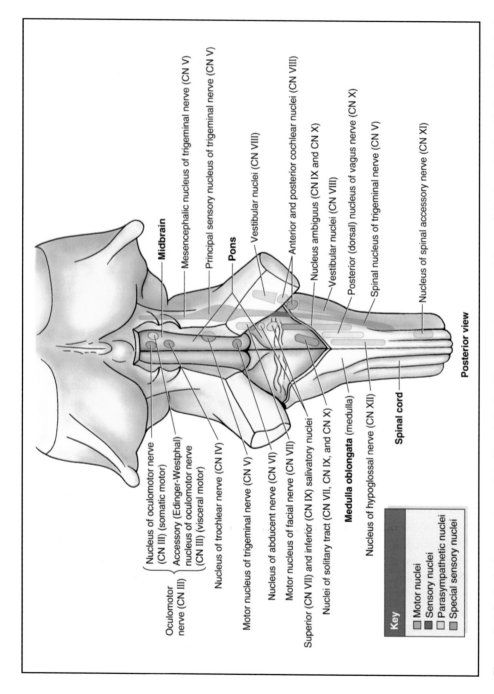

Figure 1-12. Brainstem motonuclei. (Reprinted with permission from Moore & Dalley, 2006, *Clinically Oriented Anatomy*, 5th ed., Williams and Wilkins, Baltimore, p. 1085, figure 8-23.)

Oculomotor nerve (CN III) { Nucleus of oculomotor nerve (CN III) (somatic motor)
Accessory (Edinger-Westphal) nucleus of oculomotor nerve (CN III) (visceral motor)

Nucleus of trochlear nerve (CN IV)

Motor nucleus of trigeminal nerve (CN V)

Nucleus of abducent nerve (CN VI)

Motor nucleus of facial nerve (CN VII)

Superior (CN VII) and inferior (CN IX) salivatory nuclei

Nuclei of solitary tract (CN VII, CN IX, and CN X)

Medulla oblongata (medulla)

Nucleus of hypoglossal nerve (CN XII)

Spinal cord

Posterior view

Midbrain

Mesencephalic nucleus of trigeminal nerve (CN V)

Principal sensory nucleus of trigeminal nerve (CN V)

Pons

Vestibular nuclei (CN VIII)

Anterior and posterior cochlear nuclei (CN VIII)

Nucleus ambiguus (CN IX and CN X)

Vestibular nuclei (CN VIII)

Posterior (dorsal) nucleus of vagus nerve (CN X)

Spinal nucleus of trigeminal nerve (CN V)

Nucleus of spinal accessory nerve (CN XI)

Key
- Motor nuclei
- Sensory nuclei
- Parasympathetic nuclei
- Special sensory nuclei

such as disinhibition or postinhibitory rebounds, the inhibitory connections may be at least partly responsible for the progression of the contraction wave (Jean, 2001).

Brainstem Interneurons Responsible for the Programming and Coordination of the Swallowing Sequence

The network of brainstem neurons thought to be responsible for the coordination of the pharyngeal swallowing motor sequence is made up of interneurons or premotoneurons. In general, central nervous system interneurons are identified by their connectivity with multiple areas of the brainstem and other areas of the central nervous system. Specifically, the physical connections of the central swallowing pattern generator interneurons provide an anatomic substrate for the integration of swallowing-related activities with airway-protective reflexes. The interneurons of the central swallowing pattern generator are thought to be located in two main brainstem areas, although some controversy exists regarding their exact locations. The dorsal swallowing group (DSG) of interneurons is located in the dorsal medulla within the nucleus tractus solitarius (NTS) and adjacent reticular formation. The neurons of the NTS receive and integrate sensory information. The ventral swallowing group (VSG) of interneurons is located in the ventrolateral medulla just above the nucleus ambiguus. The motor nuclei of the nucleus ambiguus control the pharyngeal muscles (Amirali, Tsai, Weisz, Schrader, & Sanders, 2001; Chiao, Larson, Yajima, Ko, & Kah-

rilas, 1994; Ezure, Oku, & Tanaka, 1993; Gestreau, Dutschmann, Obled, & Bianchi, 2005; Kessler & Jean, 1985; Larson, Yajima, & Ko, 1994).

Dorsal swallowing group interneurons are thought to be involved in triggering, shaping and timing the sequential swallowing motor pattern. These interneurons exhibit a sequential firing pattern that parallels the sequential motor pattern typical of deglutition, with considerable overlap between the sequential firing of the various neurons. The neurons in this part of the reticular formation have been shown to have direct connections with the motoneurons that drive the musculature of the pharynx involved in swallowing. Each dorsal swallowing group neuron may be directly activated by signals from peripheral afferent fibers originating in the corresponding part of the oropharynx under its control.

Stimulation of the superior laryngeal nerve results in initial activity, producing a single spike, in all of the dorsal swallowing group interneurons (see Figure 1–12). Some of the neurons in the dorsal swallowing group exhibit activity before the onset of the swallowing motor sequence which is continuous and is called "preswallowing activity." Those dorsal swallowing group interneurons that display preswallowing activity can be activated by stimulation of both the superior laryngeal nerve and the glossopharyngeal nerve. This pattern of activity observed in the dorsal swallowing group interneurons suggests that these neurons are involved in the initiation of swallowing. Cortical input into the swallowing central pattern generator has been found to involve the neurons of the dorsal swallowing group. The dorsal swallowing group neurons, therefore, receive convergent information from both cortical and peripheral inputs that trigger swallowing. Finally, the two hemicentral pattern generators located in each half of the medulla are tightly synchronized and it is thought that this connection occurs within the dorsal swallowing group of interneurons (Cunningham & Sawchenko, 2000; Jean, 2001; Kessler & Jean, 1985).

The interneurons of the ventral swallowing group are thought to be "switching" neurons that distribute and coordinate the swallowing drive to the various pools of motoneurons involved in swallowing. The firing behavior of these neurons also exhibits a sequential pattern, but with more overlap, longer latency, greater duration variability and lower frequency than the interneurons of the dorsal swallowing group. This type of firing behavior indicates that the connections between the ventral swallowing group interneurons and their afferent fibers are likely to be polysynaptic. The ventral swallowing group interneurons are probably activated by the interneurons of the dorsal swallowing group. They, in turn, are connected to all the various groups of motoneurons involved in swallowing and, within the ventral swallowing group interneurons, each neuron can project to more than one motor nucleus. The trigeminal and hypoglossal motor nuclei are connected only to the ventral swallowing group interneurons and not to the dorsal swallowing group. Swallowing motoneurons only receive input from the ipsilateral efferent fibers of the ventral swallowing interneurons (Amri, Car, & Roman, 1990; Jean, 2001; Kessler & Jean, 1985; Larson, Yajima, & Ko, 1994).

In addition to the interneurons of the ventral and dorsal swallowing groups, swallowing interneurons have been identified within the trigeminal and hypoglossal motor nuclei, or in close proximity. They may play the role of premotor neurons or be involved in the organization of the swallowing drive to the various motoneurons involved in swallowing within a single motor nucleus. They might also be involved in the bilateral coordination of the motoneuron pools (Car & Amri, 1987; Jean, 2001; Kessler & Jean, 1985; Ono, Ishiwata, Kuroda, & Nakamura, 1998).

There is also a population of interneurons, identified more rostrally in the pons, that fire during the oropharyngeal phase of swallowing. These interneurons have been classified as sensory relay neurons and are thought to provide information from the oropharyngeal receptors to the higher nervous centers (Jean, Kessler, & Tell, 1994).

In conclusion, the dorsal swallowing group interneurons are involved in initiating the swallowing sequence. They stimulate the interneurons of the ventral swallowing group which then modulate and coordinate the stimulation of the various motoneurons involved in the swallowing sequence (Bieger, 2001; Roda, Gestreau, & Biachi, 2002).

ESOPHAGEAL PHASE

The bolus is transported down the esophagus into the stomach. The esophageal phase is quite simple and consists of a peristaltic wave of contraction that propagates down the esophagus. There is considerable variability in the speed and strength of the esophageal contractile wave. Once initiated, it is not an all-or-none phenomenon, but may dissipate before reaching the lower esophageal sphincter. Sensory feedback likely plays a role in regulating the speed and intensity of the esophageal peristaltic wave, depending on the characteristics of the bolus. The lower esophageal sphincter is a site of high pressure, resulting from tonic contraction of the smooth muscle making up the sphincter. Increased pressure within the sphincter prevents reflux of stomach contents into the esophagus. During swallowing, the lower esophageal sphincter tone is inhibited, relaxing the sphincter for bolus passage into the stomach (Jean, 2001).

Secondary esophageal peristalsis is defined as peristalsis without a preceding oropharyngeal phase of swallowing. Secondary peristalsis occurs in response to stimulation of esophageal sensory receptors by distension of the esophageal lumen, and is otherwise similar in character, with regard to strength and speed of contraction, to primary esophageal peristalsis. Tertiary peristalsis of the esophagus refers to peristalsis of the smooth muscle portion of the esophagus, unrelated to extrinsic innervation (Jean, 2001).

The esophageal phase of swallowing requires both excitatory and inhibitory input to the muscles of the esophagus. At rest, the esophagus is electromyographically silent. All of the esophageal motoneurons are strongly inhibited during the oropharyngeal phase of swallowing and the contractile wave of the esophagus during the esophageal phase is preceded by inhibitory input. Once the bolus enters the esophagus, bolus movement involves the coordinated contraction of the smooth and striated muscles of the esophagus. Contraction of esophageal striated muscle is controlled by the motonuclei of the brainstem (nucleus ambiguus) while smooth muscle contraction is controlled by the autonomic nervous system. Smooth muscle of the esophagus is innervated by preganglionic fibers originating in the vagal motor nucleus. As are the muscles of the oropharynx, the muscles of the esophagus are inhibited and stimulated by motoneurons under the control of interneurons associated with the swallowing central pattern generator. Less information is available regarding the location of the central pattern generator interneurons. They regulate the esophagus and coordinate the oropharyngeal and esophageal phases of swallowing. Similarly, little is known regarding the interaction of these interneurons with the esophageal motoneurons. It is believed that fewer interneurons are involved in regulating the esophageal phase of deglutition, and that central control may be more dependent on afferent input than during oropharyngeal swallowing (Jean, 2001).

STUDY QUESTIONS

1. What are the four phases of deglutition and which are under voluntary control and which are primarily involuntary or "reflexive" in nature?
2. What are the three sphincters in the upper aerodigestive tract? Which chambers do they divide? How do they open and close?
3. What muscles are involved in bolus propulsion through the pharynx?
4. What sensory nerves are important in triggering the pharyngeal phase of swallowing and what areas of the mucosa do they supply?

5. Describe in general terms what is known about the central control of pharyngeal swallowing. What is the central pattern generator? What are the inputs to the central pattern generator? How does the central pattern generator control swallowing?

REFERENCES

Altschuler, S. M. (2001). Laryngeal and respiratory protective reflexes. *American Journal of Medicine, 111*, 90S–94S.

Altschuler, S. M., Bao, X., Bieger, D., Hopkins, D. A., & Miselis, R. R. (1989). Vicerotopic representation of the upper alimentary tract in the rat: Sensory ganglia and nuclei of the solitary and spinal trigeminal tracts. *Journal of Comparative Neurology, 283*, 248–268.

Amirali, A., Tsai, G., Weisz, D., Schrader, N., & Sanders, I. (2001). Mapping of brain stem neuronal circuitry active during swallowing. *Annals of Otology, Rhinology, and Laryngology, 110*, 502–513.

Amri, M., Car, A., & Roman, C. (1990). Axonal branching of medullary swallowing neurons projecting on the trigeminal and hypoglossal motor nuclei: Demonstration by electrophysiological and fluorescent double labeling techniques. *Experimental Brain Research, 81*, 384–390.

Barlow, S. M., & Burton, M. K. (1990). Ramp-and-hold force control in the upper and lower lips: Developing new neuromotor assessment applications in traumatically brain injured adults. *Journal of Speech and Hearing, 33*, 660–675.

Bieger, D. (2001). Rhombencephalic pathways and neurotransmitter controlling deglutition, *American Journal of Medicine, 111*, 85S–89S.

Bieger, D., & Hopkins, D. A. (1987). Viscerotopic representation of the upper alimentary tract in the medulla oblongata in the rat: The nucleus ambiguus. *Journal of Comparative Neurology, 262*, 546–562.

Broussard, D. L., & Altschuler, S. M. (2000). Central integration of swallow and airway-protective reflexes. *American Journal of Medicine, 108*, 62S–67S.

Car, A., & Amri, M. (1987).Activity of neurons located in the region of the hypoglossal motor nucleus during swallowing in sheep. *Experimental Brain Research, 69*, 175–182.

Chiao, G. Z., Larson, C. R., Yajima, Y., Ko, P., & Kahrilas, P. J. (1994). Neuronal activity in nucleus ambiguus during deglutition and vocalization in conscious monkeys. *Experimental Brain Research, 100*, 29–38.

Cunningham, E. T., & Sawchenko, P. E. (2000). Dorsal medullary pathways subserving oromotor reflexes in the rat: Implications from the central neural control of swallowing. *Journal of Comparative Neurology, 417*, 448–466.

Dodds, W. J., Stewart, E. J., & Logemann, J. A. (1990). Physiology and radiology of the normal and pharyngeal phases of swallowing. *American Journal of Roentgenology, 154*, 953–963.

Doty, R. W. (1968). Neural organization of deglutition. In *Handbook of Physiology: The alimentary Canal.* Washington, DC: American Physiology Society, sect. VI, 1861–1902.

Doty, R. W., & Bosma, J. F. (1956). An electromyographic analysis of reflex deglutition. *Journal of Neurophysiology, 19*, 44–60.

Ezure, K., Oku, Y., & Tanaka, I. (1993). Location and axonal projection of one type of swallowing interneuron in cat medulla. *Brain Research, 632*, 216–224.

Gestreau, C., Dutschmann, M., Obled, S., & Bianchi, A. L. (2005). Activation of XII motoneurons and premotor neurons during various oropharyngeal behaviors. *Respiratory Physiology Neurobiology, 147*, 159–176.

Guyton, A. C. (1981). *Textbook of medical physiology* (6th ed., pp. 803–804). Philadelphia, PA: W. B. Saunders.

Hamdy, S., Aziz, Q., Rothwell, J. C., Hobson, A., Barlow, J., & Thompson, D. G. (1997).

Cranial nerve modulation of human cortical swallowing pathways. *American Journal of Physiology, 272,* G802–G808.

Hamdy, S., Mikulis, D. J., Crawley, A., Xue, S., Lau, H., Henry, S., & Diamant, N. E. (1999). Cortical activation during human volitional swallowing: and event related fMRI study. *American Journal of Physiology: Gastrointestinal Liver Physiology, 277,* G219–G225.

Hamdy, S., Rothwell, J. C., Brooks, D. J., Bailey, D., Aziz, Q., & Thompson, D. G. (1999). Identification of the cerebral loci processing human swallowing with $H_2(15)O$ PET activation. *Journal of Neurophysiology, 81,* 1917–1926.

Hrycyshyn, A. W., & Basmajian, J. V. (1972). Electromyography of the oral sage of swallowing in man. *American Journal of Anatomy, 133,* 333–340.

Jean, A. (1990). Brainstem control of swallowing: Localization and organization of the central pattern generator for swallowing. In A. Taylor (Ed.), *Neurophysiology of the jaws and teeth* (pp. 294–321). London, UK: MacMillan.

Jean, A. (2001). Brainstem control of swallowing: Neuronal network and cellular mechanisms. *Physiological Reviews, 81,* 929–969.

Jean, A., Car, A., & Roman, C. (1975). Comparison of activity in pontine versus medullary neurons during swallowing. *Experimental Brain Research, 22,* 211–220.

Jean, A., Kessler, J. P., & Tell, F. (1994). Nucleus tractus solitarii and deglutition: Monoamines, excitatory amino acids, and cellular properties. In R. A. Baracco (Ed.), *Nucleus of the solitary tract* (pp. 362–375). Boca Raton, FL: CRC.

Kendall, K. (2002). Oropharyngeal swallowing variability. *Laryngoscope, 112,* 547–551.

Kendall, K., Leonard, R., & McKenzie, S. (2003). Sequence variability during hypopharyngeal bolus transit. *Dysphagia, 18,* 1–7.

Kendall, K., McKenzie, S., Leonard, R., Gonçalves, M., & Walker, A. (2000). Timing of events in normal swallowing: A videofluoroscopic study. *Dysphagia, 15,* 74–83.

Kessler, J. P., & Jean, A. (1985). Identification of the medullary swallowing regions in the rat. *Experimental Brain Research, 57,* 256–263.

Kidder, T. M. (1995). Esophago/pharyngo/laryngeal interrelationships: Airway protection mechanisms. *Dysphagia, 10,* 228–231.

Larson, C. R., Yajima, Y., & Ko, P. (1994). Modification in activity of medullary respiratory-related neurons for vocalization and swallowing. *Journal of Neurophysiology, 71,* 2294–2304.

Lawn, A. M. (1966). The localization in the nucleus ambiguus of the rabbit of the cells of origin of motor nerve fibres in the glossopharyngeal nerve and various branches of the vagus nerve by means of retrograde degeneration. *Journal of Comparative Neurology, 127,* 293–305.

Lawn, A. M. (1988). The nucleus ambiguus of the rabbit. *Journal of Comparative Neurology, 127,* 307–320.

McConnel, F. M. S. (1988a). Analysis of pressure generation and bolus transit during pharyngeal swallowing. *Laryngoscope, 98,* 71–78.

McConnel, F. M. S. (1988b). Timing of major events of pharyngeal swallowing. *Archives of Otolaryngology-Head and Neck Surgery, 114,* 1413–1418.

Miller, A. J. (1982). Deglutition. *Physiologic Reviews, 62,* 129–184.

Mosier, K., & Bereznaya, I. (2001). Parallel cortical networks for volitional control of swallowing in humans. *Experimental Brain Research, 140,* 280–289.

Ono, T., Ishiwata, Y., Kuroda, T., & Nakamura, Y. (1998). Swallowing-related perihypoglossal neurons projecting to hypoglossal motoneurons in the cat. *Journal of Dental Research, 77,* 351–360.

Ootani, S., Umezaki, T., Shin, T., & Murata, Y. (1995). Convergence of afferents from the SLN and GPN in cat medullary swallowing neurons. *Brain Research Bulletin, 37,* 397–404.

Roda, F., Gestreau, C., & Biachi, A. L. (2002). Discharge patterns of hypoglossal motoneurons during fictive breathing, coughing, and swallowing. *Journal of Neurophysiology, 87,* 1703–1711.

Tomomune, N., & Takata, M. (1988). Excitatory and inhibitory postsynaptic potentials in cat hypoglossal motoneurons during swallowing. *Experimental Brain Research, 71,* 262–272.

Zald, D. H., & Pardo, J. V. (1999). The functional neuroanatomy of voluntary swallowing. *Annals of Neurology, 46,* 281–286.

Zoungrana, O. R., Amri, M., Car, A., & Roman, C. (1997). Intracellular activity of motoneurons of the rostral nucleus ambigus during swallowing in sheep. *Journal of Neurophysiology, 77,* 909–922.

2

Head and Neck Physical Exam

Katherine A. Kendall

Dysphagia is the sensation that solids or liquids are not being swallowed correctly. Possible etiologies of dysphagia include neuromuscular disease involving the oral and pharyngeal musculature normally active during swallowing, altered anatomy such as occurs after surgical resections, radiation therapy, trauma, cervical osteophytes, pharyngeal diverticuli, cricopharyngeal spasm, foreign bodies, tumors, and mucosal irritation or injury.

INDICATIONS

A thorough history and head and neck examination is indicated in all patients suffering from dysphagia but may not provide enough information to gain a complete understanding of the pathophysiologic process. Flexible fiberoptic endoscopy may be required to complete the examination. A dynamic videofluoroscopic swallow study complements the physical examination and is usually indicated.

HISTORY

Chief Complaint

Symptoms of dysphagia may include a history of coughing or choking while eating. These symptoms indicate the patient may be aspirating during deglutition. Patients may have required that a Heimlich maneuver be performed on them when the airway became blocked by a food bolus. Patients may have noticed an increased need to clear their throat, and may complain of increased mucus or phlegm production or the sensation of something sitting on their vocal cords. They may note a change to a wet or gargling vocal quality as saliva or residual bolus drips onto the vocal folds. Patients may complain that foods get stuck at various locations in the pharynx. It is important to determine where this sensation occurs as it can focus the physical examination on the areas most likely to be involved or abnormal. It is also important to determine if difficulty is experienced with solids only, or with both liquids and solids. Dysphagia for solids only is often due to an obstruction or narrowing of the alimentary passage and a history of dysphagia for both liquids and solids may indicate generalized neuromuscular incoordination, or a very advanced obstructive process. Dysphagia for liquids only is often seen with poor airway protection such as occurs with a vocal fold paralysis or paresis, because liquids can flow into the airway where a solid bolus holds together better and usually causes little difficulty. A history of weight loss underscores the severity of the problem and a history of pneumonia indicates the occurrence of intolerable aspiration. Meal duration may be prolonged in these patients and they may avoid certain types of food they know to worsen their symptoms (Castell & Donner, 1987).

A sudden onset of dysphagia is more likely to occur with trauma or ingestion of a foreign body. Careful questioning of the patient may be required to elicit a history of chicken or fish in the recent diet, indicating the possiblility of a bone lodged in the aerodigestive tract.

Past Medical History

A history of heartburn, indigestion, or known gastroesophageal reflux is significant in that chronic irritation of the pharyngeal mucosa can enhance a foreign-body sensation. A long exposure of the esophageal mucosa to stomach acid may lead to poor relaxation of the upper esophageal sphincter and subsequent solid food dysphagia. Over time, failure of upper esophageal sphincter relaxation can lead to the development of pharyngeal diverticuli. Gastroesophageal reflux can also lead to aspiration of an extremely caustic nature that is not necessarily associated with swallowing (Leonard & Kendall, 1999; Shaker, 1995).

A history of neuromuscular disease is important as this may be the primary etiology of the swallowing abnormality and gives an indication of the prognosis for improvement. Past surgical procedures involving structures of the oral cavity and pharynx may be responsible for altered swallowing function. Head and neck radiation therapy can lead to fibrosis of structures whose mobility is required for adequate swallowing and will cause xerostomia (Kendall, McKenzie, & Leonard, 1998).

A detailed medication history may shed light on factors contributing to the patient's symptoms of dysphagia. Many medications cause decreased salivary production and contribute to poor bolus lubrication and clearing. These medications act primarily through their effects on the parasympathetic nervous system, responsible for the stimulation of salivation. Drugs may be "parasympathomimetic," meaning that they stimulate or simulate the parasympathetic nervous system. This results in increased salivation, occasionally to the point of drooling. Drugs that are "parasympatholytic" block or decrease parasympathetic stimulation causing a decrease in salivary output and a dry mouth. "Anticholinergic" drugs fall into this category. Antihistamines and antinausea medications commonly have anticholinergic side effects. The use of multiple drugs, a common finding in older patients, may result in drug interactions that potentiate the anticholinergic effects of those drugs. The side effect of a dry mouth can reduce the patient's ability to communicate, predispose to malnutrition, promote mucosal damage, denture misfit or dental caries, and increase the risk of serious respiratory infection secondary to the loss of antimicrobial activity of saliva (Feinberg, 1993; Narhi et al., 1992).

Other drug categories also have dry mouth as a side effect. The following is a partial list of examples. The side effects of any drug can usually be investigated by referencing any of a number of drug handbooks or the Physicians Desk Reference (Arky, 1996).

Drugs that increase brain dopamine levels by stimulating the release of dopamine may cause a dry mouth. An example of this type of medication is Symmetrel, a drug that is used in the treatment of Parkinson's disease. Antipsychotic medications that act by blocking dopamine receptors also cause a dry mouth. Tricyclic antidepressants are basic in the treatment of depression. These drugs are thought to block serotonin and norepinephrine reuptake. They include Elavil, Senequan, and Tofranil. Some patients taking this type of medication experience dry mouth as these drugs produce a significant reduction in salivary flow. Newer antidepressants that block seratonin reuptake are also known to cause dry mouth. Examples of these medications include Prozac, Zoloft, Desyrel, and Paxil. Lithium carbonate used to treat manic-depressive disorders causes a dry mouth. Benzodiazepines are drugs used to treat symptoms of anxiety. The drugs act by potentiating the effect of GABA, a brain inhibitory neurotransmitter. Dry mouth is a side effect of many of these compounds (Hunter & Wilson, 1995; Vogel & Carter, 1995).

Diabetes mellitus is also associated with reduced salivary flow. In the case of diabetes, oral dryness is not associated with a malfunction of the parasympathetic nervous system but appears to be due to disturbances in glycemic control (Sreebny, Yu, Green, & Valdini, 1992).

EXAMINATION

The patient should be sitting upright for the examination. A bright light source is required to illuminate the oral cavity, pharynx and hypopharynx. A head mirror or headlight is recommended. The patient should be seated at a level so that he or she is slightly higher than the examiner. The legs should be uncrossed and the patient should be sitting up straight, leaning slightly forward at the hip.

The face of the patient should be examined for any obvious asymmetries or outward signs of trauma. Facial musculature and sensation should be tested to rule out abnormalities of cranial nerves V and VII. The eyes and orbits should be evaluated for deficits of cranial nerves II, III, IV, or VI. Abnormalities of cranial nerve function and facial sensation may be clues to the diagnosis of central or neuromuscular disease. A nasal exam should rule out any masses that could impinge upon the soft palate and therefore preclude complete closure of the velum. The lips should be first inspected and evaluated in terms of sensation and competency. Salivary leak should be noted. Two tongue blades aid in the examination of the oral cavity. The patient is asked to open the mouth and the tongue blades are employed to move structures allowing complete inspection of all the mucosal surfaces. Upon opening, the interincisal distance can be evaluated. Trismus can be a sign of temporomandibular joint disease or pterygoid muscle abnormalities. Tumors invading the pterygoid muscles are a cause of trismus. Trismus may interfere with mastication and proper bolus preparation. The dentition should be inspected. Carious, broken, and missing teeth may also lead to difficulty with bolus preparation. The mucosal surfaces should be inspected for irregularities, lesions and moisture. Saliva quantity and quality should be noted.

Adequate tongue mobility is paramount to effective swallowing. The tongue should be inspected for any surface irregularities, fasciculations or atrophy. The patient should be asked to protrude the tongue and to move it from side to side in order to judge mobility. The lingual sulci should be examined to rule out tethering of the tongue to the inner surface of the mandible. Palpation of the tongue allows detection of any masses that are not evident on visual inspection alone.

Examination of the oral pharynx also should begin with a visual inspection of the mucosal surfaces to rule out any obvious abnormalities. The soft palate should elevate symmetrically when the patient is asked to say "ah." The presence or absence of enlarged tonsillar tissue should be noted.

The hypopharyngeal exam requires indirect laryngoscopy. This method enables the visual inspection of the tongue base as well as the larynx and region of the upper esophageal inlet. The patient must be properly positioned to carry out the examination in such a manner as to provide the best visualization with the least discomfort to the patient. The patient should be asked to sit up straight. The head of the patient should be above the head of the examiner. The patient should be asked to extend the neck anteriorly so that the mandible is forward. This position moves the tongue base anteriorly and brings the larynx into view. The patient is then asked to protrude the tongue maximally. The examiner holds the tongue with a thin gauze sponge and stabilizes the position of the patient with the same hand. A warmed mirror is introduced into the oral pharynx with the other hand using care not to touch the tongue base with the mirror. As we have previously mentioned, the tongue base is extremely sensitive and a region involved in the swallowing reflex initiation. It is also involved in airway protection and the initiation of the gag reflex. The soft palate, however, is not as sensitive and the mirror can be placed against it as it is positioned posteriorly in the oral pharynx for viewing of the hypopharynx.

The mirror can be pivoted back and forth to allow full examination of the hypopharyngeal structures. Starting with the base of the tongue, the vallecula, and the epiglottis, evaluation for any anatomic abnormalities is carried out. The presence or absence of saliva pooling in the vallecula, piriform fossae or glottic opening is then noted. Pooling of saliva suggests significant dysfunction of the swallowing mechanism and identifies patients at significant risk for aspiration. The piriform fossae are also evaluated in terms of asymmetries, mucosal lesions, or masses.

The larynx is then inspected and vocal fold mobility and closure are assessed. The patient is asked to say "ee" which closes the vocal folds and further elevates the larynx for inspection. A higher frequency "ee" will often elevate the larynx even further for viewing. Any vocal fold lesions that inhibit full vocal fold closure are noted. The patient may be asked to perform a rapid "ee-ee-ee" sequence to assess fine control of vocal fold movement and closure. The vocal folds should be evaluated during inspiration, as well, to allow visualization of the vocal fold medial surfaces that are obscured during phonation. The interarytenoid region should be evaluated for color and character of tissues, as erythema of this region may indicate irritation by chronic gastroesophageal reflux.

Once hypopharyngeal inspection has been carried out, a test of sensation in the oral pharynx can be performed. By touching the tongue base and posterior pharyngeal wall, a gag reflex should be elicited.

The final part of the physical examination involves palpation of the neck for anatomic abnormalities, especially masses.

The routine physical examination is limited in that the evaluation of the nasopharynx and hypopharyngeal sensation cannot be performed adequately. To complete these parts of the evaluation, a flexible nasopharyngoscope is used. One nostril can be spayed with topical neosynephrine (1/4%) and/or topical anesthetic such as Lidocaine (4%). The scope is lubricated and dipped in an antifog solution. It is then passed along the nasal floor to allow inspection of the nasopharynx.

All mucosal surfaces should be inspected. Palatal mobility is evaluated along with velopharyngeal closure by asking the patient to perform a forceful "sss" sound. Once this portion of the examination is complete, the patient is asked to breathe through his nose and thus open the nasopharyngeal passage for further advancement of the flexible scope and evaluation of hypopharyngeal sensation. This technique can also be employed to visually inspect the hypopharynx in patients who are unable to tolerate or have unfavorable anatomy for an indirect examination.

The tip of the flexible scope is used to touch the tongue, piriform fossae, lateral pharyngeal walls, aryepiglottic folds, laryngeal surface of the epiglottis, and the vocal folds themselves. The examination is carried out bilaterally and the two sides are compared. Patients with normal sensation will cough or swallow when touched with the scope. Abnormal sensation can contribute significantly to abnormalities of initiating a swallow and control of the bolus.

REVIEW

The head and neck physical examination allows an assessment of alterations in anatomy, motor function, and sensory function that affect a patient's ability to swallow. The following is a list reviewing the information that may be gained during the physical examination.

- Obvious tumor, surgical changes, or other anatomic abnormalities.
- Abnormalities of tongue, palatal, and vocal fold mobility.

- Inadequate sphincteric functions such as oral incompetence, velopharyngeal incompetence, and poor laryngeal closure.
- Loss of sensation.
- Pooling of secretions.

LIMITATIONS

In patients with subtle abnormalities of sensation, the gross nature of the physical examination will be inadequate to detect them. Yet, these sensory deficits may be responsible for delayed swallow reflex triggering and poor bolus control. The same problems exist in the evaluation of subtle motor deficits that may not be detected on the physical examination. The complex coordination of swallowing may be abnormal in patients with central control deficits who present with normal anatomy, sensation, and apparent muscular function. Thus, the physical examination may not provide enough information to fully understand the nature of the patient's swallowing problems. A dynamic videofluoroscopic swallow study is often required to further elucidate subtle abnormalities of the swallowing mechanism.

STUDY QUESTIONS

1. Discuss three symptoms consistent with severe dysphagia.
2. What important information is learned from the past medical history with respect to complaints of dysphagia? Name three specific examples.
3. How does gastroesophageal reflux disease cause dysphagia?

4. Describe the limitations of the physical examination and what testing can be done to complement the physical examination.

REFERENCES

Arky, R. (1996). *Physician's desk reference*. Montvale, NJ: Medical Economics.

Castell, D. O., & Donner, M. W. (1987). Evaluation of dysphagia: A careful history is crucial. *Dysphagia, 2*, 65–71.

Feinberg, M. (1993). The problems of anticholinergic adverse effects in older patients. *Drugs and Aging, 3*, 335–348.

Hunter, K. D., & Wilson, W. S. (1995). The effects of antidepressant drugs on salivary flow and content of sodium and potassium ions in human parotid saliva. *Archives of Oral Biology, 40*, 983–989.

Kendall, K., McKenzie, S., & Leonard, R. (1998). Structural mobility in deglutition after single modality treatment of head and neck carcinomas with radiation therapy. *Head and Neck, 20*, 720–725.

Leonard, R., & Kendall, K. (1999). Dysphagia secondary to cricopharyngeal achalasia. *Phonoscope: Voice-Speech-Swallowing Clinics in Head and Neck Practice, 2*, 123–128.

Narhi, T. O., Meurman, J. H., Ainamo, A., Nevalainen, J. M., Schmidt-Kaunisaho, K. G., Siudosaari, P., . . . Makila, E. (1992). Association between salivary flow rate and the use of systemic medication among 76-, 81-, and 86-year-old inhabitants in Helsinki, Finland. *Journal of Dental Research, 71*, 1875–1880.

Shaker, R. (1995). Airway protective mechanisms: Current concepts. *Dysphagia, 10*, 216–227.

Sreebny, L. M., Yu, A., Green A., & Valdini, A. (1992). Xerostomia in diabetes mellitus. *Diabetes Care, 15*, 900–904.

Vogel, D., & Carter, J. E. (1995). *The effects of drugs on communication disorders*. San Diego, CA: Singular.

3

Dysphagia in Head and Neck Cancer Patients

Katherine A. Kendall

Successful deglutition depends on the smooth and coordinated functioning of multiple structures in the head and neck region. Although the swallowing sequence can be influenced by input from higher cortical centers, it is primarily a semiautomatic mechanism. The swallowing mechanism relies on sensory input from the muscles and the mucosal surfaces of the structures involved, as they help regulate and fine-tune the sequence of muscular contractions that results in a swallow. It makes sense that disruption of the sensory, muscular or structural integrity of the oral cavity, pharynx and larynx results in dysphagia. In patients with head and neck cancer, tumor growth, changes in tissue characteristics secondary to radiation (with or without chemotherapy), and any surgical procedure involving the head and neck region have the potential to cause dysphagia. Head and neck cancer patients are the most

common head and neck population to experience dysphagia, and the concepts involved in understanding the etiology of dysphagia in this group can be generalized to other patient populations. This chapter focuses on the swallowing difficulty experienced by head and neck cancer patients.

INTRODUCTION

In patients with head and neck cancer, interference with normal swallowing may result from the growth of the tumor invading structures and impairing their functioning or from the obstructive effects of the tumor, itself, that interfere with bolus movement. Surgery to excise the tumor with a margin of normal tissue typically results in a defect with loss of structures needed for normal deglutition. The method chosen for reconstruction of the defect will subsequently influence the restoration of normal anatomic contours and function. Thus, the reconstruction impacts the character and the severity of the resultant dysphagia. When postoperative radiation therapy is added to the regimen, dysphagia may worsen secondary to xerostomia and fibrosis of soft tissues in the field of radiation exposure.

Chemoradiation therapy, now used in many cases rather than surgery, avoids removal of the tissues involved in the tumor. Administration of intravenous chemotherapeutic agents as radiation sensitizers, combined with concurrent radiation therapy achieves oncologic outcomes that are similar or better than those achieved with surgery followed by radiation therapy alone. Although tissues are not removed with chemoradiation therapy, intense inflammation of the treated tissues occurs, and ultimately results in tissue fibrosis and weakness of those tissues. The "preserved" tissues are scarred and exhibit decreased mobility, usually resulting in dysphagia.

PRETREATMENT EVALUATION

All patients diagnosed with head and neck cancer involving the oral cavity, pharynx, and larynx should be considered to be at risk for dysphagia. Prior to treatment, dysphagia can result from either tissue invasion by the tumor or from the tumor obstructing bolus flow. In both cases, the tumor prevents the normal structural displacements needed for bolus propulsion and airway protection. Tumor involvement of sensory nerves also has the potential to impair feedback mechanisms needed

for swallowing coordination and may lead to silent aspiration.

The location of the tumor in the upper aerodigestive tract influences the likelihood of pretreatment dysphagia. In a study of 67 head and neck cancer patients prior to treatment, Stenson et al. found that significantly more patients with laryngeal and hypopharyngeal tumors aspirated than did patients with oral cavity or oropharynx tumors. These authors identified a greater degree of "pharyngeal impairment" on swallowing studies in patients with laryngeal and hypopharyngeal tumors, leading to aspiration (Stenson, MacCracken, List, Haraf, Brockstein, et al., 2000). Langerman et al. found that 71% of patients with hypopharyngeal cancer, 44% of patients with oropharyngeal cancer, and 23% of patients with oral cavity tumors aspirated at baseline (Langerman, MacCracken, Kasza, Haraf, Vokes, et al., 2007). In addition to tumor location, the size of the tumor further impacts the degree of dysphagia, with larger tumors causing a greater degree of dysphagia (Frowen, Cotton, Corry, & Perry, 2010; Starmer, Gourin, Lua, & Burkhead, 2011). Although patients with tumors of the larynx and hypopharynx are at the most risk of developing aspiration, patients with tumors of the oral cavity and pharynx are more likely to report other symptoms such as pain, dysgeusia (distortion of taste), and anorexia that lead to a decrease in dietary intake before treatment (Kubrak, Olson, Jha, Jensen, & McCargar, 2010).

Determining aspiration risk in head and neck cancer patients prior to treatment is critical to optimize nutrition during treatment and to prevent possible aspiration pneumonia. Swallowing therapy directed toward correcting specific deficits can also be initiated during treatment in an attempt to minimize the long-term effects of the tumor and treatment on swallowing function. Furthermore, Frowen et al. found that the best predictor of swallowing function after treatment is swallowing at pretreatment baseline (Frowen et al., 2010). Head and neck cancer patients, therefore, must be evaluated for swallowing function before embarking on oral feeding, both during and after treatment. Patients' perceptions of the difficulty they experience may be erroneous, and they often understate their actual swallowing difficulties (Baker, Fraser, & Baker, 1991). For this reason, a bedside swallow evaluation is often insufficient, and should be followed by a dynamic videofluoroscopic swallow study to confirm and document actual swallowing function.

GASTROSTOMY TUBE PLACEMENT

The majority of head and neck cancer patients will experience worsening of swallowing function during treatment, especially if they are being treated with chemoradiation therapy (Frowen et al., 2010). Chemoradiation therapy causes severe mucositis that results in odynophagia along with anorexia, loss of taste, and xerostomia that contribute to a decrease in oral intake. During treatment, many patients are not able to maintain their nutritional requirements orally and must have a feeding tube placed. Feeding tubes have been shown definitively to decrease weight loss and the need for parenteral hydration during treatment (Chen, Li, Lau,

Farwell, Luu, et al., 2010). As treatment may last as long as 8 weeks, a percutaneous gastrostomy, when possible, is preferred over a nasogastric tube for patient comfort.

The timing of percutaneous gastrostomy (G-tube) placement is controversial. Many centers place feeding tubes in patients prior to the initiation of therapy, regardless of pretreatment weight loss or complaints of dysphagia, to minimize the chance that treatment may be interrupted for the placement of a feeding tube (Nguyen, North, Smith, Dutta, Alfieri, et al., 2006; Wiggenraad, Flierman, Goossens, Brand, Verschuur, et al., 2007). However, other centers have identified longer G-tube dependence and a higher incidence of permanent G-tube use in those patients whose G-tubes were placed prophylactically, rather than when clinically indicated by weight loss (Chen, et al., 2010; McLaughlin, Gokhale, Shuai, Diacopoulos, Carrau, et al., 2010). There may also be no significant long-term benefits of G-tube placement with respect to weight loss, as patients tend to regain lost weight after therapy. Langmore et al. found that those patients who maintained some sort of oral feeding during treatment had better long-term swallowing function than those who relied on a feeding tube (Langmore, Crisciunas, Miloro, Evans, & Cheng, 2011). Presumably, the continued movement of upper aerodigestive tract structures by swallowing during treatment decreases subsequent fibrosis and movement limitations. Further studies are needed to evaluate the impact of specific swallowing exercises during treatment in preventing long-term dysphagia, even if a patient becomes G-tube dependent during therapy. Clearly, if patients are encouraged to maintain some sort of oral intake during treatment, a pretreatment assessment is imperative to maximize airway safety.

SURGERY

Although chemoradiation therapy is now considered to be the preferred initial treatment for cancer of the oropharynx, hypopharynx, and larynx, surgery is typically still considered the mainstay of treatment for small cancers, and cancers of the oral cavity, oral tongue, and some early laryngeal cancers. Chemoradiation failures also require surgical treatment. After surgery, patients are usually NPO (nothing by mouth) for one to two weeks, to allow healing of the surgical deficit. In our center, a swallow study is done after surgery in every patient, prior to attempting oral feeding. Initially, we made an effort to perform a swallow study prior to the patient's discharge from the hospital, and this typically was post-op day 7 to 10. But patients studied this early postoperatively often have extreme difficulty with dysphagia. Many of these patients will do much better on a swallow study performed a few weeks later.

We now have modified our protocol so that patients are studied later in the postoperative course. This minimizes the number of studies performed on an individual patient and improves the chance that the patient will be well enough to participate in attempts to identify strategies for safe swallowing. Each patient must be considered on an individual basis in terms of deciding when the swallow study, and thus oral feeding, should be attempted. Healing from surgery, local edema, other medi-

cal conditions, the development of oro- or pharyngocutaneous fistulae, and the psychological condition of the patient must be factored into the decision.

Several studies have found little improvement of swallowing function when the immediate postoperative swallowing is compared to swallowing function as long as 1 year later (Baker, Fraser, & Baker, 1991; Pauloski, Logemann, & Rademaker, 1995; Pauloski, Logemann, Rademaker, McConnel, Heiser et al., 1993). However, Pauloski and colleagues were able to demonstrate some functional adaptation and the development of secondary coping strategies in patients after anterior tongue and floor of mouth resections (Pauloski, Logemann, Fox, & Colangelo, 1995).

ORAL SPHINCTER

When the lips are involved in a surgical cancer resection, the subsequent functioning of the oral sphincter is influenced by the size, sensation, and structural support of the reconstructed ostium. Up to one-half of the lower lip can be excised and closed primarily without serious cosmetic and functional consequences. If greater than one-half of the lip requires removal, local flaps are usually needed for reconstruction. When microstomia results from extensive resection of the lips, the patient will experience difficulty with bolus introduction into the oral cavity. If the resection involves the mental nerve on one or both sides, the subsequent loss of sensation of the lower lip results in difficulty in maintaining oral competence, even if the sphincter mechanism remains intact. Lip sensory deficits also cause difficulty in bolus manipulation and the patient may experience drooling or loss of the bolus during bolus preparation for swallowing. Oral incompetence creates difficulty with the development of intraoral pressures required to move the bolus from the oral cavity into the pharynx. (Try to swallow saliva with lips open to experience just how significant a problem this is!) Therefore, patients with oral incompetence often have difficulty in initiation of the pharyngeal phase of the swallow.

ANTERIOR FLOOR OF MOUTH

Floor of mouth structures important for deglutition include the muscles responsible for hyoid elevation and tongue stabilization. A lack of hyoid elevation, due to resection or dysfunction of the suprahyoid muscles in the floor of the mouth, results in an inability to open the pharyngoesophageal sphincter. This disability can be so severe that patients are completely unable to swallow. Tongue mobility in the anterior and posterior directions depends on the pliability of the floor of the mouth region and the attachments of the tongue musculature to the anterior mandible. When tissue is lost from this area, difficulty in bolus preparation and propulsion from the oral cavity into the pharynx results from a loss of tongue maneuverability (Pauloski, Logemann, Fox, & Colangelo, 1995). Furthermore, lack of contact of the tongue with the pharyngeal constrictors during the pharyngeal phase of the swallow will lead to pharyngeal residue, often aspirated after the swallow. If the lingual nerve and the hypoglossal nerve are involved in the resection, problems with tongue

sensation, taste, and tongue mobility will result.

Reconstruction of floor of mouth defects can have a significant impact on patients' functional outcomes. Any closure that results in tethering of the tongue or further loss of tongue bulk, for example when local tongue flaps are used, will amplify the disability. Surgeons must avoid closing the defect in such a way that the tongue is pulled anteriorly because this will limit posterior tongue mobility, in particular, the ability of the tongue to contact the posterior pharyngeal wall. Failure of the tongue to contact the posterior pharyngeal wall during the pharyngeal phase of swallowing will result in poor pharyngeal constriction and residue in the pharynx that will be aspirated during subsequent respiration. Similarly, if a large or bulky regional flap is inset into the defect, it may displace the tongue too far posteriorly and prevent normal oral manipulation of the bolus. In order to transfer the bolus into the pharynx, the tongue must be able to contact the palate sequentially from anterior to posterior.

Skin grafting, local nasolabial flaps, and free tissue transfer such as the radial forearm or jejunal flaps, are alternatives for closure of floor of mouth defects. Surgeons performing this type of surgery may consider the addition of a hyoid suspension procedure to permanently open the pharyngoesophageal sphincter if the suprahyoid musculature has been removed.

TONGUE

Loss of tongue bulk after tongue cancer resection can significantly impact oral and pharyngeal movement of the bolus.

The degree of impairment is influenced by the location and the extent of the resection (McConnel, Logemann, Rademaker, et al., 1994). Anterior defects are likely to lead to problems with oral bolus manipulation and difficulty in propelling the bolus into the pharynx, especially if the tongue cannot contact the palate. Loss of posterior tongue tissue affects the pharyngeal phase of the swallow and results in difficulty in generating the forces required to propel the bolus into the upper esophagus. In these cases, the dynamic videofluoroscopic swallow study demonstrates poor pharyngeal constriction with pharyngeal residue as a consequence.

Restoration of tongue mobility and bulk must be a primary consideration in the reconstruction of any tongue defect. Several options exist, including closure by secondary intention or granulation, skin grafts, regional flaps or free tissue transfer. McConnel reported that, after excision of oral tongue tumors greater than 2 cm in size without involvement of other oral cavity structures, the best swallowing results were achieved in patients who had skin graft reconstructions (McConnel & Mendelsohn, 1987; McConnel & O'Connor, 1994). For base of tongue defects, McConnel found that primary closure resulted in better swallowing function than pectoralis myocutaneous flaps or radial forearm free flaps (McConnel, 1996) (Figure 3–1). After partial glossectomy, some alteration of tongue function is likely, irrespective of the reconstructive method.

Research from our own laboratory has attempted to compare swallowing in normal controls to swallowing in patients with resections for oral cavity or oropharyngeal cancer, and across

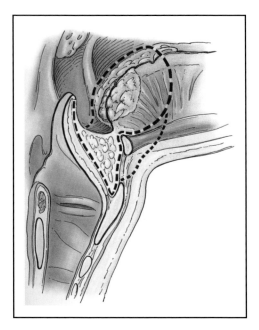

Figure 3–1. A resection of a base of tongue tumor will create difficulty with pharyngeal constriction if significant base of tongue bulk is required to be removed.

subgroups of patients with oropharyngeal resection involving the tongue (Leonard & Gonçalves, unpublished data, 1997). The resection categories are designated unilateral limited, unilateral extensive, anterior, posterior, and subtotal, according to the site and extent of glossal resection. Timing and displacement characteristics of events and structures involved in swallow have been obtained from videofluoroscopic studies performed as uniformly as possible across patient and control subjects. In a comparison of control to postoperative subjects, duration of upper esophageal sphincter opening was the only parameter that was not significantly different between the two groups. Across categories of glossectomy patients, those with unilateral limited resections generally fared better on parameters investigated, whereas those in the posterior and subtotal categories performed most poorly.

MANDIBLE

Cancer that involves the anterior floor of the mouth, the tongue or the lateral pharyngeal wall often invades the adjacent mandible, as well (Figure 3–2). Occasionally, a portion of the mandible is removed to provide an adequate margin for the tumor resection. The alveolar and the mental nerves run through the mandible and may be sacrificed along with a segment of the mandible, resulting in the loss of sensation to the remaining ipsilateral mandibular teeth and lower lip. When the angle of the mandible is removed, the contralateral masseter and medial pterygoid muscles are unopposed, resulting in jaw swing

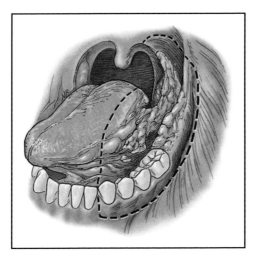

Figure 3–2. An example of a retromolar trigone tumor that involves both the lateral tongue and the adjacent alveolar ridge. A portion of the mandible will need to be resected along with a portion of the lateral tongue.

and malocclusion. If the anterior portion of the jaw is removed, a deformity results with the loss of the chin contour and oral incompetence ("Andy Gump" deformity). The hyoid elevators will have lost their attachment and consequent failure of the hyoid to elevate may produce poor pharyngoesophageal sphincter opening. The use of osseous free flaps and mandibular plates for reconstruction of the mandible has improved the outcomes in these patients in terms of the cosmetic defect. Unfortunately, the functional difficulties often remain.

PALATE

Defects of the hard palate result in oronasal fistulae. A fistula effectively enlarges the oral cavity by the area of the nasal cavity and results in an open chamber instead of a closed structure. Bolus material can readily pass into the nasal cavity during preparation for swallowing. Manipulation of the bolus is more difficult as the tongue may be unable to retrieve material from the nasal cavity. The hard palate also serves as a surface against which the tongue pushes to propel the bolus into the pharynx in preparation for swallowing. Defects in the palate cause difficulty with pressure generation and inefficient bolus transfer. In general, obturation of a hard palate defect with a prosthesis is very successful in improving the dysphagia.

Soft palate defects inhibit the dual sphincter function of the soft palate. During the oral phase of swallowing, the soft palate acts to divide the oral and pharyngeal cavities, as it is fully relaxed and resting on the tongue base. The soft palate then elevates and divides the nasopharynx from the oropharynx during the pharyngeal phase of swallowing. Any loss of palate mobility will impact these functions of the soft palate. Loss of palatal tissue further will prevent full closure of these sphincters and allow pressure and bolus material to escape inappropriately through the defect.

Soft palate defects pose difficult reconstructive challenges. Most techniques available cannot recreate the unique muscle configuration of the palate and mobility is diminished. Usually palatal bulk can be restored with local flaps. Prosthetic obturators can help position the poorly mobile palate into a position that is more favorable for the pharyngeal phase of swallowing, but nasal respiration is often comprised.

PHARYNX

Removal of portions of the pharyngeal walls, such as occurs in resections of tonsillar fossa cancer, results in the potential for weakness of the wall at the resection site. It must be kept in mind that the pharynx acts as a chamber that provides resistance to the posterior movement of the tongue base, thereby generating the pressures needed to propel the bolus through the pharyngoesophageal sphincter. The subsequent sequential contraction of the pharyngeal musculature aids in clearing the bolus from the pharyngeal cavity. Dehiscence of the pharyngeal musculature may result in diverticuli with the potential for residue in the pharynx after the swallow. Surgery that affects the posterior pharyngeal wall may also produce tethering of the pharynx to the prevertebral fascia. Although elevation of the pharyngeal cavity is not thought to be a significant requirement for deglutition, patients who experience posterior pharyngeal wall tethering complain of severe dysphagia and have poor pharyngeal constriction on the dynamic videofluoroscopic swallow study.

Reconstruction of pharyngeal wall defects is best accomplished with primary closure if the size of the defect permits. When bulky, adynamic flaps are required, dysphagia may be worsened by lack of muscular tone in the flap area or by obstruction to bolus flow by flap bulk (Zafereo, Weber, Lewin, Roberts, & Hanasono, 2010).

LARYNX

Supraglottic Laryngectomy

The supraglottic laryngectomy was designed for removal of cancers involving supraglottic structures such as the epiglottis and false vocal folds. The surgical procedure involves removal of the hyoid bone and includes resection of the structures superior to the petiole of the epiglottis and the laryngeal ventricles. To reconstruct the defect, the remaining laryngeal structures (the vocal folds) are sutured to the residual tongue base. Airway protection during swallowing is severely compromised by the removal of most of the structures responsible for directing the bolus away from the glottis and pulling the larynx under the tongue base for protection. Prevention of aspiration is accomplished by the well-timed closure of the vocal folds alone. Supraglottic laryngectomy patients must be trained in swallow techniques that insure timely vocal fold closure and, even so, are at significant risk for the development of aspiration pneumonia (Freeman, Marks, & Ogura, 1979). Some surgeons have recommended that the remaining larynx be suspended anteriorly to the mandible during the reconstruction to improve airway protection provided by the bulk of the tongue base (Calcaterra, 1971).

Supraglottic laryngectomy has largely been replaced with endoscopic supraglottic laser resection. This procedure is done transorally through a laryngoscope. A laser is used to remove the tumor with a cuff of normal tissue. The defect is allowed to close by secondary intention. This technique is usually employed for cancers involving the epiglottis and is contraindicated if the tumor extends into the pre-epiglottic space or other surrounding structures (Burns, Har-El, Shapsay, Maune, & Zeitels, 2009) (Figure 3–3). The advantage of the endoscopic technique is that the hyoid bone is not removed and the attachments of the larynx to the hyoid bone (the thyrohyoid membrane and the thyrohyoid muscles) are not removed, thus preserving the anterior displacement of the larynx under the tongue during deglutition. Swallowing results are far superior with this technique (Karatzanis, Psychogios, Zenk, Waldfahrer, Hornung, et al., 2010; Peretti, Piazza, Cattaneo, De Benedetto, Martin, et al., 2006).

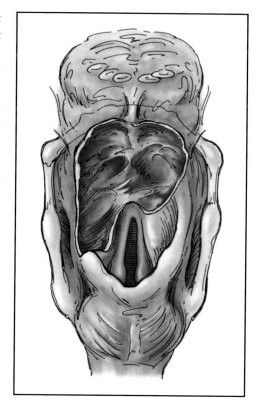

Figure 3–3. After endoscopic supraglottic laryngectomy, the defect is left to heal by secondary intention. Note the removal of the epiglottis and the left ventricular fold. Posterior view of structures involved in hypopharynx.

Partial Laryngectomy

Partial laryngeal surgeries have been designed to remove cancers involving the structures of the larynx with reconstruction of a voicing source using the residual tissues. Frequently, after reconstruction, the glottic aperture is too small to serve as an adequate airway and a permanent tracheostomy is required. The ability of the reconstructed vibratory source to prevent bolus penetration during deglutition is often incomplete. Again, these patients may require therapy to develop strategies for safe, effective swallowing. Due to these difficulties with functional outcomes, open partial laryngectomy has largely been replaced by endoscopic laser surgery. Endoscopic surgery removes the tumor with a cuff of normal tissue and the resulting defect is allowed to close by secondary intention (Hinne, Salassa, Grant, Pearson, Hayden, et al., 2007). The voice and swallowing results depend on the size and location of the resulting defect. Because there are no suture lines to heal, many surgeons recommend early oral diet. However, initial attempts at oral feeding should be done under the supervision of a speech language pathologist and a videofluoroscopic swallowing study may be required to assess the effectiveness of strategies for safe swallowing.

Total Laryngectomy

Total laryngectomy includes removal of the larynx from its attachments to the inferior pharyngeal constrictor and cricopharyngeaus muscle. The trachea in transected and brought out to the skin. The hyoid bone is removed and the hyoid attachments to the middle pharyngeal constrictor are divided. Hyoid attachments to the suprahyoid muscles are also divided (Figure 3–4). If the tumor extends beyond the larynx, various amounts of tongue base tissue or piriform sinus mucosa and pharyngeal constrictor muscle are included in the resection.

Primary closure of a laryngectomy defect typically involves vertical closure of the pharyngeal mucosa with or without a second layer in which the pharyngeal constrictors are closed together, creating a muscular tube. A cricopharyngeal myotomy may be performed simultaneously in order to decrease resistance to bolus movement into the esophagus. The tongue base is usually closed in a horizontal fashion. Contracture of this

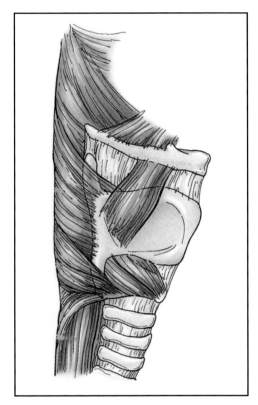

Figure 3–4. Attachments of the pharyngeal constrictor muscles to the larynx (lateral view). These are divided during a total laryngectomy. The hyoid bone is also removed during the resection. The cut end of the trachea is brought out to the skin.

incision is responsible for the development of a "pseudo-epiglottis" and pouch at the base of tongue. A "pseudo-epigottis and "vallecula," or pouch, can be difficult for the patient to clear of bolus material. Closure of the tongue base in a vertical direction can avoid this problem, but requires that ample pharyngeal mucosa be available. With large resections, residual tissues may be inadequate for closure and pedicled or free flaps are required to achieve pharyngeal closure.

After total laryngectomy, laryngeal elevation, the mechanism usually responsible for the opening of the pharyngoesophageal sphincter, is no longer possible. Laryngectomy patients must rely on the forces generated by the base of the tongue against the pharyngeal walls to drive the bolus inferiorly. A "pumping" action of the tongue is often observed in these patients to help generate the increased pressures required to compensate for lack of pharyngoesophageal sphincter opening. If significant tongue tissue resection is required for adequate cancer removal, patients can be expected to experience significant dysphagia. Laryngectomy reconstruction, however, results in complete separation of the airway from the digestive tract and obviates any concerns for aspiration (Maclean, Szczesniak, Cotton, Cook, & Perry, 2011).

The true incidence of swallowing difficulties after a total laryngectomy is not known. This, in part, is due to variability in defining what constitutes "dysphagia" in a patient population with no risk of aspiration. In a survey of laryngectomees from New South Wales, Australia, Maclean et al. found that 72% of respondents reported some difficulty with swallowing. Many of the patients reporting swallowing problems (71%) had made modifications of their diet (most commonly avoiding meat) and 86% of them required liquids to wash solids down (Maclean, Cotton, & Perry, 2009).

BASE OF THE SKULL

When head and neck cancers invade the base of the skull, the impact on swallowing is often due primarily to the loss of cranial nerve function. Because of the anatomic proximity of the cranial nerves at the skull base, multiple nerve deficits are usually present (Jennings, Sirocky, & Jackson, 1992; Kronenberger, & Meyers, 1994). Tumors in the region of the infratemporal fossa, near the foramen ovale, can be expected to impact the trigeminal nerve. The muscles of mastication and sensation to the tongue and soft palate will be impaired, thus affecting oral bolus preparation and manipulation. Tumors near the jugular foramen may involve the glossopharyngeal nerve and the vagus. Because the glossopharyngeal nerve provides sensation to the posterior one third of the tongue, swallow initiation may be delayed.

Both the glossopharyngeal and the vagus nerves provide innervation to the muscles of the pharynx. Once the pharyngeal swallowing sequence is initiated, weakness of the pharynx due to tumor involvement of the vagus and glossopharyngeal nerves results in poor pharyngeal contraction with poor pharyngeal clearing. In extreme cases, the patient is unable to propel the bolus into the pharyngoesophageal sphincter. An ipsilateral vocal fold paralysis is usually present in these already severely compromised patients. As tumors near the jugular foramen enlarge, the hypoglossal nerve will become involved. The resultant tongue weakness has significant impact on both the oral and pharyngeal phases of swallowing.

POSTOPERATIVE AND PRIMARY RADIATION THERAPY

The addition of postoperative radiation therapy to surgical treatment will likely worsen dysphagia (Nguyen, Frank, Moltz, Millar, Smith, et al., 2009). During the radiation treatment period, patients experience significant mucositis resulting in pain, swelling, mucus production, and xerostomia. Oral feeding may be extremely difficult. Acute effects of radiation therapy usually last for approximately 8 to 12 weeks after the final treatments. Swallowing therapy may be limited during this period by the patient's inability to participate. Generally, the use of exercises during this radiation has not yet been shown to be effective in limiting the resulting dysphagia. However, further study of the effects of swallowing therapy in this patient population is needed.

The long-term effects of radiation therapy involve the fibrosis of residual soft tissues and xerostomia. Tissue fibrosis of the muscles involved in deglutition limits the normal range of muscle motion, resulting in decreased tongue mobility and lack of larynx and hyoid elevation. Xerostomia will further predispose to dental caries as well as diminished lubrication of the bolus.

A study of 20 patients treated for head and neck cancer with radiation therapy alone revealed that the most common abnormality identified 1 year after the completion of therapy on the dynamic videofluoroscopic swallow study was poor pharyngeal constriction, likely secondary to a decrease of tongue range of motion (Kendall, McKenzie, & Leonard, 1998).

CHEMORADIATION THERAPY

In recent years, tumors of the oropharynx have been preferentially treated with a combination of chemotherapy given concurrently with radiation. Tumors of the base of tongue, tonsil, posterior pharyngeal wall, and palate are included in this group. Hypopha-ryngeal tumors are also commonly treated with this approach and include tumors of the piriform fossa, supraglottic larynx, and larynx (without cartilage invasion). Dysphagia is a frequent side effect of this type of therapy. Swallowing problems are likely caused by radiation-induced edema and muscular fibrosis. Some patients experience permanent lymphedema resulting in long-term swelling of supraglottic structures. Clinical factors that increase the risk for permanent dysphagia after chemoradiation therapy include increasing age, location of the tumor in the larynx or hypopharynx, and increasing size of the tumor (Caudell, Schaner,Desmond, Meridith, Spencer, et al., 2010).

The rationale behind chemoradiation therapy as primary treatment rather than surgery followed by radiation, is that "organ sparing" treatment rather than removal of tissues with cancer by surgery, should improve functional outcomes. Unfortunately, as the intensity of these treatments has increased to improve oncologic outcomes, the incidence of long-term dysphagia experienced by this patient population is also increasing. In a retrospective review of 132 patients, Teguh et al. found poor scores of swallowing function on swallowing related quality of life questionnaires in approximately 30% of tongue base cancer patients and in approximately 20% of tonsillar fossa cancer patients. This group of investigators was also able to demonstrate a relationship between the dose of radiation received by the superior constrictor muscles and the degree of dysphagia (Teguh, Levendag, Noever, Van Rooij, Voet, et al., 2008). Other investigators have found that the dose of radiation received by the larynx and supraglottis also has significant influence on the degree of dysphagia (Roe, Carding, Dwivedi, Kazi, Rhys-Evans, et al., 2010; Teguh, Levendag, Noever, Van Rooij, Voet, et al., 2008).

Intensity-Modulated Radiation Therapy (IMRT) has been developed to decrease radiation scatter and concentrate the radiation to the tumor site. However, to date, there has been no significant evidence that this approach is able to reduce the dose received by the pharyngeal constrictors, and thus reduce dysphagia (Caudell et al., 2010; Roe et al., 2010).

In a retrospective study of 83 patients treated with IMRT for head and neck cancer, Caudell et al. found that at one year after treatment, 22% of patients remained gastrostomy tube dependent and 45% of patients demonstrated aspiration on a swallowing study. Twenty percent of patients developed a pharyngoesophageal stenosis severe enough to require dilation. Increasing radiation dose was again found to be associated with a higher risk of developing any of these problems, but the use of IMRT versus more conventional radiation methods did not significantly lower the risk. In a well-designed study of IMRT and swallowing function, Feng et al. prospectively evaluated 73 patients with oropharyngeal cancer treated with chemoradiation using IMRT to avoid exposure of the pharyngeal constrictors. This study (Caudell et al., 2010) demonstrated excellent oncologic results (>90% survival at one year) and 94% of patients were eating a normal diet at one year after treatment. Interestingly, despite a preponderance of dietary normalcy, 26% of patients demonstrated aspiration on a videofluoroscopic study of swallowing and 60% of those that

aspirated did so silently or with an ineffective cough response (Feng, Hyungjin, Lyden, Haxer, & Worden, et al., 2010). These results support the hypothesis that patient perception of function after chemoradiation therapy may not be consistent with the findings of more objective means of evaluation.

Most head and neck chemoradiation patients report a deterioration of swallowing function from baseline during the 3- to 6-month posttreatment time frame. Those patients who had dysphagia prior to treatment will experience more severe dysphagia during and posttreatment (Agarwal, Baccher, Budrukkar, Chaturvedi, Chaukar, et al., 2010; Feng et al., 2010). Swallowing studies performed during this period may document aspiration in up to 69% of patients. Langerman et al. found a greater incidence of aspiration in patients with laryngeal and hypopharyngeal tumors compared to other tumor locations (Langerman et al., 2007). Nguyen et al. found that the risk of aspiration after completion of treatment increased with increasing size of the initial tumor (Nguyen, Frank, Moltz, Vos, Smith, et al., 2009). Despite complaints of dysphagia symptoms and a high incidence of deteriorating function, it is during this time frame that patients are typically encouraged to start eating an oral diet. Careful evaluation, prior to attempts at oral eating, has the potential to decrease the risk of aspiration by determining if swallowing strategies and consistency modifications are beneficial. Referral of all head and neck chemoradiation patients to a speech pathologist is therefore recommended.

Many patients treated with primary chemoradiation therapy will also undergo a neck dissection to address metastatic disease to the cervical lymph nodes. In the past, patients with bulky neck disease were scheduled for a neck dissection irrespective of response of the disease to chemoradiation therapy. In recent years, however, more and more patients are assessed with Positron Emission Tomography (PET) scans prior to neck dissection. Only those patients with an incomplete response to chemoradiation therapy in the cervical lymph nodes, as identified on PET, will undergo a neck dissection. Typically, neck dissections are performed 3 to 6 months after completion of the chemoradiation therapy. This is a time when dysphagia is also a significant problem for the patient. Concerns that the addition of a neck dissection to treatment will increase long-term problems with dysphagia have been raised, but so far studies done to determine the impact of neck dissection on long-term swallowing function report conflicting results (Chapuy, Annino, Snavely, Li, Tishler, et al., 2011; Lango, Egleston, Ende, Feigenberg, D'Ambrosio, et al., 2010).

Despite a large body of literature that documents significant dysphagia in patients after treatment with chemoradiation therapy, little is known about the specific physiologic changes that occur in swallowing function. An understanding of such changes would be extremely helpful in designing swallowing therapy protocols for patients during and immediately after chemoradiation treatment. The vast majority of studies done to evaluate swallowing in chemoradiation therapy patients have used subjective assessment tools completed by the patient or the presence or absence of gastrostomy tube to measure swallowing function. Those studies that have used a videofluoro-

scopic study of swallowing typically report only the presence or absence of aspiration rather than an in-depth analysis of the physiologic changes that lead to poor swallowing. One exception is the work done by researchers at Northwestern University in Chicago. In evaluating physiologic swallowing function with videofluoroscopy, Pauloski et al. analyzed 132 head and neck cancer patients to determine if patient complaints of dysphagia correlate with physiologic abnormalities. The study found that patients who complain of dysphagia were more likely to have abnormalities on the swallowing study. Interestingly, the estimate of percent bolus swallowed, a crude method of judging pharyngeal constriction, was the most likely to correlate with complaints of dysphagia. Unfortunately, this study did not report on the incidence of swallowing abnormalities in patients who did not complain of dysphagia (Pauloski, Rademaker, Logemann, Lazarus, Newman, et al., 2002).

In a follow-up study of 53 patients before treatment and at three months after treatment completion (when dysphagia is likely to be the most severe), an in-depth analysis of swallowing physiology was done. The most common physiologic abnormality was "reduced tongue base retraction," seen in approximately 95% of patients with tumor located in oropharynx and larynx at three months after treatment. Overall, the studies were judged to demonstrate significant changes in structural mobility, but despite this, dramatic change in the timing of swallowing gestures was not identified. In comparing pretreatment swallowing to post-treatment swallowing, the authors concluded that patients did not develop new dysfunction after treatment, but abnormalities that were mild before therapy became more severe after therapy (Logemann, Rademaker, Pauloski, Lazarus, Mittal, et al., 2006). Based on these results, successful individualized therapy protocols could be formulated for physiologic abnormalities identified on pretreatment swallowing studies. Even if no clear abnormality is identified on a pretreatment swallowing study, therapy could be based on the most common abnormalities identified to date: pharyngeal residue (consistent with poor pharyngeal constriction needed to clear the bolus from the pharynx) and poor tongue base retraction (an important component of adequate pharyngeal constriction). Furthermore, in a study of 11 head and neck cancer patients using simultaneous videofluoroscopy and manometry, these researchers subsequently confirmed poor pharyngeal constriction to be a significant component of swallowing dysfunction (Pauloski, Rademaker, Lazarus, Boeckxstaens, Kahrilas, et al., 2009).

QUALITY OF LIFE

The lingering effects of head and neck cancer treatment have an impact on overall quality of life. Especially when more than one treatment modality exists and both provide equal oncologic outcome, it is important to determine the impact of each treatment on overall functioning and therefore, quality of life. In the instance of head and neck cancer treatment, surgery followed by radiation therapy and primary chemoradiation therapy with and without a neck dissection result in equal overall prognosis for cure. The impact of these treatments on swallowing function, however, determines their effect on long-term quality of life.

Most studies of quality of life in head and neck cancer patients have demonstrated a decrease in nearly all parameters of health-related quality of life during and immediately after chemoradiation treatment, with improvements beginning around six months later, when the acute affects of therapy are diminishing. Studies looking specifically at swallowing function, however, note a deterioration of swallowing function at three months with little improvement at the 12-month posttreatment point (Wilson, Carding, & Patterson, 2011). Long-term quality of life studies in head and neck cancer patients are relatively few but have documented persistent swallowing dysfunction. In a study of 62 head and neck cancer patients treated with chemoradiation therapy who had survived at least five years after their diagnosis, Campbell et al. found that 44% of the patients demonstrated at least some aspiration on a videofluorscopic swallowing study and 21% silently aspirated. Aspiration was significantly associated with diminished quality of life scores for chewing, swallowing, and normalcy of diet (Campbell, Spinelli, Marbella, Myers, Khun, et al., 2004). A more recent study of 337 similar patients revealed that less than half of the patients reported normal or near-normal functioning for eating (Funk, Karnell, & Christensen, 2012).

When quality of life studies are conducted directly comparing patients treated by laryngectomy and postoperative radiation therapy to patients treated with chemoradiation therapy for laryngeal cancer, the results indicate that laryngectomy patients report diminished satisfaction in the domains of speech and shoulder functioning and that chemoradiation therapy patients report worse satisfaction in the domains of chewing and swallowing (Lotempio, Wang, Sadeghi, Celacure, Juillard, et al., 2005). One might conclude that patients undergoing total laryngectomy are more impacted by their speech rehabilitation challenges than by any swallowing difficulties and that patients treated with chemoradiation therapy, while maintaining excellent speech capabilities, may suffer significantly with dysphagia. Patient treatment options, taking into account the location and size of the tumor, will be clearer, as further studies bring to light the potential long-term effects of each treatment option.

CONCLUSION

The variability inherent in head and neck cancer patients, with respect to location and size of the tumor, as well as treatment modality, creates significant difficulty when categorizing patients into groups for comparison of outcome studies involving deglutition. Each patient must be considered individually. Other factors, including the overall medical condition, social situation and support system, will likely impact the patient's ability to achieve adequate safe oral intake and to maintain nutritional requirements.

As clinicians, our goal is to optimize the functioning of each individual patient after first effectively eradicating the cancer. Surgeons must continue to take into account the structures involved in the tumor and thoughtfully reconstruct defects in such a way

to minimize functional deficits and obstruction to bolus flow. Radiation oncologists must continue to evaluate strategies for minimizing radiation scatter and determine the minimal dose required for effective treatment of any given tumor. Speech-language pathologists must be involved with the care of these patients before they begin treatment. Swallowing function must be assessed prior to treatment and strategies for safe, effective swallowing during treatment must be determined. Swallowing exercises must be initiated, and if possible, continued during treatment. Patients should be monitored closely in the post-treatment period and encouraged as they begin to expand their oral intake.

There is still substantial research to be done in the area of swallowing function after treatment for head and neck cancer. In particular, objective data on the effect of swallowing exercises during treatment on long-term swallowing outcomes are needed. The potential to improve the long-term swallowing function, and thus the quality of life, in head and neck cancer patients is significant.

STUDY QUESTIONS

1. How does tongue tethering impact swallowing function? For example, if the tongue is tethered to the anterior oral cavity (as in primary closure of an anterior floor-of-mouth defect), how does that affect the movement of the bolus through the pharynx?
2. What are the consequences (for swallowing) of a palatal defect?
3. What reconstructive options are available to repair a tongue defect

and what is the potential impact of each option on swallowing function?

4. How does poor hyoid bone elevation impact swallowing function?

5. What pretreatment factors best predict the likelihood of developing dysphagia after treatment for head and neck cancer?

6. Discuss the use of non-oral feeding during chemoradiation therapy. What are the pros and cons?

7. What structures are removed during an open supraglottic laryngectomy? What are the implications for swallowing function?

8. What clinical factors increase the risk of dysphagia after chemoradiation therapy?

9. What treatment factors increase the risk of developing dysphagia after chemoradiation therapy?

10. What is the incidence of aspiration in long-term (greater than five years) survivors of head and neck cancer?

REFERENCES

Agarwal, J., Baccher, G., Budrukkar, A., Chaturvedi, P., Chaukar, D., & D'Cruz, A. (2010). Prospective subjective evaluation of swallowing function and dietary pattern in head and neck cancer treated with concomitant chemo-radiation. *Journal of Cancer Research and Therapeutics, 6,* 15–21.

Baker, B. M., Fraser, A. M., & Baker, C. D. (1991) Long-term postoperative dysphagia in oral/pharyngeal surgery patients: Subjects' perceptions vs. videofluoroscopic observations. *Dysphagia, 6,* 11–16.

Burns, J. A., Har-El, F., Shapsay, S., Maune, S., & Zeitels, S. M. (2009). Endoscopic laser resection of laryngeal cancer: Is it oncologically safe? *Annals of Otology, Rhinology, and Laryngology, 118,* 399–404.

Calcaterra, T. (1971). Laryngeal suspension after supraglottic laryngectomy. *Archives of Otolaryngology, 94,* 306–309.

Campbell, B. H., Spinelli, K., Marbella, A. M., Myers, K. B., Khun, J. C., & Layde, P. M. (2004). Aspiration, weight loss, and quality of life in head and neck cancer survivors. *Otolaryngology-Head and Neck Surgery, 130,* 110–1103.

Caudell, J. J., Schaner, P. E, Desmond, R. A., Meridith, R. F., Spencer, S. A., & Bonner, J. A. (2010). Dosiemetric factors associated with long-term dysphagia after definitive radiotherapy for squamous cell carcinoma of the head and neck. *International Journal of Radiation-Oncology-Biology-Physics, 76,* 403–409.

Chapuy, C. I., Annino, D. J., Snavely, A., Li, Y., Tishler, R. B., Norris, . . . Goguen, L. A. (2011). Swallowing function following postchemoradiotherapy neck dissection: Review of findings and analysis of contributing factors. *Otolaryngology-Head and Neck Surgery, 145,* 428–434.

Chen, A. M., Li, B. Q., Lau, D. H., Farwell, D. G., Luu, Q., Stuart, K., . . . Vijayakumar, S. (2010). Evaluating the role of prophylactic gastrostomy tube placement prior to definitive chemoradiotherapy for head and neck cancer. *International Journal of Radiation-Oncology-Biology-Physics, 136,* 126–133.

Feng, F. Y., Hyungjin, M. K., Lyden, T. H., Haxer, M. J., Worden, F. P., Feng, M., . . . Eisbruch, A. (2010). Intensity-modulated chemoradiotherapy aiming to reduce dysphagia in patients with oropharyngeal cancer: Clinical and functional results. *Journal of Clinical Oncology, 28,* 2732–2738.

Freeman, R. B., Marks, J. E., & Ogura, J. H. (1979). Voice preservation in treatment of carcinoma of the piriform sinus. *Laryngoscope, 89,* 1855–1863.

Frowen, J., Cotton, S., Corry, J., & Perry, A. (2010) Impact of demographics, tumor characteristics, and treatment factors on swallowing after chemoradiation therapy for head and neck cancer. *Head and Neck, 32*, 513–528.

Funk, G., Karnell, L. H., & Christensen, A. J. (2012). Long-term health-related quality of life in survivors of head and neck cancer. *Archives of Otolaryngology-Head and Neck Surgery, 138*, 123–133.

Hinne, M. L., Salassa, J. R., Grant, D. G., Pearson, B. W., Hayden, R. E., Martin, A., . . . Steiner, W. (2007). Transoral laser microsurgery for advanced laryngeal cancer. *Archives of Otolaryngology-Head and Neck Surgery, 113*, 1198–1204.

Jennings, K. S., Sirocky, D., & Jackson, C. G. (1992). Swallowing problems after excision of tumors of the skull base: Diagnosis and management in 12 patients. *Dysphagia, 7*, 40–44.

Karatzanis, A. D., Psychogios, G., Zenk, J., Waldfahrer, F., Hornung, J., Velegrakis, G. A., & Heinrich, I. (2010). Evaluation of available surgical management options for early supraglottic cancer. *Head and Neck, 32*, 1048–1055.

Kendall, K. A., McKenzie, S. W., & Leonard, R. J. (1998). Structural mobility in deglutition after single modality treatment of head and neck carcinomas with radiation therapy. *Head and Neck, 20*, 720–725.

Kronenberger, M. B., & Meyers, A. D. (1994). Dysphagia following head and neck cancer surgery. *Dysphagia, 9*, 236–244.

Kubrak, C., Olson, K., Jha, N., Jensen, L., McCargar, L., Seikaly, H., . . . Parliament, M., & Baracos, V. E. (2010). Nutrition impact symptoms: key determinants of reduced dietary intake, weight loss, and reduced functional capacity of patients with head and neck cancer before treatment. *Head and Neck, 32*, 290–300.

Langerman, A., MacCracken, E., Kasza, K., Haraf, D. J., Vokes, E. E., & Stenson, K. M. (2007). Aspiration in chemoradiated patient with head and neck cancer. *Archives of Otolaryngology-Head and Neck Surgery, 133*, 1289–1295.

Langmore, S., Crisciunas, G. P., Miloro, K. V., Evans, S. R., & Cheng, D. M. (2011). Does PEG use cause dysphagia in head and neck cancer patients? *Dysphagia.* [Epub ahead of print]

Lango, M. N., Egleston, B., Ende, K., Feigenberg, S., D'Ambrosio, D. J., Cohen, R. B., . . . Ridge, J. A. (2010). Impact of neck dissection on long-term feeding tube dependence in patients with head and neck cancer treated with primary radiation or chemoradiation. *Head and Neck, 32*, 341–347.

Logemann, J. A., Rademaker, A. W., Pauloski, B. R., Lazarus, C. L., Mittal, B. B., Brockstein, B., . . . Liu, D. (2006). Site of disease and treatment protocol as correlates of swallowing function in patients with head and neck cancer treated with chemoradiation. *Head and Neck, 28*, 64–73.

Lotempio, M. M., Wang, K. H., Sadeghi, A., Celacure, M. D., Juillard, G. F., & Wang, M.B. (2005). Comparison of quality of life outcomes in laryngeal cancer patients following chemoradiation vs. total laryngectomy. *Otolaryngology-Head and Neck Surgery, 132*, 948–953.

Maclean, J., Cotton, S., & Perry, A. (2009). Post-laryngectomy: It's hard to swallow. *Dysphagia, 24*,172–179.

Maclean, J., Szczesniak, M., Cotton, S., Cook, I., & Perry, A. (2011). Impact of a laryngectomy and surgical closure technique on swallow biomechanics and dysphagia severity. *Otolaryngology-Head and Neck Surgery, 144*, 21–28.

McConnel, F. M. S. (1996). *Evaluation of the reconstruction of the oropharynx with modified barium swallow and manofluorography.* Presented at the First International Neurolaryngology Symposium October 3, 1996, Bethesda, MD.

McConnel, F. M. S., Logemann, J. A., Rademaker, A. W., Pauloski, B. R., Baker, S.R., Lewin, J., . . . Baker, T. (1994). Surgical variables affecting postoperative swallowing efficiency in oral cancer patients: A pilot study. *Laryngoscope, 104*, 87–90.

McConnel, F. M. S., & Mendelsohn, M. (1987). The effects of surgery on pharyngeal deglutition. *Dysphagia, 1*, 145–151.

McConnel, F. M. S., & O'Connor, A. (1994). Dysphagia secondary to head and neck cancer surgery. *Acta Otorhinolaryngologica Belgium, 48*, 165–170.

McLaughlin, B. T., Gokhale, A. S., Shuai, Y., Diacopoulos, J., Carrau, R., Heron, D. E., . . . Argiris, A. (2010). Management of patients treated with chemoradiotherapy for head and neck cancer without prophylactic feeding tubes: The University of Pittsburgh experience. *Laryngoscope, 120*, 71–75.

Nguyen, N. P., Frank, C., Moltz, C. C., Millar, C., Smith, H. J., Dutta, S., . . . Sallah S. (2009). Aspiration risk and postoperative radiation for head and neck cancer. *Cancer Investigation, 27*, 47–51.

Nguyen, N. P., Frank, C., Moltz, C. C., Vos, P., Smith, H. J., Nguyen, P. D., . . . Sallah, S. (2009). Analysis of factors influencing aspiration risk following chemoradiation for oropharyngeal cancer. *British Journal of Radiology, 82*, 675–680.

Nguyen, N. P., North, D., Smith, H. J., Dutta, S., Alfieri, A., Karlsson, U., . . . Sallah, S. (2006). Safety and effectiveness of prophylactic gastrostomy tubes for head and neck cancer patients undergoing chemoradiation. *Surgical Oncology, 15*, 199–203.

Pauloski, B. R., Logemann, J. A., Fox, J. C., & Colangelo, L. A. (1995). Biomechanical analysis of the pharyngeal swallow in postsurgical patients with anterior tongue and floor of mouth resection and distal flap reconstruction. *Journal of Speech and Hearing Research, 38*, 110–123.

Pauloski, B. R., Logemann, J. A., Rademaker, A. W., McConnel, F. M. S., Stein, D., Beery, Q., . . . Baker, T. (1995). Speech and swallowing function after oral and oropharyngeal resections: One-year follow-up. *Head and Neck, 16*, 313–322.

Pauloski, B. R., Rademaker, A. W., Lazarus, C., Boeckxstaens, G., Kahrilas, P. J., & Logemann, J. A. (2009). Relationship between manometric and videofluoroscopic measures of swallow function in healthy adults and patients treated for head and neck cancer with various modalities. *Dysphagia, 42*, 196–203.

Pauloski, B. R., Rademaker, A. W., Logemann, J. A., Lazarus, C. L., Newman, L., Hamner, A., . . . Tachowiak, L. (2002). Swallow function and perception of dysphagia in patients with head and neck cancer. *Head and Neck, 24*, 555–565.

Pauloski, B. R., Logemann, J. A., Rademaker, A. W., McConnel, F. M. S., Heiser, M. A., Cardinale, S., . . . Baker, T. (1993). Speech and swallowing function after anterior tongue and floor of mouth resection with distal flap reconstruction. *Journal of Speech and Hearing Research, 36*, 267–276.

Peretti, G., Piazza, C., Cattaneo, A., De Benedetto, L., Martin, E., & Nicolai, P. (2006). Comparison of functional outcomes after endoscopic versus open-neck supraglottic laryngectomies. *Archives of Otology, Rhinology, and Laryngology, 115*, 827–832.

Roe, J. W. G., Carding, P. N., Dwivedi, R. C., Kazi, R. A., Rhys-Evans, P. H., Harrington, K. J., & Nutting, C. M. (2010). Swallowing outcomes following intensity modulated radiation therapy (IMRT) for head and neck cancer: A systematic review. *Oral Oncology, 46*, 727–733.

Starmer, H. H., Gourin, C. G., Lua, L. L., & Burkhead, L. (2011). Pretreatment swallowing assessment in head and neck cancer patients. *Laryngoscope, 121*, 1208–1211.

Stenson, K. M., MacCracken, E., List, M., Haraf, D. J., Brockstein, B., Weichselbaum, R., & Vokes, E. E. (2000). Swallowing function in patients with head and neck cancer prior to treatment. *Archives of Otolaryngology-Head and Neck Surgery, 126*, 371–377.

Teguh, D. N., Levendag, P. C., Noever, I., Van Rooij, P., Voet, P., Van der Est, H., . . . Schmitz, P. I. M. (2008). Treatment techniques and site considerations regarding dysphagia-related quality of life in cancer of the oropharynx and nasopharynx. *International Journal of Radiation-Oncology-Biology-Physics, 72*, 1119–1127.

Wiggenraad, R. G., Flierman, L., Goossens, A., Brand, R., Verschuur, H. P., Croll,

G. A., . . . Vriesendorp, R. (2007). *Clinical Otolaryngology, 32*, 384–390.

Wilson, J. A., Carding, P. N., & Patterson, J. M. (2011). Dysphagia after nonsurgical head and neck cancer treatment: Patients' perspective. *Otolaryngology-Head and Neck Surgery, 145*, 767–771.

Zafereo, M. E., Weber, R. S., Lewin, J. S., Roberts, D. B., & Hanasono, M. M. (2010). Complications and functional outcomes following complex oropharyngeal reconstruction. *Head and Neck, 32*, 1003–1011.

4

Neurogenic Dysphagia

Jacqui Allen

Neurogenic disorders are among the most common etiologies responsible for swallowing dysfunction. A heterogeneous group of pathologies must be considered, that span acute onset central disorders such as stroke, progressive, insidious disorders such as amyotrophic lateral sclerosis (ALS) and peripheral neuromyogenic dysfunction as seen in inflammatory myositis (Table 4–1). The effects of neuromyogenic dysfunction may also manifest in a variety of ways including end organ weakness or failure, incoordination of gestures or total failure of central patterning. The underlying etiology determines which aspect of deglutition is most prominently affected and therefore which therapies may be effective in rehabilitating swallow or preventing complications of dysphagia. More than three quarters of cases of oropharyngeal dysphagia are due to neurological disorders (Diniz, Vanin, Xavier, & Parente, 2009; White, O'Rourke, Ong, Cordato, & Chan, 2008). In order to offer the best diagnostic and treatment

options to patients we must understand basic pathophysiological mechanisms in these disorders and the most vulnerable portions of deglutition in each case.

This chapter briefly presents the most common neuromyogenic disorders related to dysphagia, characteristics of dysphagia and videofluoroscopic findings specific to each and optimum assessment of the patient: crucial in both making the correct diagnosis and in advising safe dietary and rehabilitative regimens.

ASSESSMENT

The test battery approach in a multidisciplinary environment offers the best diagnostic accuracy and will provide the most useful information regarding diagnosis, prognosis, compensatory strategies, and dietary safety. Multiple methods are available to assess the dysphagic patient and each provides complementary information that can be crucial to treatment planning in a

Table 4–1. Etiology of Neurogenic Dysphagia

CENTRAL		PERIPHERAL	
Nondegenerative	**Degenerative**	**Neuromuscular**	**Myopathy**
Cerebrovascular Accident

Brain Injury

Medication

Neoplasm

Congenital— cerebral palsy, syringobulbia, Arnold Chiari malformation | Dementia— Alzheimer's disease, multi-infarct

Parkinson's disease

Multiple sclerosis

Huntington's disease

Supranuclear palsy | Myasthenia gravis

Polio, Post-polio syndrome

Amyotrophic lateral sclerosis | Muscular dystrophies: Oculopharyngeal muscular dystrophy (OPMD), Myotonic (MD), Duchenne (DMD)

Polymyositis, Dermatomyositis, Inclusion body myositis |
| | | **Neuropathy** | **Iatrogenic** |
| | | Guillain-Barré syndrome | Post surgery or radiotherapy of the head and neck |

team setting (Rugiu, 2007). Many of these strategies are discussed in this book. A thorough clinical evaluation by a trained swallowing professional such as a speech pathologist is the first step. Although this is invaluable in identifying struggling patients and developing rapport, multiple studies have demonstrated that patients with neuromyogenic conditions frequently present with silent aspiration and cannot, by definition, be identified by bedside evaluation (Diniz et al., 2009; Gonzalez-Fernandez & Daniels, 2008; Kang, Kim, Seo, & Seo, 2011; Ramsey, Smithard & Kalra, 2003; Rugiu, 2007; White et al., 2008). Sensitivity of the bedside examination ranges from 40 to 80% and specificity ranges from 59 to 91% (Ramsey, Smithard, & Kalra, 2003; Rugiu, 2007; Gonzalez-Fernandez & Daniels, 2008). Instrumental examina-tion is invaluable in detecting silent aspirators and most commonly consists of a dynamic videofluoroscopic swallowing study (VFSS), also called a dynamic swallow study (DSS). The dynamic swallow study (Chapters 14 to 17) provides objective and quantitative data which can elaborate the nature and severity of a swallowing problem, provide insights into prognosis in individual patients, and be used to develop remedial treatment programs. It has been considered the "gold standard" in instrumental assessment (Gonzalez-Fernandez & Daniels, 2008; Kang, Kim, Seo, & Seo, 2011; Ney, Weiss, Kind, & Robbins, 2009; Rugiu, 2007). However, this radiographic study is two dimensional and requires exposure to ionizing radiation (approximately that of two cervical spine x-rays) and specialized equipment and personnel are not always available to the assessing clinician. Consequently, the use and timing of the DSS must be considered with respect to minimizing both diagnostic costs and x-ray exposure, particularly in patient populations that experience frequent and significant change, sometimes rapid and for the better, sometimes prolonged and for the worse. An instrumental flexible endoscopic evaluation of swallowing (FEES; Chapter 11) may also identify aspiration, provide distinct laryngopharyngeal anatomic information that may complement the DSS, be performed at the bedside (useful in those patients unable to be transported to a radiology suite) and avoids the consequent risks of radiation exposure (most pertinent in young, elderly or multiply injured patients). Information from FEES is complementary to videofluoroscopic study information and both studies may be useful in any given patient (Gonzalez-Fernandez & Daniels, 2008; Rugiu, 2007). A battery of diagnostic strategies that permits the most efficacious collection of information in a practical and safe way should be the aim when assessing swallowing problems in neurogenic patients.

CENTRAL NERVOUS SYSTEM DISORDERS

Cerebrovascular Accident (CVA)

Dysphagia is found in 29 to 80% of those presenting with an acute stroke (Diniz et al., 2009; Garon, Sierzant, & Ormiston, 2009; Gonzalez-Fernandez & Daniels, 2008; Kang et al., 2011; Kumar, Selim, & Caplan, 2010; Ney et al., 2009; Rugiu, 2007). In many cases (50 to 90%)

rapid improvement may be expected over the short to medium term but persistent dysphagia is seen in approximately 20 to 50% of patients (Diniz et al., 2009; Garon et al., 2009; Gonzalez-Fernandez & Daniels, 2008; Rugiu, 2007; White et al., 2008). Around half of those with acute strokes develop aspiration and 35% develop aspiration pneumonia (Ney et al., 2009). Even a year later 15 to 20% of post-CVA patients develop pneumonia and almost half of CVA patients are malnourished (Ney et al., 2009). Swallowing function has bilateral cortical representation with interconnecting crossed pathways at the level of the brainstem (Gonzalez-Fernandez & Daniels, 2008; White et al., 2008). Insults to the internal capsule, thalamus, basal ganglia, and midbrain structures such as the cerebral peduncles may also affect deglutition. Dysphagia is therefore a prominent feature of brainstem and both right and left cortical insults (Kumar et al., 2010; Ney et al., 2009; Paliwal, Kalita, & Misra, 2009) and usually affects the oropharyngeal phase of deglutition (Donner, Bosma, & Robertson, 1985; Rugiu, 2007). Sensory deficits (particularly if they affect the pharynx) also lead to significant dysfunction and may be a cause of silent aspiration. Therefore, injury at many sites can result in swallowing difficulties.

Dysphagia after stroke is associated with development of aspiration pneumonia (3 to 11-fold increased risk) (Altman, Yu, & Schaefer, 2010; Gonzalez-Fernandez & Daniels, 2008; Kumar, Selim, & Caplan, 2010; Ney, Weiss, Kind, & Robbins, 2009; Rugiu, 2007; White, O'Rourke, Ong, Cordato, & Chan, 2008). Silent aspiration is common after stroke (2 to 66%) and may manifest only as recurrent pulmonary complications (Gonzalez-Fernandez & Daniels, 2008; Ramsey, Smithard, & Kalra, 2003; Ney, Weiss, Kind, & Robbins, 2009; Rugiu, 2007). Aspiration pneumonia is the most common cause of re-hospitalization in acute stroke patients and contributes to more than 50% of post-CVA deaths in the first 30 days (Ney et al., 2009). Silent aspiration (by definition) is not detected by bedside evaluation and therefore a high index of suspicion is required. Consequences of aspiration in stroke patients are severe. Aspiration pneumonia is the leading cause of death post-stroke and reduced oxygenation resulting from pneumonia may exacerbate neurological injury and slow recovery (Kang et al., 2011; White et al., 2008). It is estimated that 5 to 15% of community acquired pneumonia is caused by aspiration (White et al., 2008).

Due to the high prevalence of dysphagia in stroke patients, screening for swallowing problems should be considered and a high index of suspicion should be maintained in all patients, even those with no overt signs of dysphagia. Initially, a bedside assessment by a speech pathologist or trained clinician should be performed. In most cases involving hemispheric or brainstem sites, an instrumental evaluation is indicated due to the high rate of silent aspiration (Gonzalez-Fernandez & Daniels, 2008; Ney et al., 2009; Ramsey, Smithard & Kalra, 2003, 2005; Rugiu, 2007). Patients presenting with additional risk factors for aspiration (based on site of lesion, comorbidities, age, pulmonary health, head and neck cancer, dementia, and cervical spine abnormalities) should be identified and also undergo instrumental evaluation regardless of findings of bedside or clinical

evaluations. Instrumental examination may consist of videofluoroscopy (DSS), endoscopy (FEES) or both. DSS and FEES both demonstrate high sensitivity and specificity in identifying aspiration (>85%) (Ramsey, Smithard, & Kalra, 2005; Rugiu, 2007). The DSS will also demonstrate pharyngoesophageal and oesophageal phase abnormalities. Fluoroscopic studies help delineate the mechanism of dysphagia, allow assessment of compensatory maneuvers and contribute to planning of safe swallow strategies. Visualization of the vocal folds is not possible with DSS, though mobility may be appreciated with a voicing task performed in the anterior-posterior view. FEES permits ready examination of the vocal folds, and, like fluoroscopy, allows assessment of asymmetry (e.g., unilateral weakness or obstruction) that will assist in devising compensatory strategies. Therefore information obtained from these studies is complementary and often both are required to devise the best treatment strategy.

Clinical factors that suggest the need for evaluation with a DSS include: (a) aspiration pneumonia, (b) cough, "wet voice" and "wet lung" following swallowing, and (c) inability to maintain oral hydration and nutrition. The DSS is of value in identifying the presence of aspiration, and the effects of various remedial strategies, even with no quantitative assessment. Our experience, however, suggests that the extra time and expense associated with obtaining objective displacement and timing measures can contribute significantly to patient care. Our research has demonstrated that a pharyngeal transit time of greater than 5 seconds (normal 1.00 ± 0.15 sec) is highly associated with aspiration pneumonia risk in stroke patients, whereas a time of less than 2 seconds has a low association (Johnson & McKenzie, 1992, 1993a).

Timing of Evaluations

Following a cerebrovascular accident, a patient's symptoms may undergo rapid change. Timing of evaluations and frequent reassessment therefore is critical. Early speech pathology assessment is required within the first week in order to evaluate the patient's ability to handle oral intake and to provide a baseline for consistent follow-up assessment. Speech pathology and nursing personnel are then prepared to watch for evidence of aspiration, assess the need for more definitive diagnostic studies, and rational progression of dietary intake. Instrumental evaluations are performed based on clinical history, risk factors, and findings of the bedside assessment. In many cases of acute stroke, dysphagia improves rapidly. Factors that suggest a prolonged period of dysphagia (>2 weeks) include failure to cleanly swallow 50 mL of water, modified Barthel Index <20, dysphasia, insular or frontal cortex involvement, Parramatta Hospitals' Dysphagia Index Score <70 (White et al., 2008). As the DSS exposes the patient to radiation, one must be careful to utilize the study at the appropriate time and maximize the amount of information obtained from each study (Chau & Kung, 2009). Early fluoroscopic examination may be necessary for identification of silent aspiration and pharyngeal residue or suspected cricopharyngeal or esophageal problems. Subsequent examinations may be scheduled after a therapeutic trial, when significant motor improvements have been noted (or deterioration seen), or when sensory changes have occurred. FEES examinations may be performed more frequently if trained staff are available, as this does not expose the patient to radiation. FEES also offers the possibility of visual feedback to the patient, which can be of great value in teaching compensatory strategies, if a viewing screen is utilized.

DSS Findings

Stroke often affects the nucleus ambiguus in the brainstem which provides motor output to the pharynx and esophagus resulting in pharyngoesophageal abnormalities. Pharyngeal weakness, prolonged pharyngeal transit time, aspiration, cricopharyngeal dysfunction, and esophageal dysmotility are common findings (Rugiu, 2007). Tongue dysfunction may be noted if the hypoglossal nucleus, situated more caudally in the brainstem, has been involved. Cortical strokes may produce facial asymmetry and weakness that can result in oral incompetence and poor oral bolus control. This may manifest with significant oral and pharyngeal residue which increases the risk of aspiration (Johnson, McKenzie, Rosenquist, Sievers, & Lieberman, 1992; Rugiu, 2007). Johnson et al. (1992) demonstrated that prolongation of pharyngeal transit times over 1s was associated with a significant increase in airway penetration and aspiration and with occurrence of aspiration pneumonia. This was also the finding in Kang et al's study of 39 post-CVA patients (Kang et al., 2011). Pharyngeal transit times longer than 1s were associated with significantly increased abnormalities on DSS, demonstrated using mixed consistency food and barium. Because stroke also results in depression of the immune system, aspiration occurring post-CVA may be less well tolerated, increasing the rate of aspiration pneumonia (White et al., 2008).

Summary

CVA is a leading cause of oropharyngeal and esophageal dysphagia. Dysphagia may be short-lived but in approximately 50% of patients it will be prolonged >2 weeks. Dysphagia is the primary risk factor for aspiration pneumonia which is the leading cause of death after stroke. Aspiration may be silent in up to two-thirds of patients after stroke. Instrumental evaluation is therefore critical in assessing these patients. DSS provides reliable information about the swallow from oral cavity to stomach. It may be complemented by information from other instrumental evaluations. The DSS provides accurate quantitative data that can be used to formulate treatment and rehabilitative strategies and demonstrate change over time. Thoughtful performance of DSS and careful post study analysis will maximize the benefit obtained from fluoroscopic evaluation.

Parkinson's Disease

Dysphagia is almost universal in patients suffering from Parkinson's disease (PD), a progressive motor system disease caused by failed dopamine production. Along with voice deterioration, dysphagia is often one of the presenting symptoms of PD. Altman et al. (2010) demonstrated that admission to hospital with a symptom of dysphagia was significantly associated with Parkinson's disease (relative risk = 4.5) compared to age and sex-matched patients admitted without dysphagia. Solids are often more problematic than liquids and the suprahyoid musculature may be significantly affected (Gonzalez-Fernandez & Robbins, 2008). Hypokinesia that characterizes limb and truncal movements in PD appears to slow initiation of the swallow sequence at the oral cavity and then prolong laryngeal and esophageal movements (Gonzalez-Fernandez & Robbins, 2008; Rugiu, 2007). Stasis and residue may be seen. Electrophysiological studies of patients with PD have demonstrated marked delay in triggering swallow, extremely prolonged pharyngeal swallow durations and normal cricopharyngeal muscle contractions (Ertekin, Tarlaci, Aydogdu, Kiylioglu, Yuceyar, Secil, & Esmeli, 2002).

Amyotrophic Lateral Sclerosis (ALS)

ALS causes dysfunction at both bulbar and spinal levels and dysphagia is a common manifestation (Ertekin, Aydogdu, Yuceyar, Kiylioglu, Tarlaci, & Uludag, 2000; Gonzalez-Fernandez & Daniels, 2008; Rugiu, 2007). ALS is a progressive, neurodegenerative disease that destroys nerve cells in the brain and spinal cord. Over time dysphagia becomes almost ubiquitous, leading to aspiration pneumonia in around 15% of patients (Ertekin et al., 2000; Gonzalez; Fernandez & Daniels, 2007). Solid food dysphagia is usually the first manifestation of swallowing difficulty, but symptoms may eventually be more global, with frequent pharyngeal residue, penetration and aspiration. Dysphagia affects quality of life in ALS patients and is a significant source of morbidity (Ertekin et al., 2000). Patients may describe a globus sensation due to poor pharyngeal transit and transphincteric flow due to UES dysfunction (Ertekin et al., 2000; Rugiu, 2007). Poor oral and tongue control (muscle may fasciculate or atrophy), delayed pharyngeal transit and UES dysfunction are often present and well delineated by DSS (Ertekin et al., 2000). These investigators performed EMG studies in 43 ALS patients and demonstrated prolonged hyolaryngeal elevation, reduced and uncoordinated UES opening, and loss of voluntarily-initiated swallow sequence. Both structural and functional swallow disorders are therefore present, and contribute to airway violation prior to, during and after swallow. Because both timing impairments and structural impairments may occur, the DSS will be invaluable in guiding rehabilitative and compensatory strategies and texture modifications. DSS may also suggest the need for non oral nutrition when swallowing safety is grossly compromised. Early assessment by videofluoroscopy should be considered in patients presenting with ALS even in the absence of reported dysphagia. Patients that demonstrate combined timing and structural abnormalities on DSS should be referred for neurological assessment if this has not been carried out already.

Brain Injury

Prevalence of dysphagia following brain injury seems to vary but may affect 20 to 70% of patients (Kang et al., 2011; Rugiu, 2007). Brain injury can occur as a result of targeted intervention (surgery or radiotherapy) or after trauma, vascular insult or metabolic disorder. Traumatic brain injury (TBI) is commonly caused by motor vehicle accidents, cycle accidents or falls. It affects both children and adults. Typically, onset of dysphagia is acute and recovery may occur following initial injury, making reassessment vital in determining ongoing dietary recommendations and modifications. Impairments often involve voluntary phases of deglutition and incoordination of gestures. These can be highlighted well using the DSS timing measures described here (see Chapters 14 to 17). Oropharyngeal deficits are also seen following traumatic brain injury (TBI) and may be accompanied by primitive reflexes (tongue pumping, sucking, tongue extrusion) (Rugiu, 2007). In patients who have been mechanically ventilated following TBI 65% failed bedside swallowing safety evaluations. TBI increased the likelihood of failing a BSE by 3.2 times. The risk of failing a swallowing survey was increased further if the patient was elderly (>70 yr) or had a tracheostomy (Brown, Hejl, Mandaville, Chaney, Stevenson, & Smith, 2011). In children, severe TBI causes a high rate of dysphagia (68 to 76%) but rapidly improves, usually over 3 months (Morgan, 2010). Given the prevalence of traumatic brain injuries in children (listed as high as 280 per 100,000), there will be a significant number of children requiring both assessment and treatment for swallowing problems (Morgan, 2010). The inherent risks of radiation exposure from videofluoroscopy must be weighed against the invaluable information that can be gained from the study that might direct dietary modifications, swallowing rehabilitation and removal of enteral feeding tubes or tracheostomies. Other factors that should be considered in children following TBI are associated motor disorders, level of cognition (ability to appreciate their dysphagia) and postural issues (Morgan, 2010). These may compound dysphagia and its management. DSS may show typical adult post-TBI findings such as tongue pumping, residue, bolus spill or delayed swallow but may also demonstrate additional findings not seen in adults such as primitive reflexes (suckle, tongue protrusions). In a prospective study of 18 children with TBI assessed by videofluoroscopy a month after injury, 17% (3/18) aspirated: about two-thirds silently (Morgan, 2010).

Multiple Sclerosis

Multiple sclerosis is a progressive demyelinating disease that involves both central and peripheral nerves (Tassorelli, Bergamaschi, Buscone, Bartolo, Funari, Crivelli, et al., 2008). Plaques form in nerve sheaths that result in significant conduction delays and eventual loss of function. As the number of plaques increases in the central nervous system the likelihood of dysphagia increases, as the dominant swallow hemisphere is more likely to have been involved (Tassorelli et al., 2008). Dysphagia occurs in 24 to 43% of patients with multiple sclerosis (MS) but is much more common as disability increases (up to 80% in advanced disease) (Gonzalez-Fernandez & Daniels, 2008; Rugiu,

2007; Tassorelli et al., 2008). Lesions in the anterior insula or opercular area (including sensorimotor and premotor cortices), in particular, can be involved in manifestation of swallow problems. The oral and pharyngeal phases are often affected and upper esophageal sphincter dysfunction is reported frequently (100% of patients in one study) (Abraham & Yun [in Gonzalez-Fernandez & Daniels, 2008]; Rugiu, 2008; Tassorelli et al., 2008). In a study of 23 MS patients, 40% were silent aspirators and more than 80% had some changes in either swallow safety or efficiency as assessed by DSS (Terre-Boliart, Orien-Lopez, Guevara-Espinosa, Ramona-Rona, Bernabeu-Guitart, & Clave-Civit, 2004). A further recent study of 101 MS patients using only a patient screening questionnaire (Northwestern Dysphagia Patient Check Sheet), demonstrated pharyngeal swallowing abnormalities in 30% and aspiration in 7% of patients. Dysphagia was associated with longer disease duration, cerebellar involvement and increasing disability (Calcagno, Ruoppolo, Grasso, De Vincentis, & Paolucci, 2002; Pooravid, Derakhshandeh, Etemadafir, Soleymani, Minagar, & Maghzi, 2010; Tassorrelli et al., 2008). Calcagno and colleagues (2002) followed 143 MS patients using FEES and also found that advanced disease and cerebellar involvement portended a higher rate of dysphagia. However, 17% of patients with milder disease also demonstrated dysphagia. This emphasizes the need to screen, with videofluoroscopy or FEES, patients suspected of aspiration, having pulmonary problems or with advanced disease. Recently, Bergamaschi and coleagues (2009) validated the DYMUS questionnaire for assessment of dysphagia in multiple sclerosis. This 10-item questionnaire is subdivided into two scales: dysphagia with solids and dysphagia with liquids, both of which demonstrated good internal validity and consistency. Each item is scored dichotomously (yes or no) and the survey may be completed within a few minutes, making the DYMUS a good screening tool for identifying those patients needing instrumental evaluation and dietary management.

Cerebral Palsy

Cerebral palsy (CP) is a nonprogressive neurological motor and processing disorder that arises following injury to the fetal or infant brain. Although thought of as a childhood disease, most people (>85%) with CP will now survive well into adulthood, particularly if there are no additional disabilities present (Haak, Lenski, Hidecker, Li, & Paneth, 2009). CP presents disorders of communication and deglutition, as well as cognition, sensation, and behavior. Swallowing problems can be both sensory and motor in nature. Spasticity that accompanies the musculoskeletal changes of CP may result in disordered swallow, unusual posturing, difficulty transferring food and fluids to the oral cavity and penetration or aspiration (Haak et al., 2009). Cough with food or fluids and choking episodes, and silent aspiration have been described in CP patients (Rogers, Arvedson, Buck, Smart, & Msall, 1994). Severity of the disorder is related to presence of other disabilities. Rogers et al.

demonstrated marked abnormalities of deglutition on DSS in 86 children with CP and concomitant other disabilities. 93% of children were nonambulatory, 90% were mentally retarded and 29% had gastrostomies placed for feeding. In patients where CP is the only disorder present, swallowing may be far more functional (Haak et al., 2009). DSS will identify which aspect of swallow is affected and direct therapy. Due to global musculoskeletal problems positioning during DSS may be difficult and need to be altered.

Dementia—Alzheimer's Disease

Dementia is characterized by an overall decline in intellectual function and memory. Motor skills, particularly sequenced activity, are also affected. Multi-infarct dementia is due to repeated vascular insults. Alzheimer's disease is due to deposition of protein that impairs neural function. Other forms of dementia may be associated with particular disorders, for example, Huntington's chorea and Pick's disease. Medications, particularly polypharmacy seen in the elderly, drugs, and alcohol can all cause dementia and cognitive decline. Swallowing problems are common in dementia. One-third of Alzheimer's disease sufferers may aspirate (on videofluoroscopy) and pneumonia is the most common cause of death in this population (Gonazalez-Fernandez & Daniels, 2008). Poor cognition, poor memory, and inability to feed oneself also contribute to eating dysfunction. Oral and oropharyngeal dysfunction both occur and can be seen on DSS. Laryngeal deficits such as poor vocal fold mobility, weak cough, and prolonged swallow gestures increases the likelihood that mismanaged bolus will result in airway violation. Institutionalization also impacts diet and mortality, as does oral hygiene, in these patients. Swallowing safety may be the most important aspect assessed by DSS as teaching rehabilitative strategies may be limited by lost memory function and caregiver input.

Medication Effects

Many medications have a detrimental effect on swallowing. Medication can cause clouding of mentation, extrapyramidal effects (mimicking Parkinsonian features) and delayed neuromuscular responses. Many medications also cause xerostomia that can exacerbate dysphagia. Many elderly individuals are on multiple medications, thus compounding drug effects (Ney et al., 2009). Pill esophagitis is not uncommon in the elderly where salivary flow is decreased and dysphagia is increased. Pills lodged in the upper esophagus can cause serious ulceration and discomfort. Many medications reduce lower esophageal sphincter pressures promoting reflux and worsening dysmotility (Tutuian, 2010). Large tablets or capsules may be particularly difficult to swallow and reformulation of medications to liquids can improve swallowing safety. A 13-mm barium tablet is often given as part of the DSS protocol (anterior-posterior view) to assess for subtle esophageal irregularities not detected with liquid boluses. This also mimics the patient taking their regular medication and may demonstrate the difficulties that they are experiencing.

Once the esophageal lumen is reduced below 13 mm solid food dysphagia may occur.

PERIPHERAL NEUROMUSCULAR DISORDERS

Inflammatory Myositis— Polymyositis (PM), Dermatomyositis (DM), Inclusion Body Myositis (IBM)

The inflammatory myopathies include polymyositis, dermatomyositis and inclusion body myositis and are due to infiltration of skeletal muscle by inflammatory cells (B-cell predominant in DM, T-cell predominant in PM and IBM) (Ebert, 2009; Mastaglia, 2008). Proximal musculature is primarily affected in PM and DM whereas IBM affects smaller peripheral muscle groups (Ebert, 2009; Mastaglia, 2008). Most cases are idiopathic; however, treatment with proton-pump inhibitor has been associated with cases of PM (Ebert, 2009). Inflammatory myopathy may present with dysphagia in 25 to 80% of patients, and during the course of disease more than 60% of those with inflammatory myopathies experience some dysphagia (Langdon, Mulcahy, Shepherd, Low, & Mastiglia, 2012; Mulcahy, Langdon & Mastaglia, 2012; Williams, Grehan, Hersch, Andre, & Cook, 2003). Williams et al. (2003) reported radiographic abnormalities in 69% of 13 myositis patients studied. During videofluoroscopy 8 of 13 aspirated and 9 of 13 had obstructive pharyngoesophageal segments (Williams et al., 2003). Approximately half of myositis patients also demonstrated pharyngeal weakness on manometry

(Langdon et al., 2012; Williams et al., 2003). Mulcahy et al. (2012) studied 18 patients with IM and found overall 78% of patients had abnormalities on videofluoroscopy, including ALL those with IBM (*n* = 8). Cox, Vershuuren, Verbist, Nik, Winzen, and Badrising (2009) studied 43 patients with IBM and 79% showed abnormal fluoroscopic swallows. Upper oesophageal sphincter opening was significantly reduced compared to neurogenic controls and age-matched healthy controls in a study by Williams et al., 2003. This was demonstrated well on videofluoroscopy, as was aspiration in those affected patients. Cox et al. (2009) also found 37% of patients with IM demonstrated UES dysfunction, with 8/43 demonstrating a diverticulum . Other DSS findings separating myositis from central neurological disorders have been debated. Williams et al. (2003) found that there was preservation of normal timing sequences and pharyngeal transit times in their cohort of 13 patients, whereas Ebert (2009) reported prolonged pharyngeal transit times. Pooling of bolus in the piriform fossae, reduced tongue base excursion, repeated swallows and impaired hyolaryngeal elevation have also been described in DSS performed in those suffering IM (Cox et al., 2009; Mulcahy et al., 2012). Due to prolonged outlet obstruction at the PES the pharynx proximally may respond in a number of ways: increased muscle effort, pharyngeal dilatation or "blow-out" formation of a hypopharyngeal diverticulum (Cox et al., 2009; Mulcahy et al., 2012; Williams et al., 2003). Pharyngeal dilatation can be measured on DSS by the pharyngeal constriction ratio ("PCR," described in Chapter 17), and a diver-

ticulum is readily diagnosed on fluoroscopy. The diagnosis of inflammatory myopathy can be difficult to make and significant delay may occur (>4 yrs). DSS may provide vital clues to diagnosing this group of patients. In a series of 529 cases of oropharyngeal dysphagia reported by Williams et al. (2003), only 5.7% were attributed to myopathy. Although a small patient group, treatment of the underlying disorder may improve muscle function and assist in resolution of dysphagic symptoms, and therefore this diagnosis should be considered in all patients with unexplained oropharyngeal dysphagia. Around half of myositis patients with outlet obstruction will respond to directed treatment such as cricopharyngeal dilation or myotomy (Williams et al., 2003).

Muscular Dystrophies— Duchene, Spinal Muscle Atrophy, Myotonic, Oculopharyngeal

Duchene Muscular Dystrophy (DMD)

DMD, the most common muscular dystrophy, is caused by a genetic defect that prevents the production of the normal muscle protein, dystrophin. DMD sufferers demonstrate oral and pharyngeal phase muscle weakness leading to poor bolus control, pharyngeal residue, and post-swallow penetration and aspiration (Gonzalez-Fernandez & Daniels, 2008). Choking may become more common with age and dietary modifications are often implemented to make swallowing easier. PES opening and hyoid displacement are typically normal. Respiratory muscle weakness may contribute to poor lung clearance making aspiration more significant in these patients and should be an indicator for early DSS assessment.

Oculopharyngeal Muscular Dystrophy

Oculopharyngeal muscular dystrophy (OPMD) is an adult onset, progressive, genetic degenerative muscular dystrophy resulting in ptosis and dysphagia. Patients may compensate for ptosis by neck extension, which can compound swallowing difficulty. Patients experience prolonged meal times, solid and dry food dysphagia followed by liquid dysphagia as the disease progresses (Manjaly, Vaughan-Shaw, Dale, Tyler, Corlett, & Frost, 2011). Cricopharyngeal dysfunction is common (>75%) and aspiration occurs late in disease. The cricopharyngeus muscle is often affected, and may be targeted through behavioral therapy, balloon dilation, and/or cricopharyngeal myotomy. Videofluoroscopic examination plays an important role in assessment and surveillance in this disorder. Manjaly et al. (2011) reviewed 9 patients with OPMD treated by repeat bougienage. The average number of dilatations per patient was 7. All patients reported subjective improvement in swallow disability (as measured by the Sydney Swallowing Questionnaire) and there were no adverse reactions to dilatation. All patients remain on oral diet and the authors' suggest that dilatation may be considered instead of surgery in some patients. DSS will identify UES dysfunction, residue, and pharyngeal changes due to prolonged outlet obstruction. This may assist in treatment planning, particularly in determining timing of cricopharyngeal intervention, as early

intervention may prevent pharyngeal dilatation and failure, formation of hypopharyngeal pseudodiverticuli or respiratory complications.

Myotonic Dystrophy

Myotonic dystrophy (MD) is the most common muscular dystrophy that can begin in adulthood. It is characterized by myotonia, or prolonged muscle contractions, as well as progressive muscle wasting and weakness. It is often associated with dysphagia (25 to 80%). The pharynx and UES are worst affected and intradeglutitive and postdeglutitive aspiration of bolus leads to pneumonia. Delayed swallowing gestures increase transit time which is associated with increased risk of aspiration (Leonard, Kendall, Johnson, & McKenzie, 2001). Pharyngeal muscle weakness contributes to poor bolus transit and can be seen on DSS as an increasing pharyngeal constriction ratio (Leonard, Rees, Belafsky, & Allen, 2011). If outlet obstruction is suspected, then early DSS examination may be useful to direct treatment and prevent pharyngeal deterioration.

Myasthenia Gravis

Myasthenia gravis (MG) is an autoimmune disorder of the neuromuscular junction resulting in inadequate acetylcholine in the junction and poor muscle contraction. This muscle weakness can affect bulbar muscles causing dysphagia. In fact, dysphagia may be the presenting complaint in a quarter of patients with MG (Colton-Hudson et al., 2002). Dysphagia is a source of significant morbidity and mortality in

MG, particularly if the underlying disorder is unrecognized. Aspiration may occur and be silent, risking pulmonary health. DSS findings include abnormal oral control of bolus with early spill, residue in the oral and oropharyngeal cavities, slow pharyngeal transit, reduced pharyngeal constriction ratio, penetration and aspiration (Colton-Hudson et al., 2002). In 20 MG patients complaining of dysphagia, 13 demonstrated penetration during swallow, 7 demonstrated aspiration of which 4 were silent aspiration (Colton-Hudson, Koopman, Moosa, Smith, Bach, & Nicolle, 2002). Normal rehabilitative strategies such as exercises are not effective in MG due to muscle fatigue and therefore positioning and dietary modifications may be more appropriate and should be guided by DSS examination. Medical therapy is indicated in MG and assessment on medication should be considered so that diet may be adapted for optimal function.

6. Do patients with neurological causes of oropharyngeal dysphagia respond to swallowing therapy?
7. Do patients with neurological causes of oropharyngeal dysphagia respond to surgical therapy?
8. Can DSS help identify who might benefit most from surgery to the upper esophageal sphincter in patients with inclusion body myositis?
9. If a DSS is recommended for a patient with Parkinson disease, what might the clinician want to consider in scheduling it?
10. Are there differences in the onset time of swallowing disorders in patients with polymyositis/dermatomyositis as compared to patients with limb girdle syndrome?
11. Are the effects of postpolio syndrome thought to be solely related to aging that renders compensatory mechanisms previously developed by a patient less effective?

STUDY QUESTIONS

1. What types of stroke produce dysphagia?
2. Which is more likely to be affected by stroke, oropharynx or hypopharynx function for swallowing?
3. What is the most optimal time for DSS in an acute stroke patient? Should DSS be repeated in acute stroke patients and if so when?
4. What are typical features of dysphagia in head injured patients?
5. Have significant features of swallowing difficulty been identified for patients with muscular dystrophy? Multiple sclerosis? Polymyositis or dermatomyositis?

REFERENCES

Altman, K. W., Yu, G. P., & Schaefer, S. D. (2010). Consequence of dysphagia in the hospitalized patient. *Archives of Oto-laryngology-Head and Neck Surgery, 136,* 784–789.

Bergamaschi, R., Rezzani, C., Minguzzi, S., Amato, M. P., Patti, F., Marrosu, M. G., . . . Solaro, C. (2009). Validation of the DYMUS questionnaire for the assessment of dysphagia in multiple sclerosis. *Functional Neurology, 24,* 159–162.

Brown, C. V. R, Hejl, K., Mandaville, A. D., Chaney, P. E., Stevenson, G., & Smith, C. (2011). Swallowing dysfunction after mechanical ventilation in trauma patients. *Journal of Critical Care, 26,* 108. e9–108.e13.

Calcagno, P., Ruoppolo, G., Grasso, M. G., De Vincentis, M., & Paolucci, S. (2002). Dysphagia in multiple sclerosis—prevalence and prognostic factors. *Acta Neurologica Scandinavica, 105,* 40–43.

Chau, K. H. T., & Kung, C. M. A. (2009). Patient dose during videofluoroscopy swallowing studies in a Hong Kong public hospital. *Dysphagia, 24,* 387–390.

Colton-Hudson, A., Koopman, W. J., Moosa, T., Smith, D., Bach, D., & Nicolle, M. (2002). A prospective assessment of the characteristics of dysphagia in myasthenia gravis. *Dysphagia, 17,* 147–151.

Cox, F. M., Vershuuren, J. J., Verbist, B. M., Niks, E. H., Winzen, A. R., & Badrising, U. A. (2009). Detecting dysphagia in inclusion body myositis. *Journal of Neurology, 256,* 2009–2013.

Diniz, P. B., Vanin, G., Xavier, R., & Parente, M. A. (2009). Reduced incidence of aspiration with spoon-thick consistency in stroke patients. *Nutrition in Clinical Practice, 24,* 414–418.

Donner, M., Bosma, J., & Robertson, D. (1985). Anatomy and physiology of the pharynx. *Gastrointestinal Radiology, 10,* 196–212.

Ebert, E. C. (2009). The gastrointestinal complications of myositis. *Alimentary Pharmacology and Therapeutics, 31,* 359–365.

Ertekin, C., Aydogdu, I., Yüceyar, N., Kiylioglu, N., Tarlaci, S., & Uludag, B. (2000). Pathophysiological mechanisms of oropharyngeal dysphagia in amyotrophic lateral sclerosis. *Brain, 123,* 125–140.

Ertekin, C., Tarlaci, S., Aydogdu, I., Kiylioglu, N., Yuceyar, N., Secil, Y., & Esmeli, F. (2002). Electrophysiological evaluation of pharyngeal phase of swallowing in patients with Parkinson's disease. *Movement Disorders, 17,* 942–949.

Garon, B. R., Sierzant, T., & Ormiston, C. (2009). Silent aspiration: Results of 2000 videofluoroscopic evaluations. *Journal of Neuroscience Nursing, 41,* 178–187.

González-Fernández, M., & Daniels, S. K. (2008). Dysphagia in stroke and neurologic disease. *Physical Medicine Rehabilitation Clinics of North America, 19,* 867–888.

Haak, P., Lenski, M., Hidecker, M. J. C., Li, M., & Paneth, N. (2009). Cerebral palsy and aging. *Developmental Medicine and Child Neurology, 51*(Suppl. 4), 16–23.

Johnson, E., & McKenzie, S. (1993). Aspiration pneumonia after stroke. *Archives of Physical Medicine and Rehabilitation, 74,* 973–976.

Johnson, E., McKenzie, A., Rosenquist, C., Sievers, A., & Liberman, J. (1992). Dysphagia following stroke: Quantitative evaluation of pharyngeal transit times. *Archives of Physical Medicine and Rehabilitation, 73,* 419–423.

Kang, S. H., Kim, D. K., Seo, K. M., & Seo, J. H. (2011). Usefulness of videofluoroscopic swallow study with mixed consistency food for patients with stroke and other brain injuries. *Journal of Korean Medical Science, 26,* 425–430.

Kumar, S., Selim, M. H., & Caplan, L. R. (2010). Medical complications after stroke. *Lancet Neurology, 9,* 105–118.

Langdon, P. C., Mulcahy, K., Shepherd, K. L., Low, V. H., & Mastaglia, F. (2012). Pharyngeal dysphagia in inflammatory muscle diseases resulting from impaired suprahyoid musculature. *Dysphagia, 27,* 408–417.

Leonard, R. J., Kendall, K. A., Johnson, R., & McKenzie, S. (2001). Swallowing in myotonic muscular dystrophy: A videofluoroscopic study. *Archives of Physical Medicine and Rehabilitation, 82,* 979–985.

Leonard, R., Rees, C. J., Belafsky, P., & Allen, J. (2011). Fluoroscopic surrogate for pharyngeal strength: The pharyngeal constriction ratio (PCR). *Dysphagia, 26,* 13–17.

Manjaly, J. G., Vaughan-Shaw, P. G., Dale, O. T., Tyler, S., Corlett, J. C. R., & Frost, R. A. (2011). Cricopharyngeal dilation for the long-term treatment of dysphagia in oculopharyngeal muscular dystrophy. *Dysphagia, 27,* 216–220.

Mastaglia, F. (2008). Inflammatory muscle diseases. *Neurology India, 56,* 263–270.

Morgan, A. T. (2010). Dysphagia in childhood traumatic brain injury: A reflection on the evidence and its implications for practice. *Developmental Neurorehabilitation, 13,* 192–203.

Mulcahy, K. P., Langdon, P. C., & Mastaglia, F. (2012). Dysphagia in inflammatory myopathy: Self-report, incidence and prevalence. *Dysphagia, 27,* 64–69.

Ney, D., Weiss, J., Kind, A., & Robbins, J. (2009). Senescent swallowing: Impact, strategies and interventions. *Nutrition in Clinical Practice, 24,* 395–413.

Paliwal, V. K., Kalita, J., & Misra, U. K. (2009). Dysphagia in a patient with bilateral medial medullary infarcts. *Dysphagia, 24,* 349–353.

Pooriavad, M., Derakhshandeh, F., Etemadifar, M., Soleymani, B., Minagar, A., & Maghzi, A. H. (2010). Oropharyngeal dysphagia in multiple sclerosis. *Multiple Sclerosis, 16,* 362–365.

Ramsey, D. J. C., Smithard, D. G., & Kalra, L. (2003). Early assessments of dysphagia and aspiration risk in acute stroke patients. *Stroke, 34,* 1252–1257.

Ramsey, D., Smithard, D., & Kalra, L. (2005). Silent aspiration: What do we know? *Dysphagia, 20,* 218–225.

Rogers, B., Arvedson, J., Buck, G., Smart, P., & Msall, M. (1994). Characteristics of dysphagia in children with cerebral palsy. *Dysphagia, 9,* 69–73.

Rugiu, M. G. (2007). Role of videofluoroscopy in evaluation of neurologic dysphagia. *Acta Otorhinolaryngologica Italia, 27,* 306–316.

Tassorelli, C., Bergamaschi, R., Buscone, S., Bartolo, M., Furnari, A., Crivelli, P., . . . Nappi, G. (2008). Dysphagia in multiple sclerosis: From pathogenesis to diagnosis. *Neurological Sciences, 29,* S360–363.

Terre-Boliart, R., Orient-Lopez, F., Guevara-Espinosa, D., Ramon-Rona, S., Bernabeu-Guitart, M., & Clave-Civit, P. (2004). Oropharyngeal dysphagia in patients with multiple sclerosis. *Revista de Neurologia, 39,* 707–710.

Tutuian, R. (2010). Adverse effects of drugs on the esophagus. *Best Practice Research Clinical Gastroenterology, 24,* 91–97.

White, G. N., O'Rourke, F., Ong, B. S., Cordato, D. J., & Chan, D. K. Y. (2008). Dysphagia: Causes, assessment, treatment and management. *Geriatrics, 63,* 15–20.

Williams, R. B., Grehan, M. H., Hersch, M., Andre, J., & Cook I. J. (2003). Biomechanics, diagnosis and treatment outcome in inflammatory myopathy presenting as oropharyngeal dysphagia. *Gut, 52,* 471–478.

5

Esophageal Phase Dysphagia

Peter C. Belafsky
Catherine J. Rees Lintzenich

INTRODUCTION

The esophageal phase of deglutition begins with passage of the food bolus through the most distal aspect of the pharyngoesophageal segment. Gravity and esophageal peristalsis are responsible for moving the bolus 25 cm along the esophageal body, through the lower esophageal sphincter, and into the proximal stomach. An esophageal etiology of dysphagia can be found in 60% of individuals presenting to an outpatient tertiary swallowing center and gastroesophageal reflux is the most common cause of swallowing dysfunction. Up to 30% of individuals with an oropharyngeal swallowing disorder may have comorbid esophageal pathology. Patients are not always successful at localizing the site of their swallowing problem (Roeder, Murray, & Dierkhising, 2004) and an individual pointing to the suprasternal notch may, in fact, have distal esophageal pathology responsible for their cervical swal-

lowing complaint. A thorough knowledge of the causes of esophageal phase dysphagia is necessary to adequately care for individuals with swallowing complaints.

ESOPHAGITIS

The most common cause of esophageal phase dysphagia is gastroesophageal reflux disease (GERD). Reflux has been estimated to affect over 59 million Americans. Up to 50% of individuals with GERD suffer from dysphagia. Dysphagia in persons with GERD appears to be more prevalent as the severity of esophagitis increases (Vakil, Traxler, & Levine, 2004) (Figure 5–1). The cause of dysphagia is likely secondary to edema and diminished esophageal body motility caused by the chronic inflammation. The swallowing difficulty will resolve in over 80% of individuals after 4 weeks of anti-reflux therapy with proton-pump inhibitors. Persistent dysphagia

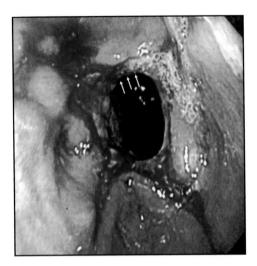

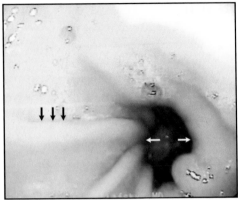

Figure 5-2. Endoscopic view of a hiatal hernia in a person with solid food dysphagia. The rugae can be seen sliding above the diaphragm (*black arrows*). Compression on the hernia sac from the diaphragm (*white arrows*) can cause solid food dysphagia. The dysphagia resolved after surgical reduction of the hernia.

Figure 5-1. High grade erosive esophagitis (Grade D) in a person presenting with solid food dysphagia. There is stricture formation (*white arrows*) at the esophagogastric junction.

indicates failed healing of the esophagitis (Wetscher, Glaser, Wieschemeyer, Gadenstaetter, Prommegger, et al., 1997). Dysphagia in persons with GERD may also be due to the presence of a peptic stricture or a hiatal hernia (HH). Although esophageal stenosis from peptic injury has declined dramatically since the disseminated use of proton-pump inhibitors, stricture must still be considered in the differential diagnosis of esophageal phase dysphagia. Most HHs do not cause dysphagia. Hernias, however, can cause swallowing dysfunction through impingement of the hernia sac by the diaphragm (Figure 5-2). Large sliding HHs and paraesophageal HHs are more likely to be associated with greater swallowing difficulty. Surgical repair of a symptomatic HH can relieve dysphagia in over 90% of individuals (Kaul, DeMeester, Oka, Ball, Stein, et al., 1990).

Gastroesophageal reflux is not the only cause of esophageal inflammation. Infection, pills and other foreign bodies, allergy, chemotherapy and radiation therapy, and caustic injury can all result in esophagitis, as well as dysphagia and stricture. Infection with *Candida albicans* is the most common cause of infectious esophagitis. Patients may present solely with the complaint of dysphagia or odynophagia, that is, pain on swallowing, and some may report symptoms such as throat clearing, globus (food sticking), or excessive throat mucus. Fiberoptic laryngoscopy may display pharyngeal candidiasis but is often normal. A fluoroscopic swallow evaluation is usually unremarkable. Esophagoscopy with biopsy is necessary to confirm the diagnosis (Figure 5-3). Risk factors for esophageal candidiasis include diabetes mellitus, corticosteroid use (inhaled, oral, and

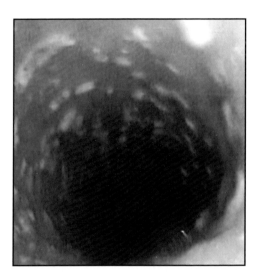

Figure 5–3. Florid esophageal candidiasis in a person presenting with solid food dysphagia and globus.

Table 5–1. Medications That Relax the Lower Esophageal Sphincter and Promote Reflux

- Oral contraceptives
- Ethanol
- Tobacco
- Theophylline
- Alpha-antagonists
- Anticholinergic agents
- Dopamine
- Nitrates
- Meperidine
- Morphine
- Calcium channel blockers
- Diazepam

injected), immunodeficiency, and a history of chemotherapy or radiation therapy. Esophageal *Candida* infection may be present, however, in the absence of these risk factors. Other less common causes of infectious esophagitis include histoplasmosis, actinomycetes, cytomegalovirus, and herpes simplex virus.

Pills can produce esophageal phase dysphagia through their systemic effects or by directly causing caustic injury. Medications may systemically cause dysphagia by inducing reflux, by impairing esophageal motility and clearance, and by compromising the immune system and predisposing the individual to esophageal infection. Table 5–1 displays a list of medications that relax the lower esophageal sphincter (LES) and promote reflux. With prolonged esophageal mucosal contact, many pills can cause caustic esophageal injury and dysphagia. In a study of 98 consecutive upper gastrointestinal radiologic examinations, over 50% of barium tablets taken by individuals while supine remained in the esophagus for more than 5 minutes (Evans & Roberts, 1976). This is ample time for many medications to produce esophageal injury. Medications most likely to cause pill-induced esophagitis include slow-release potassium, the tetracyclines, nonsteroidal anti-inflammatory drugs (NSAIDS), and alendronate (Fosamax). In order to prevent pill-induced esophagitis, patients should be instructed to take pills with a relatively large quantity of water (120 cc), take pills upright, avoid a double swallow if possible (to avoid deglutitive inhibition), and avoid lying down for 30 minutes after consumption.

Eosinophilic esophagitis (EE) is an emerging cause of esophageal phase dysphagia in children and adults. It has risen from near obscurity to become the most common cause of esophageal food impaction in children and adults. Although the exact etiology of EE is unknown, the disorder is believed to be atopic in nature. Persons typically present with dysphagia and/or odynophagia that is unresponsive to antireflux medication. Forty percent may suffer from food impactions. Most individuals have a prior history of allergic rhinitis, eczema, or asthma. Endoscopy may reveal a corrugated, ringed, or "trachealized" esophagus (Figure 5–4). Esophageal strictures are common. The diagnosis is made by demonstrating >20 eosinophils per high-powered field on esophageal biopsy. The mucosa can often look normal so it is important to emphasize the need to biopsy an ordinary appearing esophagus in an individual with dysphagia and no other apparent cause. Treatments with topical and systemic corticosteroids, montelukast, proton-pump inhibitors, histamine antagonists, and cromolyn sodium have all shown varying degrees of success. Esophageal dilation may

occasionally be necessary but should be performed with caution, as the mucosa is often extremely friable (easily torn, fragile) with an increased risk of perforation and laceration. Referral to an allergist with expertise in food allergy is indicated and repeat endoscopy is necessary to confirm the resolution of esophageal inflammation after initiation of an appropriate elimination diet.

ESOPHAGEAL WEBS AND RINGS

Esophageal webs and rings are another frequent cause of esophageal phase dysphagia. An esophageal B-ring or Schatzki's ring is one of the most common causes of solid food dysphagia in adults (Figure 5–5). Schatzki's rings can be found in up to 14% of patients

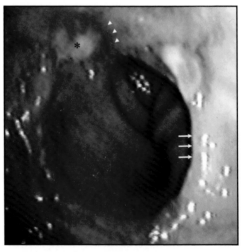

Figure 5–5. Schatzki's B-ring (*white arrows*) in an individual with solid food dysphagia. Also present are high-grade esophagitis (*white arrowheads*) with ulceration (*black asterisk*) and a small hiatal hernia. Treatment with proton-pump inhibitors resolved the dysphagia and healed the esophagitis. Dilation and surgical reduction of the hernia was not necessary.

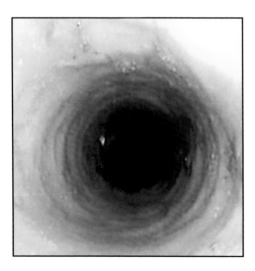

Figure 5–4. Endoscopic view of a corrugated, trachealized mid-esophagus in a person with eosinophilic esophagitis.

on fluoroscopic swallow evaluations (DeVuAlt & Kenneth, 1996). They occur at the gastroesophageal junction and have squamous esophageal mucosa on the proximal margin and columnar gastric mucosa on the distal margin of the ring. They usually occur in the presence of a hiatal hernia and frequently become symptomatic when the diameter of the lumen is <13 mm. Esophageal dilation is the treatment of choice. In comparison to the B-ring, which is membranous and occurs at the gastroesophageal junction (GEJ), the esophageal A-ring is a thick muscular ring that is present 2 cm above the GEJ (Figure 5–6). It marks the upper border of the lower esophageal sphincter. Esophageal A-rings are an infrequent cause of dysphagia. Treatment with dilation is usually unsuccessful, and the treatment of choice is injection of botulinum toxin into the muscular ring.

Esophageal webs are mucosal constrictions that occur above the gastro-

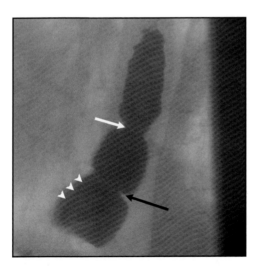

Figure 5-6. Barium esophagram displaying a esophageal A-ring (*white arrow*). Also present is a hiatal hernia (*white arrowheads*) and a Schatzki's B-ring (*black arrow*).

esophageal junction. Unlike a Schatzki's ring, they have squamous mucosa on both sides. An esophageal web usually occurs in the proximal esophagus. A web in the postcricoid region may be associated with Plummer-Vinson syndrome. Dilation is curative. Other less frequent causes of esophageal dysphagia include vascular rings, diverticula, and large esophageal varices.

ESOPHAGEAL MOTILITY DISORDERS

Occasionally esophageal endoscopy and fluoroscopy fail to reveal an etiology of the solid food dysphagia. In these cases esophageal body and LES manometry is essential in identifying the causative disorder. Manometric causes of dysphagia include ineffective esophageal motility (IEM), a hypertensive LES, distal esophageal spasm (DES), nutcracker esophagus, and achalasia.

Ineffective esophageal motility is defined as low amplitude (<30 mm Hg) but peristaltic esophageal contractions in >30% of swallows tested on manometry. IEM is the most common esophageal motor abnormality in persons with GERD. Although many clinicians suspect that reflux causes IEM, the precise cause and effect relationship has not been defined. A diagnosis of IEM does not guarantee ineffective passage of barium on fluoroscopic swallow study. Forty-five percent of persons with manometric IEM will have normal transit of barium through the esophagus (Shakespear, Blom, Huprick, & Peters, 2004).

A hypertensive LES (HTLES) is defined as a LES resting pressure >45 mm Hg. Symptoms associated with a

HTLES include dysphagia, regurgitation, heartburn, and chest pain (Gockel, Lord, Bremner, Crookes, Hamrah, & Demeester, 2003). Unlike achalasia, which is associated with absent esophageal body motility and incomplete LES relaxation, a HTLES is associated with ineffective or normal esophageal body peristalsis and complete LES relaxation. Manometric parameters suggest the hypertensive sphincter is causing outlet obstruction. An association with GERD has been reported. Treatment options include peppermint and sildenafil (which have been shown to relax the LES), botulinum toxin, dilation, and surgical myotomy.

Nutcracker esophagus is defined as high amplitude (>180 mm Hg) **peristaltic** esophageal contractions. Presenting symptoms include dysphagia and atypical chest pain (Csendes, Carcamo, & Henriquez, 2004). An association with GERD has been reported although causality remains uncertain. Antireflux medication is utilized to treat comorbid GERD, although it has not been shown to have a significant effect on pain relief (Borjesson, Rolny, Mannheimer, & Pilhall, 2003). Sildenafil has been shown to decrease the amplitude of peristaltic contractions in persons with nutcracker esophagus and may be considered a treatment option (Lee, Park, Kim, Lee, & Conklin, 2003).

In comparison to nutcracker esophagus, which displays high amplitude **peristaltic** contractions, distal esophageal spasm (DES) is characterized by high amplitude **nonperistaltic** or **simultaneous** contractions. Presenting symptoms include dysphagia and atypical chest pain. The pain is often worse with the consumption of food at extremes of temperature. The pain may be indistinguishable from that of a heart attack. The simultaneous hyperkinetic esophageal contractions can give the appearance of a "corkscrew esophagus" on barium esophagram (Figure 5–7). The diagnosis is made by a combination of manometry and radiography. Treatment options include botulinum toxin, smooth muscle relaxants such as sildenafil, nitrates, and calcium channel blockers, and surgical myotomy. Variable success with pain control has been reported with tricyclic antidepressants, selective serotonin reuptake inhibitors, and trazodone. Comorbid GERD is treated with anti-reflux medication. DES may progress to achalasia in some individuals.

Achalasia is a disorder of unknown etiology characterized by the absence of esophageal peristalsis and by failure of lower esophageal sphincter relaxation. Patients present with a history of slowly progressive dysphagia. Regurgitation and weight loss are also frequent.

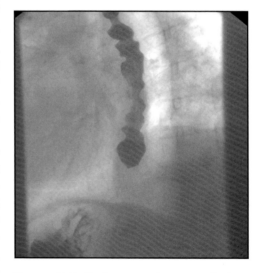

Figure 5–7. Barium esophagram displaying a corkscrew esophagus in an individual with distal esophageal spasm.

Diagnosis is made by barium esophagram and esophageal manometry. The esophagram shows a dilated tortuous esophagus with a "bird's beak" appearance at the LES (Figure 5–8). Manometry shows an absence of esophageal peristalsis and failure of LES relaxation. Endoscopy is performed to exclude cancer that can produce a similar appearance on fluoroscopy (pseudoachalasia). Treatment options include endoscopic injection of botulinum toxin to relax the LES, dilation, and surgical myotomy.

SYSTEMIC CAUSES OF ESOPHAGEAL PHASE DYSPHAGIA

There are various connective tissue diseases that can affect the esophagus. Systemic sclerosis (scleroderma), polymyositis, dermatomyositis, and systemic lupus erythematosus can all affect esophageal motility to varying degrees. Scleroderma affects the smooth muscle portion of the esophagus while sparing the proximal skeletal portion. The LES is often affected and may become hypotensive and incompetent. Severe GERD is frequent. In contrast to scleroderma, the inflammatory myopathies affect the proximal skeletal muscle portion of the esophagus. The cricopharyngeus and pharyngeal musculature may be involved. The distal esophagus and LES are spared. For this reason, associated GERD is less common than with scleroderma.

Patients with Sjögren's syndrome (an autoimmune disease that affects moisture-producing glands) often complain of dysphagia. Although esophageal peristalsis may be affected, patients often develop severe swallowing problems as a result of xerostomia. Pills, breads and other dry foods can be extremely difficult to consume. Salivary bicarbonate is important in neutralizing even physiologic amounts of reflux. All persons with Sjögren's syndrome can lack this important buffering capacity and are prone to develop severe GERD.

Other systemic diseases affecting the esophagus include diabetes mellitus, Parkinson's disease, and hypothyroidism. The autonomic dysfunction associated with diabetes can result in esophageal dysmotility with delayed esophageal emptying and in gastroparesis with delayed gastric emptying. Parkinson's disease can result in oropharyngeal and esophageal phase swallowing problems. Hypothyroidism can produce esophageal dysmotility and LES dysfunction that should normalize with appropriate thyroid replacement therapy (Eastwood, Braverman, White, & Vander, 1982).

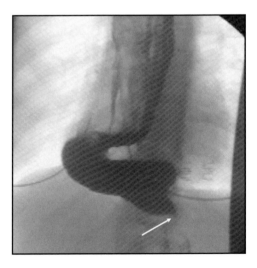

Figure 5–8. Barium esophagram displaying a dilated, tortuous esophagus with a "bird's beak" appearance at the lower esophageal sphincter (*white arrow*) in an individual with achalasia.

ESOPHAGEAL NEOPLASMS

The majority of esophageal tumors are malignant. Squamous cell carcinoma used to be the most common esophageal cancer. Adenocarcinoma, however, has now overrun squamous cell cancer as the most frequent esophageal malignancy. In fact, adenocarcinoma of the esophagus is the most rapidly expanding cancer in the United States. Early diagnosis by endoscopy and biopsy is critical. Benign esophageal tumors include leiomyomas, papillomas, cysts, fibrovascular polyps, lipomas, hemangiomas, and granular cell tumors. The most common presenting symptom for all esophageal tumors is dysphagia. Patient localization for the site of dysphagia is often inaccurate. We advocate esophagoscopy for all persons with solid food dysphagia in order to rule out esophageal neoplasia and its premalignant precursors.

CONCLUSION

The causes of esophageal phase dysphagia are diverse, and a detailed understanding of esophageal pathology is necessary to properly evaluate and manage patients presenting with dysphagia. Even patients complaining of suprasternal dysphagia symptoms localized in the neck may have esophageal pathology. Esophageal manometry and fluoroscopic studies can be useful in detecting anatomic and motility abnormalities. A low threshold for esophageal endoscopy should be maintained so that neoplasms or potentially treatable infectious causes are not missed. Endoscopy is mandatory in any patient with solid food dysphagia to rule out esophageal carcinoma.

STUDY QUESTIONS

1. What is the most common cause of esophagitis?
2. Match each of the following esophageal motility disorders with the description that best fits:

   a. Achalasia   c. DES
   b. IEM   d. Nutcracker

   (1) High amplitude nonperistaltic esophageal contractions.
   (2) Lower esophageal sphincter (LES) hypertension; absence of esophageal peristalsis.
   (3) High-amplitude esophageal contractions, peristaltic.
   (4) Low-amplitude esophageal contractions, peristaltic.

3. Does scleroderma affect the proximal esophagus?
4. What is one medication that is a common cause of pill-induced esophagitis?

REFERENCES

Borjesson, M., Rolney, P., Mannheimer, C., & Pilhall, M. (2003). Nutcracker esophagus: A double-blind, placebo-controlled, crossover study of the effects of lansoprazole. *Alimentary Pharmacology Therapy, 18*, 1129–1135.

Csendes A., Carcamo, C., & Henriquez, A. (2004). Nutcracker esophagus: Analysis of 80 patients. *Revista Medica de Chile, 132*, 160–164.

DeVault, K. R. (1996). Lower esophageal (Schatzki's) ring: Pathogenesis, diagnosis and therapy. *Digestive Diseases, 14*, 323–329.

Eastwood, G. L., Braverman, L. E., White, E. M., & Vander Salm, T. J. (1982). Reversal of lower esophageal sphincter hypotension and esophageal aperistalsis after treatment for hypothyroidism. *Journal of Clinical Gastroenterology, 4*, 307–310.

Evans, K. T., & Roberts, G. M. (1976). Where do all the tablets go? *Lancet, 2*, 1237.

Gockel, I., Lord, R. V., Bremner, C. G., Crookes, P. F., Hamrah, P., & DeMeester, T. R. (2003). The hypertensive lower esophageal sphincter: A motility disorder with manometric features of outflow obstruction. *Journal of Gastrointestinal Surgery, 7*, 692–700.

Kaul, B. K., DeMeester, T. R., Oka, M., Ball, C. S., Stein, H. J., Kim, C. B., & Cheng, S. C. (1990). The cause of dysphagia in uncomplicated sliding hiatal hernia and its relief by hiatal herniorrhaphy: A roentgenographic, manometric, and clinical study. *Annals of Surgery, 211*, 406–410.

Lee, J. I., Park, H., Kim, J. H., Lee, S. I., & Conklin, J. L.(2003). The effect of sildenafil on oesophageal motor function in healthy subjects and patients with nutcracker oesophagus. *Neurogastroenterology and Motility, 15*, 617–623.

Roeder, B. E., Murray, J. A., & Dierkhising, R. A. (2004). Patient localization of esophageal dysphagia, *Digestive Diseases and Sciences, 49*, 697–701.

Shakespear, J. S., Blom, D., Huprich, J. E., & Peters, J. H. (2004). Correlation of radiographic and manometric findings in patients with ineffective esophageal motility. *Surgical Endoscopy, 18*, 459–462.

Vakil, N. B., Traxler, B., & Levine, D. (2004). Dysphagia in patients with erosive esophagitis: Prevalence, severity, and response to proton pump inhibitor treatment. *Clinical Gastroenterology and Hepatology, 2*, 665–668.

Wetscher, G. J., Glaser, K., Wieschemeyer, T., Gadenstaetter, M., Prommegger, R., & Profanter, C. (1997). Tailored antireflux surgery for gastroesophageal reflux disease: Effectiveness and risk of postoperative dysphagia. *World Journal of Surgery, 21*, 605–610.

6

Laryngopharyngeal Reflux

Catherine J. Rees Lintzenich
Peter C. Belafsky

DEFINITION AND NOMENCLATURE OF LARYNGOPHARYNGEAL REFLUX (LPR)

Laryngopharyngeal reflux (LPR) is the backflow of stomach contents into the laryngopharynx (Koufman, Aviv, Casiano, & Shaw, 2002). LPR has been implicated in the pathophysiology of numerous disorders of the upper aerodigestive tract, including dysphonia, laryngeal granulomas, and subglottic stenosis. Although laryngopharyngeal reflux is currently the term endorsed by the American Academy of Otolaryngology-Head and Neck Surgery, multiple synonyms are used, including reflux laryngitis, posterior laryngitis, laryngeal reflux, gastroesophagopharyngeal reflux, esophagopharyngeal reflux, pharyngoesophageal reflux, gastroesophageal-laryngeal reflux, atypical reflux, silent reflux, and supraesophageal reflux. Perhaps the most common synonym for LPR is extraesophageal reflux (Belafsky, 2003; Koufman, Belafsky, Bach, Daniel, & Postma, 2002).

The idea that acidic gastric contents can affect structures above the upper esophageal sphincter was put forth in 1968 (Cherry & Marguilies, 1968; Delahunty & Cherry, 1968; Koufman, 2002a). At this time, LPR was postulated to relate to contact ulcers and granulomas, and the mechanism was felt to be vagally mediated from acidic contents contacting the lower esophagus. Although this theory has not entirely lost favor, actual drops in the pH of the pharynx in patients with LPR symptoms were demonstrated in 1987 and 1989 (Wiener, Koufman, & Wu, 1987; Wiener, Koufman, Wu, Cooper, Richter, et al., 1989). These findings suggested that the physical presence of gastric contents in the laryngopharynx was to blame in the disease process. It is likely that both theories of causality play a role in LPR disease.

EPIDEMIOLOGY OF REFLUX

The incidence of laryngopharyngeal reflux is not clearly understood, but it has been estimated that up to 4% to 10% of patients with otolaryngologic complaints have underlying LPR (Toohill, Mushtag, & Lehman, 1990). In a community cohort of 100 patients without any history of voice or laryngeal complaints, 35% had symptoms of LPR and 64% demonstrated one or more physical finding of LPR on laryngoscopic examination (Reulbach, Belafsky, Blalock, Koufman, & Postma, 2001). This study suggested that physical findings and symptoms of LPR frequently are found in the general population and that some degree of LPR may be normal. In a prospective cohort of 113 new patients with laryngeal and voice disorders, 50% were found to have abnormal results on 24-hour dual-pH probe testing (Koufman, Amin, & Panetti, 2000, 2001). LPR was highest in patients presenting with laryngeal neoplasia (88%) and muscle tension dysphonia (70%).

Reflux to a certain degree is ubiquitous in adults, and clinical disease only occurs in the presence of excessive reflux and/or a breakdown of mucosal defenses. In the lower esophagus, up to 50 reflux episodes at or below pH 4 in a 24-hour period is considered normal (Demeester, Johnson, Joseph, Toscano, Hall, et al., 1976). In the pharynx, the normal or physiologic limit of reflux is not as clear. Generally, up to two episodes of reflux with pH less than 4 may be seen in healthy controls without LPR disease (Merati, Lim, Ulualp, & Toohill, 2005; Vincent, Garrett, Radionoff, Reussner, & Stasney, 2000; Ylitalo, Lindestad, & Ramel, 2001; Ylitalo & Ramel, 2002a, 2002b). However, animal studies have suggested that as few as three pharyngeal reflux episodes per week are sufficient to produce laryngeal damage in the face of a pre-existing mucosal injury (Koufman, 1991).

DIFFERENCE BETWEEN LPR AND GERD

Laryngopharyngeal reflux must be distinguished from classic gastroesophageal reflux disease (GERD). The primary characteristics of GERD include heartburn and esophagitis. The majority of patients with LPR deny heartburn (70%), (Koufman, Aviv, et al., 2002) and the incidence of esophagitis is only about 25% in the LPR population (Koufman, 1991; Koufman et al., 2002; Koufman, Belafsky, et al., 2002; Koufman, Sataloff, & Toohill, 1996; Wiener et al., 1989). GERD patients tend to have primarily nighttime supine reflux, whereas LPR patients tend to have daytime upright reflux. Episodes of pathologic esophageal reflux may be prolonged, but LPR episodes are typically brief. Patients with GERD are more frequently obese, whereas body mass index is not related to LPR prevalence (Halum, Postma, Johnston, Belafsky, & Koufman, 2005). GERD is thought to be a result of lower esophageal sphincter dysfunction and/or esophageal dysmotility, but this does not appear to be true for LPR. Esophageal acid clearance is better in LPR patients than in classic GERD patients, (Postma, Tomek, Belafsky, & Koufman, 2001a) and LPR may be related to dysfunction of the upper esophageal sphincter (Celik, Alkan, & Ercan, 2005; Gerhardt, Shuck, Bordeaux, & Winship, 1978; Helm, Dodds, Riedel, Teeter, Hogan, & Arndorfer,

1983; Koufman, 2002a; Koufman, Belafsky, et al., 2002; Orsmeth & Wong, 1999; Ulualp, Toohill, Kern, & Shaker, 1998).

In the healthy adult, the esophagus is well-equipped to handle intermittent exposure to acidic gastric contents (Koufman, 1991). Lower esophageal sphincter competence is physically supported by: the muscular diaphragm; the acute angle of entry of the esophagus into the stomach (i.e., the cardiac angle); and the high abdominal pressure imposed on the intra-abdominal segment of the esophagus. LES pressure is also regulated by hormonal mechanisms and in response to alkalinization of gastric contents.

Primary peristalsis clears the majority of a distal esophageal bolus, and secondary peristalsis as a result of repeat swallows every 30 to 60 seconds allows for improved clearance as well as buffering by saliva. Salivary bicarbonate bathing the esophagus helps to neutralize refluxate within the esophageal lumen. Increased acid in the distal esophagus stimulates an increase in salivary production in the normal individual (Koufman, 1991).

The esophageal lining displays innate tissue resistance to physiologic reflux events. Mucus lining the esophageal lumen prevents the penetration of large molecules such as pepsin. The "unstirred water layer" below is rich in bicarbonate and buffers the environment adjacent to the esophageal mucosal cells. Furthermore, the esophageal epithelium itself is capable of blocking both acid and pepsin with cell membranes and intracellular bridges. Local blood flow is increased in the event of esophageal injury to facilitate recovery (Orlando, 1986).

In stark contrast, the larynx is poorly protected from injury by gastric refluxate, specifically acid and pepsin (Axford, Sharp, Ross, Pearson, & Dettmar, 2001; Johnston et al., 2003; Koufman, 1991). The upper airways are exquisitely sensitive to acid and especially to activated pepsin. Pepsin has been shown to be active above pH 4, suggesting that a smaller drop in pH is required to cause laryngeal injury than esophageal injury (Johnston, Knight, Dettmar, Lively, & Koufman, 2004). As noted above, very few episodes of pharyngeal reflux (three per week) can damage the larynx in the setting of a mucosal injury (Koufman, 1991; Little, Koufman, Kohut, & Marshall, 1985). The larynx is not protected by salivary bicarbonate, endogenous tissue buffering, or peristalsis. The larynx has poor intrinsic tissue defenses as well. Carbonic anhydrase isoenzyme III (CA III) is an enzyme with buffering capacity that is increased in the esophagus in response to acid. However, CA III is actually reduced in laryngeal tissue damaged by acid and pepsin, further decreasing laryngeal protection (Axford et al., 2001; Johnston et al., 2003, 2004).

DIAGNOSIS OF LPR PATIENT SYMPTOMS

The diagnosis of LPR is primarily based on a constellation of clinical signs and physical findings. In a 2002 survey sent to 415 members of the American Broncho-Esophagological Association, the responders were in agreement about certain symptoms of LPR (Book, Rhee, Toohill, & Smith, 2002). These include throat clearing (98%), chronic cough (97%), globus (95%), dysphonia (95%), and postnasal drip (57%). The Reflux Symptom Index (RSI) has been shown to be a reliable and valid patient-administered questionnaire for identifying patient symptoms (Table 6–1) (Belafsky, Postma, & Koufman, 2002b). One group, however, has reported sensitivity and specificity for the RSI of 80.7% and 37.5%, respectively, in patients with hypopharyngeal reflux documented by pH studies (Park, Choi, Kwon, Yoon, & Kim, 2006).

The most common complaint of LPR patients appears to be dysphonia, followed by chronic throat clearing, cough, globus sensation, and dysphagia (Koufman, 1991; Woo, Noordzij, & Ross, 1996). Most LPR patients do not complain of heartburn. LPR has been implicated in the etiology of a multitude of otolaryngologic disorders, including subglottic stenosis, chronic sinusitis, chronic otitis media, laryngeal granulomas, paroxysmal laryngospasm, Reinke's edema, Zenker's diverticulum, and laryngeal carcinoma (Cohen, Bach, Postma, & Koufman, 2002; DelGaudio, 2005; Koufman, 1991; Lewin et al., 2003; Maronian, Azadeh, Waugh, & Hillel, 2001; Sasaki, Ross, & Hundal, 2003).

Physical Findings

Laryngeal examination with a flexible or rigid laryngoscope is essential to the diagnosis of LPR. Findings associated with LPR include erythema, laryngeal and vocal fold edema, subglottic edema/pseudosulcus vocalis, ventricular obliteration, posterior commissure hypertrophy, laryngeal granulomas, lymphoid hypertrophy, and excessive

Table 6-1. Reflux Symptom Index (maximum score 45)

Within the past month, how did the following problems affect you?	0 = No problem 5 = Severe problem					
Hoarseness or a problem with your voice	0	1	2	3	4	5
Clearing your throat	0	1	2	3	4	5
Excess throat mucus or postnasal drip	0	1	2	3	4	5
Difficulty swallowing food, liquids, or pills	0	1	2	3	4	5
Coughing after you ate or after lying down	0	1	2	3	4	5
Breathing difficulties or choking episodes	0	1	2	3	4	5
Troublesome or annoying cough	0	1	2	3	4	5
Sensations of something sticking in your throat or a lump in your throat	0	1	2	3	4	5
Heartburn, chest pain, indigestion, or stomach acid coming up	0	1	2	3	4	5

Source: From Belafsky, P. C., Postma, G. N., & Koufman, J. A. (2002b). Validity and reliability of the reflux symptom index (RSI). *Journal of Voice, 16,* 274–277. Reproduced with permission.

pharyngeal mucus. Endoscopic findings can be succinctly described with the Reflux Findings Score (RFS) (Table 6–2), which is an indicator of overall laryngeal inflammation.

It is important to recognize that the diagnosis is based on a constellation of findings rather than any one finding. For example isolated posterior commissure hypertrophy does not correlate well with LPR, but it is felt to be an important sign of LPR when associated with other laryngeal findings listed in the RFS. Laryngeal erythema has been described in LPR (Hanson, Jiang, & Chi, 1998), but this may be highly variable

Table 6–2. Reflux Findings Score (maximum score 26)

Pseudosulcus (infraglottic edema)	0 = Absent 2 = Present
Ventricular obliteration	0 = None 2 = Partial 4 = Complete
Erythema/hyperemia	0 = None 2 = Arytenoids only 4 = Diffuse
Vocal fold edema	0 = None 1 = Mild 2 = Moderate 3 = Severe 4 = Polypoid
Diffuse laryngeal edema	0 = None 1 = Mild 2 = Moderate 3 = Severe 4 = Obstructing
Posterior commissure hypertrophy	0 = None 1 = Mild 2 = Moderate 3 = Severe 4 = Obstructing
Granuloma/granulation	0 = Absent 2 = Present
Thick endolaryngeal mucus	0 = Absent 2 = Present
	Total

Source: From Belafsky, P. C., Postma, G. N., & Koufman, J. A. (2001b). Validity and reliability of the reflux findings score (RFS). *Laryngoscope, 111*, 1313–1317. Reproduced with permission.

depending on the examiner's video equipment. Diffuse laryngeal erythema is thought to be a stronger indicator of LPR than erythema localized to the arytenoids (Belafsky, 2003).

Endoscopic findings isolated to the true vocal folds can range from mild edema to Reinke's edema, also known as polypoid degeneration or polypoid corditis (Figure 6–1) (Belafsky, 2003). Obliteration of the laryngeal ventricle is the result of edema of the true and false vocal folds (Figure 6–2). This may be one of the first signs to improve after the initiation of antireflux therapy. Posterior commissure hypertrophy, or posterior laryngeal edema, is graded from mild, producing a mus-

tachelike appearance of the posterior larynx, to severe, producing an actual obstruction of the posterior airway by the edematous mucosa (Figure 6–3). Patients with LPR and posterior laryngeal edema appear to have a higher incidence of laryngeal sensory deficits on functional endoscopic evaluation of swallowing with sensory testing (FEEST), which improves with LPR treatment (Aviv, Liu, Parides, Kaplan, & Close, 2000). Pseudosulcus vocalis is also known as infraglottic edema (Figure 6–4) (Koufman, 1995). This finding represents edema of the ventral surface of the vocal folds and extends along the entire length of the true vocal fold. This detail differentiates pseudosulcus vocalis from sulcus vergeture, which stops at the vocal process rather than extending to the posterior larynx. The presence of pseudosulcus is at least 70% sensitive and 77% specific for LPR (Belafsky, Postma, & Koufman, 2002a; Hickson, Simpson, & Falcon, 2001).

Vocal fold granulomas are typically seen on the vocal process and have a high recurrence rate (Figure 6–5). LPR has recently been identified as an eti-

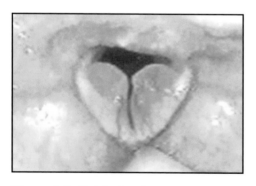

Figure 6–1. Reinke's edema.

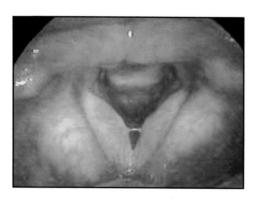

Figure 6–2. Ventricular obliteration and Reinke's edema.

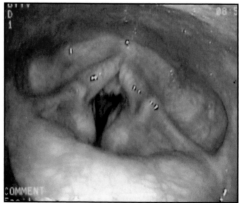

Figure 6–3. Posterior commissure hypertrophy.

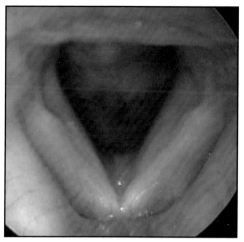

Figure 6–4. Pseudosulcus vocalis.

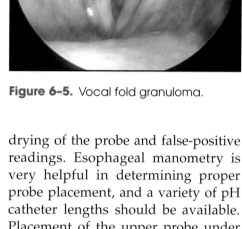

Figure 6–5. Vocal fold granuloma.

ologic factor in the development of granulomas. Lymphoid hyperplasia, especially seen as hypertrophy of the lingual tonsils (Mamede, De Mello-Filho, Vigario, & Dantas, 2000) and cobblestoning of the posterior pharyngeal wall, can also be related to LPR, although these findings are nonspecific. Finally, LPR may be associated with the sensation of increased mucus in the throat, which can often be confused with postnasal drip (Belafsky, 2003).

pH Monitoring

Twenty-four hour dual-probe pH testing is currently the gold standard for diagnosis of LPR. The upper pH probe should be in the hypopharynx above the upper esophageal sphincter, not in the proximal esophagus. The lower probe is ideally 5 cm above the lower esophageal sphincter, which is the standard position used by gastroenterologists. The hypopharyngeal probe should be no more than 2 cm above the upper esophageal sphincter (UES) to prevent

drying of the probe and false-positive readings. Esophageal manometry is very helpful in determining proper probe placement, and a variety of pH catheter lengths should be available. Placement of the upper probe under endoscopic visualization does not allow confirmation of the lower probe position (Harrell et al., 2005; Postma, Belafsky, Aviv, & Koufman, 2002).

Although up to 50 episodes of reflux in the distal esophagus are normal, when these reflux events reach the pharynx, the diagnosis of LPR may be made. In a recent meta-analysis of 24-hour dual-probe pH monitoring, the technique was found to be consistent between multiple studies. Up to 20% of normal subjects had brief reflux events at the upper probe when the probe was in the hypopharynx, and this number increased when the probe was at the UES (Merati et al., 2005).

The exact cutoff for number of reflux events in the pharynx is controversial (Richardson, Heywood, Sims, Stoner, & Leopold, 2004). It is clear that in the setting of mucosal airway injury, even one episode of LPR is enough to exacerbate the injury (Little et al., 1985). However, in an asymptomatic individual without voice or airway concerns, one or two episodes of LPR may be physiologic rather than clinically significant. The results of 24-hour pH monitoring should be reviewed on an individual patient basis. Intake of meals and beverages will give false readings and must be considered in interpretation of pH studies. Finally, both number of LPR events and acid exposure time should be considered. Although pH 4 or less is the accepted cutoff for reflux events in the esophagus, it has been suggested that pH 5 or less may be clinically important in the laryngopharynx, given the persistent activation of pepsin at this pH (Postma, 2000). Impedance tesing overcomes some of the pitfalls of pH-testing described here.

Impedance testing overcomes some of the pitfalls of pH-testing described above. Multichannel intraluminal impedance testing describes anterograde or retrograde bolus or air movement in the esophagus, allowing the clinician to more easily differentiate between swallow and reflux events. This also allows for testing of reflux disease independent of the pH of the refluxate. Impedance testing is often combined with simultaneous pH studies.

Other Diagnostic Studies

Cinefluoroscopy is used as an adjunct by some clinicians to diagnose LPR. Esophageal reflux can often be seen with this study, but LPR may be missed.

Many clinicians also believe that an evaluation of the esophagus, either by the otolaryngologist or the gastro-enterologist, is critical in any patient diagnosed with LPR. This recommendation is based on findings of esophageal pathology, in particular Barrett's esophagus, in a significant proportion of patients with LPR (Postma et al., 2005). LPR symptoms may be more predictive of esophageal adenocarcinoma than typical GERD symptoms (Reavis, Morris, Gopal, Hunter, & Jobe, 2004). Esophageal adenocarcinoma is a devastating disease with an often delayed diagnosis, and evaluation of the esophagus when LPR is present may result in earlier diagnosis in some patients.

TREATMENT OF LPR

Patients with suspected LPR should be counseled about the standard lifestyle changes recommended for GERD patients (Table 6–3). Perhaps the most

Table 6-3. Recommended Lifestyle Modifications in LPR

Elevate head of bed 6 inches
Smoking cessation
Low-fat diet
Weight loss
Avoid lying down within 3 hours of eating
Eat small frequent meals
Avoid refluxogenic foods:
Alcohol
Chocolate
Peppermint
High-fat foods
Tomato-based products
Spicy foods
Citrus

important of these recommendations are smoking cessation and alcohol avoidance. Chewing gum has been shown to increase both pharyngeal and esophageal pH because of an increase in salivary bicarbonate, salivary flow, and swallowing frequency. Bicarbonate gum is an even more effective adjunctive antireflux therapy (Smoak & Koufman, 2001). Over-the-counter antacids and liquid alginate certainly have a role in mild GERD, but their effectiveness in treating LPR is not clear. Liquid alginate, especially the formulation available in Europe, forms a physical barrier to help prevent reflux (Mandel, Daggy, Brodie, & Jacoby, 2000).

Most patients with symptomatic LPR require pharmacologic treatment with H2-receptor antagonists and/or proton-pump inhibitors. According to the position statement on LPR by the American Academy of Otolaryngology-Head and Neck Surgery, LPR treatment should be more aggressive and of longer duration than GERD treatment. Mild symptoms may be appropriately treated with lifestyle modifications and H2-receptor antagonists.

Most LPR patients require twice-daily proton-pump inhibitor (PPI) therapy, although this therapy has not been well supported in placebo-controlled trials (Koufman, Aviv, et al., 2002; Noordzij et al., 2001; Park et al., 2005; Postma & Johnson, 2002; Steward et al., 2004;). Twice-daily dosing is important because none of the PPIs suppress gastric acid for more than 16 hours (Peghini, Katz, Bracy, & Castell, 1998). Some investigators suggest using high dose H2-receptor antagonists at night in addition to twice daily PPI therapy, but the efficacy of this approach is controversial (Pan, Wang,

& Guo, 2004; Tutuian & Castel, 2004). More than 2 months therapy may be necessary for LPR symptom improvement, and more than 6 months therapy may be required to see resolution of laryngeal findings (Belafsky, Postma, & Koufman, 2001a). Patients should be carefully counseled about the need for prolonged therapy and the proper timing of medication doses. PPIs should be taken 30 to 45 minutes before a meal for maximum efficacy. Resistance to PPI therapy should be considered in patients without improvement after 6 months therapy, and this can be documented by repeat pH testing while on medication (Amin, Postma, Johnson, Digges, & Koufman, 2001).

In refractory LPR, especially in life-threatening cases such as subglottic stenosis, surgical therapy may be considered as an alternative to PPIs. There are limited data supporting endoscopic antireflux procedures in LPR at this point. LPR symptoms often improve after Nissen fundoplication or hiatal hernia repair (Lindstrom, Wallace, Loehrl, Merati, Toohill, et al., 2002; Westcott, Hopkins, Bach, Postman, Belafsky, et al., 2004; Wright & Rhodes, 2003).

CONCLUSION

Laryngopharyngeal reflux should be considered as a contributing factor in most disorders of the upper aerodigestive tract. LPR is different from classic gastroesophageal reflux disease in that most patients do not experience heartburn or have findings or esophagitis. A constellation of patient symptoms and physical findings are important in diagnosing LPR. Twenty-four-hour dual-probe pH monitoring with the upper probe in the hypopharynx is the gold standard for LPR diagnosis. Twice-daily proton-pump inhibitor therapy for at least 6 months is the mainstay of LPR therapy.

STUDY QUESTIONS

1. Which is most damaging to tissues: pepsin, acid, or both combined?
2. Describe the mechanism of reflux.
3. What is the most typical sign of laryngopharyngeal reflux (LPR)?
4. What is more important in the diagnosis of reflux, a single sign, or a constellation of signs? What would constitute a constellation of signs?
5. Is any reflux in the esophagus considered normal?
6. In the treatment of reflux, which typically improve first, signs or symptoms?

REFERENCES

Amin, M. R., Postma, G. N., Johnson, P., Digges, N., & Koufman, J. A. (2001). Proton pump inhibitor resistance in the treatment of laryngopharyngeal reflux. *Otolaryngology-Head and Neck Surgery, 125*, 374–378.

Aviv, J. E., Liu, H., Parides, M., Kaplan S. T., & Close, J. G., (2000). Laryngopharyngeal sensory deficits in patients with laryngopharyngeal reflux and dysphagia. *Annals of Otology, Rhinology and Laryngology, 1099*, 1000–1006.

Axford, S. E., Sharp, N., Ross, P. E., Pearson, J. P., Dettmar, P. W., Panetti, M., & Koufman, J. A. (2001a). Cell biology of laryngeal epithelial defenses in health and disease: Preliminary studies. *Annals of Otology Rhinology and Laryngology, 110*, 1099–1108.

Belafsky, P. C. (2003). Abnormal endoscopic pharyngeal and laryngeal findings attributable to reflux. *American Journal of Medicine, 115*, 90S–96S.

Belafsky, P. C., Postma, G. N., & Koufman, J. A. (2001a). Laryngopharyngeal reflux symptoms improve before changes in physical findings. *Laryngoscope, 111*, 979–981.

Belafsky, P. C., Postma, G. N., & Koufman, J. A. (2001b). Validity and reliability of the reflux findings score (RFS). *Laryngoscope, 111*, 1313–1317.

Belafsky, P. C., Postma, G. N., & Koufman, J. A. (2002a). The association between laryngeal pseudosulcus and laryngopharyngeal reflux, *Otolaryngology-Head and Neck Surgery, 126*, 649–652.

Belafsky, P. C., Postma, G. N., & Koufman, J. A. (2002b). Validity and reliability of the reflux symptom index (RSI). *Journal of Voice, 16*, 274–277.

Book, D. T., Rhee, J. S., Toohill, R. J., & Smith T. L. (2002). Perspectives in laryngopharyngeal reflux: An international survey. *Laryngoscope, 112*, 1399–1406.

Celik, M., Alkan, Z. S., & Ercan, I. (2005). Cricopharyngeal muscle electromyography in laryngopharyngeal reflux. *Laryngoscope, 115*, 138–142.

Cherry, J., & Margulies, S. I. (1968). Contact ulcer of the larynx. *Laryngoscope, 78*, 1937–1940.

Cohen, J. T., Bach, K. K., Postma, G. N., & Koufman, J. A. (2002). Clinical manifestations of laryngopharyngeal reflux. *Ear Nose and Throat Journal, 81*(Suppl. 2), 19–23.

Delahunty, J. E., & Cherry, J. (1968). Experimentally produced vocal cord granulomas. *Laryngoscope, 78*, 1941–1947.

DelGaudio, J. M., (2005). Direct nasopharyngeal reflux of gastric acid is a contributing factor in refractory chronic sinusitis. *Laryngoscope, 115*, 946–956.

Demeester, T. R., Johnson, L. F., Joseph, G. J., Toscano, M. S., Hall, A. W., & Skinner, D. B. (1976). Patterns of gastroesophageal reflux in health and disease. *Annals of Surgery, 184,* 459–470.

Gerhardt, D. C., Shuck, T. J., Bordeaux, R. A., & Winship, D. H. (1978). Human upper esophageal sphincter. Response to volume, osmotic, and acid stimuli. *Gastroenterlogy, 75,* 268–274.

Halum, S. L., Postma, G. N., Johnston, C., Belafsky, P. C., & Koufman, J. A. (2005). Patients with isolated laryngopharyngeal reflux are not obese. *Laryngoscope, 115,* 1042–1045.

Hanson, D. G., Jiang, J., & Chi, W. (1998). Quantitative color analysis of laryngeal erythema in chronic posterior laryngitis. *Journal of Voice, 12,* 78–83.

Harrell, S., Evans, B., Goudy, S., Winstead, W., Lentsch, E., Koopman, J., & Wo, J. M. (2005). Design and implementation of an ambulatory pH monitoring protocol in patients with suspected laryngopharyngeal reflux. *Laryngoscope, 115,* 89–92.

Helm, J. F., Dodds, W. J., Riedel, D. R., Teeter, B. C., Hogan, W. J., & Arndorfer, R. C. (1983). Determinants of esophageal acid clearance in normal subjects. *Gastroenterology, 85,* 607–612.

Hickson, C., Simpson, C. B., & Falcon, R. (2001). Laryngeal pseudosulcus as a predictor of laryngopharyngeal reflux. *Laryngoscope, 111,* 1742–1745.

Hill, R. K., Simpson, C. B., Velazquez, R., & Larson, M. (2004). Pachydermia is not diagnostic of active laryngopharyngeal reflux disease. *Laryngoscope, 114,* 1557–1561.

Johnston, N., Bulmer, D., Gill, G., Panetti, M., Ross, P. E., Pearson, J. P., . . . Koufman, J. A. (2003). Cell biology of laryngeal epithelial defenses in health and disease: Further studies. *Annals of Otology, Rhinology, and Laryngology, 112,* 481–491.

Johnston, N., Knight, J., Dettmar, P. W., Lively, M. O., & Koufman, J. A. (2004). Pepsin and carbonic anhydrase isoenzyme III as diagnostic markers for laryngopharyngeal reflux disease. *Laryngoscope, 114,* 2129–2134.

Koufman, J. A. (1991). The otolaryngologic manifestations of gastroesophageal reflux disease (GERD): A clinical investigation of 225 patients using ambulatory 24-hour pH monitoring and an experimental investigation of the role of acid and pepsin in the development of laryngeal injury. *Laryngoscope, 101*(Suppl. 53), 1–78.

Koufman, J. A. (1995). Gastroesophageal reflux and voice disorders. In J. S. Rubin, R. T. Sataloff, & G. Korovin (Eds.), *Diagnosis and treatment of voice disorders* (pp. 161–175), New York, NY: Igaku-Shoin.

Koufman, J. A. (2002a). Laryngopharyngeal reflux is different from classic gastroesophageal reflux disease. *Ear Nose and Throat Journal, 81*(Suppl. 2), 7–9.

Koufman, J. A. (2002b). Laryngopharyngeal reflux 2002: A new paradigm of airway disease. *Ear Nose and Throat Journal, 81*(Suppl. 2), 2–6.

Koufman, J. A., Amin, M. R., & Panetti, M. (2000, 2001) Prevalence of reflux in 113 consecutive patients with laryngeal and voice disorders. *Otolaryngology-Head and Neck Surgery, 123,* 385–388. Erratum in: *Otolaryngology Head and Neck Surgery, 124,* 104.

Koufman, J. A., Aviv, J. E., Casiano, R. R., & Shaw, G. Y. (2002). Laryngopharyngeal reflux: Position statement of the Committee on Speech, Voice, and Swallowing Disorders of the American Academy of Otolaryngology-Head and Neck Surgery. *Otolaryngology-Head and Neck Surgery, 127,* 32–35.

Koufman, J. A., Belafsky, P. C., Bach, K. K., Daniel, E., & Postma, G. N. (2002). Prevalence of esophagitis in patients with pH-documented laryngopharyngeal reflux. *Laryngoscope, 112,* 1606–1609.

Koufman, J. A., Sataloff, R. T., & Toohill, R. (1996). Laryngopharyngeal reflux: Consensus report. *Journal of Voice, 10,* 215–216.

Koufman, J. A., Weiner, G. J., & Wu, W. C., Cooper, J. B., Richter, J. E., & Castell,

D. O. (1988). Reflux laryngitis and its sequelae: The diagnostic role of ambulatory 24-hour pH monitoring. *Journal of Voice, 2*, 78–89.

Lewin, J. S., Gillenwater, A. M., Garrett, J. D., Bishop-Leone, J. K., Nguyen, D. D., Callender, D. L., Ayers, G. D., & Myers, J. N. (2003). Characterization of laryngopharyngeal reflux in patients with premalignant and early carcinomas of the larynx. *Cancer, 97*, 1010–1014.

Lindstrom, D. R., Wallace, J., Loehrl, T. A., Merati, A. L, & Toohill, R. J. (2002). Nissen fundoplication surgery for extraesophageal manifestation of gastroesophageal reflux (EER). *Laryngoscope, 112*, 1762–1765.

Little, F. B., Koufman, J. A., Kohut, R. I., & Marshall, R. B. (1985). Effect of gastric acid on the pathogenesis of subglottic stenosis. *Annals of Otology, Rhinology and Laryngology, 94*, 516–519.

Mamede, R. C., De Mello-Filho, F. V., Vigario, L. C., & Dantas, R. O. (2000). Effect of gastroesophageal reflux on hypertrophy of the base of tongue. *Otolaryngology-Head and Neck Surgery, 122*, 607–610.

Mandel, K. G., Daggy, B. P., Brodie, D. A., & Jacoby, H. I. (2000). Review article: Alginate-raft formulations in the treatment of heartburn and acid reflux. *Alimentary Pharmacology Therapy, 14*, 669–690.

Maronian, N. C., Azadeh, H., Waugh, P., & Hillel, A., (2001). Association of laryngopharyngeal reflux disease and subglottic stenosis. *Annals of Otology, Rhinology and Laryngology, 110*, 606–612.

Merati, A. L., Lim, H. J., Ulualp, S. O., & Toohill, R. J. (2005). Meta-analysis of upper probe measurements in normal subjects and patients with laryngopharyngeal reflux. *Annals of Otology, Rhinology, and Laryngology, 114*, 177–182.

Noordzij, J. P., Khidr, A., Evans, B., Desper, E., Mittal, R. K., Reibel, J. F., & Levine, P. A. (2001). Evaluation of omeprazole in the treatment of reflux laryngitis: A prospective, placebo-controlled, randomized, double-blind study. *Laryngoscope, 111*, 2147–2151.

Orlando, R. C. (1986). Esophageal epithelial resistance. *Journal of Clinical Gastroenterology, 8*(Suppl. 1), 12–16.

Orsmeth, E. J., & Wong, R. K. H. (1999). Reflux laryngitis: Pathophysiology, diagnosis, and management. *American Journal of Gastroenterology, 94*, 2812–2817.

Pan, T., Wang, Y., & Guo, Z. (2004). Additional bedtime H2-receptor antagonist for the control of nighttime gastric acid breakthrough. *Cochrane Database System Review, 4*, CD004275.

Park, K. H., Choi, S. M., Kwon, S. U., Yoon, S. W., & Kim, S. U. (2006). Diagnosis of laryngopharyngeal reflux among globus patients. *Otolaryngology-Head and Neck Surgery, 134*, 81–85.

Park, W., Hicks, D. M., Khandwala, F., Richter, J. E., Abelson, T. I., Milstein C., & Vaezi, M. F. (2005). Laryngopharyngeal reflux: Prospective cohort study evaluating optimal dose of proton-pump inhibitor therapy and pretherapy predictors of response. *Laryngoscope, 115*, 1230–1238.

Peghini, P. L., Katz, P. O., Bracy, N. A., & Castell, D. O. (1998). Nocturnal recovery of gastric acid secretion with twice-daily dosing of proton pump inhibitors. *American Journal of Gastroenterology, 93*, 763–767.

Postma, G. N. (2000). Ambulatory pH monitoring methodology. *Annals of Otology, Rhinology and Laryngology, 109*, 10–14.

Postma, G. N., Belafsky, P. C., Aviv, J. E., & Koufman, J. A. (2002). Laryngopharyngeal reflux testing. *Ear, Nose, and Throat Journal, 81*(Suppl. 2), 14–18.

Postma, G. N., Cohen, J. T., Belafsky, P. C., Halum, S. L., Gupta, S. K., Bach, K. K., & Koufman, J. A. (2005).Transnasal esophagoscopy: Revisited (over 700 consecutive cases). *Laryngoscope, 115*, 321–323.

Postma, G. N., & Johnson, L. F. (2002). Treatment of laryngopharyngeal reflux. *Ear Nose and Throat Journal, 81*(Suppl. 2), 24–26.

Postma, G. N., Tomek, M. S., Belafsky, P. C., & Koufman, J. A. (2001). Esophageal motor function in laryngopharyngeal reflux is superior to that in classic gastroesophageal reflux disease. *Annals of Otology, Rhinology and Laryngology, 110,* 114–116.

Reavis, K. M., Morris, C. D., Gopal, D. V., Hunter, J. G., & Jobe, B. A. (2004). Laryngopharyngeal reflux symptoms better predict the presence of esophageal adenocarcinoma than typical gastroesophageal reflux symptoms. *Annals of Surgery, 239,* 849–858.

Reulbach, T. R., Belafsky, P. C., Blalock, P. D., Koufman, J. A., & Postma, G. N. (2001). Occult laryngeal pathology in a community-based cohort. *Otolaryngology-Head and Neck Surgery, 124,* 448–450.

Richardson, B. E., Heywood, B. M., Sims, H. S., Stoner, J., & Leopold, D. A. (2004). Laryngopharyngeal reflux: Trends in diagnostic interpretation criteria. *Dysphagia, 19,* 248–255.

Sasaki, C. T., Ross, D. A., & Hundal, J. (2003). Association between Zenker diverticulum and gastroesophageal reflux disease: Development of a working hypothesis. *American Journal of Medicine, 18* (Suppl. 3A), 169S–171S.

Smoak, B. R., & Koufman, J. A. (2001). Effects of gum chewing on pharyngeal and esophageal pH. *Annals of Otology, Rhinology and Laryngology, 110,* 1117–1119.

Steward, D. L., Wilson, K. M., Kelly, D. H., Patil, M. S., Schwartzbauer, H. R., Long, J. D., & Welge, J. A. (2004). Proton pump inhibitor therapy for chronic laryngopharyngitis: Randomized placebo-control trial. *Otolaryngology-Head and Neck Surgery, 131,* 342–350.

Toohill, R. J., Mushtaq, E., & Lehman, R. H. (1990). Otolaryngologic manifestations of gastroesophageal reflux. In T. Sacristan, J. J. Alvarez-Vincent, & J. Bartual (Eds.), *Proceedings of XIV World Congress of Otolaryngology-Head and Neck Surgery* (pp. 3005–3009). Amsterdam, The Netherlands: Kugler & Ghedini.

Tutuian, R., & Castell, D. O. (2004). Nocturnal acid breakthrough—approach to management. *Medscape General Medicine, 6,* 11.

Ulualp, S. O., & Toohill, R. J. (2000). Laryngopharyngeal reflux: state of the art diagnosis and treatment. *Otolaryngology Clinics of North America, 33,* 785–802.

Ulualp, S. O., Toohill, R. J., Kern, M., & Shaker, R. (1998). Pharygo-UES contractile reflux in patients with posterior laryngitis. *Laryngoscope, 108,* 1354–1357.

Vincent, D. A., Jr., Garrett, J. D., Radionoff, S. L., Reussner, L. A., & Stasney, C. R. (2000). The proximal probe in esophageal pH monitoring: Development of a normative database. *Journal of Voice, 14,* 247–254.

Wiener, G. J., Koufman, J. A., & Wu, W. C. (1987). The pharyngo-esophageal dual ambulatory pH probe for evaluation of atypical manifestations of gastroesophageal reflux (GER). *Gastroenterology, 92,* 1694.

Wiener, G. J., Koufman, J. A., Wu, W. C., Cooper, J. B., Richter, J. E., & Castel, D. O. (1989). Chronic hoarseness secondary to gastroesophageal reflux disease: Documentation with 24-h ambulatory pH monitoring. *American Journal of Gastroenterology, 84,* 1503–1508.

Westcott, C. J., Hopkins, M. B, Bach, K., Postma, G. N., Belafsky, P. C., & Koufman, J. A. (2004). Fundoplication for laryngopharyngeal reflux disease. *Journal of the American College of Surgery, 199,* 23–30.

Woo, P., Noordzij, P., & Ross, J. (1996). Association of esophageal reflux and globus symptom: Comparison of laryngoscopy and 24-hour pH manometry. *Otolaryngology-Head and Neck Surgery, 115,* 502–507.

Wright, R. C., & Rhodes, K. P. (2003). Improvement of laryngopharyngeal reflux symptoms after laparoscopic Hill repair. *American Journal of Surgery, 185,* 455–461.

Ylitalo, R., Lindestad, P. A., & Ramel, S. (2001). Symptoms, laryngeal findings, and 24-hour pH monitoring in patients with suspected gastroesophago-pharyngeal reflux. *Laryngoscope, 111,* 1735–1741.

Ylitalo, R., & Ramel, S. (2002a & 2002b). Gastroesophagopharyngeal reflux in patients with contact granuloma: A prospective controlled study. *Annals of Otology, Rhinology and Laryngology, 111,* 178–183; Corrected and republished in: *Annals of Otology, Rhinology and Laryngology, 111* (5 Pt. 1), 441–446.

7

Nursing Evaluation and Care of the Dysphagic Patient

Ann E. F. Sievers

Early identification of patients with dysphagia is important to maintain nutritional requirements, to protect the airway during swallow and to prevent untoward complications. In a hospitalized patient, a nurse may be the first person to recognize the signs and symptoms of dysphagia. The nurse also plays a major role in implementing ongoing strategies for treatment, particularly as these relate to alternative feeding methods or monitoring of dietary recommendations and restrictions. Communication of pertinent information to the physician managing the patient's care, other professionals, the patient, and his or her family members or significant others in the patient's life is an integral part of the nurse's responsibility. It therefore is incumbent on the dysphagia team nurse and the staff nurse, to be knowledgeable about the person with dysphagia, including symptoms, risk factors, complications, and overall plan of care. This chapter addresses,

first, the role of the nurse in observing and evaluating patients with, or at risk for, dysphagia and, second, the role of the nurse in the ongoing care and monitoring of dysphagic patients, particularly as it relates to hospitalized patients.

INDICATIONS

Patients at Risk for Dysphagia Discussion

Patients at risk for dysphagia may have an underlying medical condition that predisposes them to difficulty swallowing, such as head or chest trauma, neuromuscular disease, brain tumor, head and neck cancer, or stroke. More difficult to identify are dysphagic patients with conditions that may not clearly signal dysphagia. Patients recovering from stroke, patients with dementia or other mental debilitation, elderly patients, and malnourished or deconditioned patients may fall into this category. All critically ill patients are at risk for dysphagia due to altered levels of consciousness, and general deconditioning. This includes weakness of musculature involved in both bolus propulsion and preparation and airway protection during deglutition. Poor oral care and the influences of intubation, changes in oral flora with bacterial overgrowth, and poor dentition lead to ventilator associated pneumonias (VAP) (Minei, 2006; Munroe, 2004; Niederman, 2005; Trieger, 2004).

Deconditioned patients lack breath support and have a poor cough in response to airway penetration by food or liquid, making them less able to respond effectively to even mild aspiration. Evidence of repeated fevers or pneumonia in a patient should also stimulate concern if there is a possibility these symptoms could be related to aspiration. This constellation of symptoms including a tachycardia, and tachypnea may alert a SIRS (Systemic Inflammatory Response Syndrome) protocol for aggressive early treatment of potential sepsis. Early sepsis intervention has been proven to save lives and decrease hospital days (ACCP 1992).

Pulmonary Risk Factors (Table 7-1)

Patients with pre-existing pulmonary disease who become dysphagic have a diminished ability to tolerate even mild aspiration. Aspiration insults are very poorly tolerated by an already compromised pulmonary system. Pulmonary diseases include all the smoking-related lung diseases, for example, emphysema, Chronic Obstructive Pulmonary

Table 7-1. Risk Factors for Aspiration

- Decreased level of consciousness.
- Supine position.
- Presence of a nasogastric tube.
- Tracheal intubation and mechanical ventilation.
- Bolus or intermittent feeding delivery methods.
- Malpositioned feeding tube.
- Vomiting.
- High-risk disease and injury conditions.
- Neurologic disorders.
- Major abdominal and thoracic trauma/surgery.
- Diabetes mellitus.
- Poor oral health.
- Inadequate R.N. staffing levels.
- Advanced age.

Source: Metheny, N. A. (2002). Risk factors for aspiration. *Journal of Parenteral and Enteral Nutrition, 26*(Suppl. 6), S26–S33.

disease (COPD) chronic bronchitis, or even lung cancer. Patients with cardiopulmonary pathologies such as cardiomyopathies, pulmonary hypertension, and cardiovascular diseases are also at heightened risk for pulmonary complications from dysphagia.

Aspiration Pneumonia

True aspiration pneumonia has a typical radiographic pattern. The pattern demonstrates infiltration or consolidation first in the right lower lobe, next most often in the right upper lobe, and less frequently in the left lower lobe.

Rarely, are all three lobes involved at the same time. This distribution is a consequence of the angle of the tracheobronchial takeoff into the parenchyma of the right lung. The right lower lobe represents a straight line of descent from the trachea and right main stem bronchus. In a patient who is supine, or lying on the right side, the right upper lobe takeoff from the right main stem bronchus represents a dependent position. The left lobe is in a dependent position in the left side-lying position. These common sites of aspiration are influenced largely by gravity and human anatomy.

Symptoms of aspiration pneumonia in a patient are diagnosed both clinically and radiographically. To ensure appropriate treatment, pneumonia related to dysphagia, or difficulty eating and drinking must be differentiated from a pneumonia related to a single aspiration event or a community acquired pneumonia from other etiologies. Aspiration pneumonia may be a result of material entering the lungs during a period of altered level of consciousness, such as can occur in trauma, diabetic coma, or acute myocardial infarction with loss of consciousness. Aspiration may occur when patients who have been instructed to remain NPO (non per os, nothing by mouth) before surgery do not comply with the instructions. Under general anesthesia, or even conscious sedation, the patient is unable to fully protect their airway. Reflux occurs as the lower esophageal sphincter is relaxed and the patient can potentially reflux and aspirate. Similarly, individuals who have eaten a meal and then experience a traumatic event leading to unconsciousness are at very high risk for aspiration. This aspiration is preceded by vomiting or reflux, and may have devastating consequences for their lungs.

Repeated aspiration occurs when the airway is unable to maintain its normal physiologic hygiene. Long-term endotracheal intubation heightens a patient's risk for repeated aspiration by the presence of an artificial tube that interferes with the normal cough, impairs the ciliary action of the lining of the trachea, and precludes the normal filtration and humidification of the nose and mouth. The presence of an artificial airway changes the normal bacterial flora in the mouth. Aggressive oral hygiene may prevent oral contamination to the lungs. Even with cuffed endotracheal tubes and tracheostomy tubes, microaspiration into the tracheobronchial tree does occur. This is a consequence of the constant expansion and contraction of the trachea during normal respiration and subsequent movement of the artificial airway cuff in the lumen of the trachea.

Repeated aspiration may also be related to a cognitively intact and awake patient's ongoing inability to protect the airway during oral nutrition. For example, a larynx that is incompetent as a consequence of paralysis or radiation effects may not be able to close quickly or completely enough to prevent aspiration. An insensate larynx, caused by stroke or laryngeal paralysis, may precipitate aspiration of foods, liquids, as well as the patient's own secretions. "Silent" aspiration can be particularly difficult to diagnose (Horner & Massey, 1988). In one study, only 42% (18 of 43) of a group of inpatients with documented aspiration on videofluoroscopy were identified as aspirating on bedside swallow evaluations (Splaingard, Hutchins, Sulton, & Chaudhuri, 1988).

Patients who chronically aspirate may become undernourished and unable to maintain their weight, and are diagnosed as failure to thrive. Immunological risk is heightened because of the lack of adequate protein, albumin, and fat stores to maintain normal body function. Laryngeal cancer patients often initially present with aspiration and cachexia. Both occurring at the same time portend for a poor outcome as both their fat and protein stores are depleted (Esper, 2005).

Clinical findings of aspiration include fever, shortness of breath, weakness, and cough. Sputum may be thick, colored, and difficult to expel by coughing. Chest auscultation may reveal rhonchi in the large airways, and the person with true pneumonia may have characteristic egophony, or "E" to "A" changes on auscultation, that is, when patient produces the vowel "ee," sound heard through stethoscope sounds like "a," as in "bait," due to abnormally increased lung density. Breath sounds are decreased over the consolidated lung (solidification of the lung secondary to pneumonia) and may even sound hollow (Bickley, 2009).

Both an episode of severe, acute aspiration and chronic, repeated aspiration can cause pneumonia and is best treated with appropriate antibiotic therapy combined with aggressive respiratory therapy. Coughing, deep breathing, oxygen, and medication support is indicated. If not treated promptly, or with the correct antibiotic regimen, the patient can become dangerously ill. Today, some pneumonia variants may not be so easily treated because of the rise in resistant microorganisms. In a patient whose immune system has been threatened as a consequence of chemo-

therapy, significant deconditioning, or AIDS, pneumonia of any origin may be lethal.

If aspiration pneumonia is diagnosed, the dysphagia team must be able to differentiate its etiologies. A distinction should be made between aspiration caused by an inability to protect the airway during eating and swallowing due to motor and/or sensory factors, and aspiration from other causes. Whatever the etiology, early correct detection is tantamount to correct treatment and, ultimately, to recovery.

DESCRIPTION OF NURSING EVALUATION

One goal of the nursing evaluation is to determine if a patient is able to maintain normal oral nutrition or if it has been impaired or altered. The evaluation also attempts to determine if aspiration is likely, possibly necessitating nonoral feeding as a precautionary measure until further diagnostic studies, such as comprehensive bedside swallow study, FEES, and or videofluoroscopy, can be completed. Components of the nursing assessment include the following.

History/Medical Record Review

Comprehensive review of the patient's medical history should provide information about risk factors for dysphagia (Table 7–2). Significant flags for possible dysphagia include cranial nerve deficits, structural anomalies, or medical or surgical conditions that may contribute to a swallowing abnormality. All medical diagnoses are noted, specifically those pertaining to a recent change in

Table 7–2. Patient History

- Identification of the Individual
- Chief Complaint
- HPI History of Present Illness
  Onset, symptoms, chronology
- PMH Past Medical History
  Illnesses, child, adult
  Hospital admits
  PHM medical
  PHM surgical
  Immunizations
  Health maintenance
- Allergies
  Medications, food, other
- Medications
  Type and diagnosis
- Social History
  Smoking
  ETOH
  Lifestyle
  Occupation
  Education
  Marital Status
  Diet
  Exercise
- Family History
- OB-GYN History

the health profile of the patient (Bickley, 2009). Surgical procedures are also noted, for example, carotid endarderectomy, thyroid, or open heart surgery may incur damage to the vagus nerve, cranial nerve X, as it courses through the neck and chest. Surgery on the cervical spine may be implicated in the onset of dysphagia, due to cranial nerve and cervical nerve impairment. Chart review must include documentation of the patient's dietary status, height and weight over time, and recent daily calorie counts. (See Chapter 10 for further details regarding appropriate calorie counts.) The inability to maintain caloric and protein goals may portend a significant nutritional problem. Document the patient's height, weight, BMI, usual weight, and the amount of weight loss or gain and over what period of time. Standard laboratory assessment of hematocrit, hemoglobin, electrolytes, trace elements, albumin, and protein also aids in the evaluation. Dietetic professionals play an indispensable role in the evaluation and treatment of individuals diagnosed with head and neck cancer as well as individuals who are at increased risk such as the elderly, those with cachexia, or multiple trauma (Dixon, 2005).

It may be helpful to organize medical history-taking or chart documentation according to a review of systems, in particular, cardiovascular, gastrointestinal, genitourinary, neurologic, skeletal, and endocrine. Consideration of this comprehensive overview makes it less likely that details that have implications for swallowing function will be overlooked. Pertinent information regarding systems should be documented in the patient's medical records, and can be reviewed with the physician managing the patient's care (Table 7–3).

Physical Exam

A hospitalized patient with dysphagia is monitored by a physician and the medical support team managing care. When the patient's condition is subject to significant and/or frequent change, a comprehensive nursing evaluation includes a physical exam directed to

Table 7–3. Review of Symptoms

• General
    Height, weight, usual weight
    Pain related to specific area
• HEENT
    Head, Eyes, Ears, Nose, Throat
    Head
    Eyes and vision
    Nose, sinuses
    Mouth, dentition
    Throat
    Larynx
• Cardiovascular
    Chest pain
    SOB (Shortness of Breath)
• Respiratory
    Cough
    SOB
    Sputum
• Endocrine
    Weight, obesity, cachexia
    Weight increase or decrease
    from normal
• Gastrointestinal
    Mouth odynophagia, dysphagia
    Swallowing
    Reflux, heartburn
    Stomach complaints
    Bowel habits
• Genitourinary
    Urine frequency, complaints
    Male genetalia
    OB-GYN
    Breast
• Hematology-Oncology
    Pallor, red, bruising, bleeding
	• Musculoskeletal
	    Posture
	    Muscle aches
	    Back/neck/hip pain
	    Bone pain
	• Neurological
	    Headache
	    LOC (loss of consciousness)
	    Dizziness vertigo
	    Seizures
	    Behavior
	    Memory
	    Thought content
	    Speech
	    Balance-gait
	    Sensation
	• Psychiatric
	    Personality
	    Affect
	    Depression
	    Anxiety
	• Skin
	    Color-turgor
	    Lesions
	    Masses
	    Rashes
	• Pain
	    Character
	    Location
	    Cause
	    Onset/duration
	    Intensity (1–10 scale)
	    Treatment
	       Medications, other Rx

the patient's nutritional status. This includes food management, oral care, swallowing issues, weight fluctuations, and airway protection. A particular focus of this assessment is on correlating the patient's current level of alertness (or level of consciousness) with swallowing function and determining how changes in physical status, that is, pulmonary, neurologic, and gastrointestinal, may impact additional diagnostic tests, such as bedside swallow or videofluoroscopy, and the patient's ability to cooperate with the objectives of these tests.

Patient Interview

It is important to have the patient, if possible, and their significant others, describe his or her own complaints and experiences with swallowing and food management. Patient complaints may be related to a single pathologic process, or may suggest multiple problems. An important distinction is whether the patient experiences difficulty swallowing or pain on swallowing, or rather describes symptoms suggesting penetration or aspiration of materials into the airway with a resultant cough. Examples of patient complaints which may be significant include:

Food sticking: Reflecting possible inability to propel bolus material properly, failure of the upper esophageal sphincter to relax, changes in mucosal integrity, esophageal conditions, or repeated reflux.

Changes in taste: Suggesting altered sensation in the oral cavity chemoreceptors may be related to neurogenic factors, alterations in oral or pharyngeal mucosa, medications and/or treatment programs, and chemotherapy or radiation therapy.

Cough with food or liquid before, during or after the swallow: Most likely due to aspiration, but may be due to pulmonary disease.

Cough at rest/between feedings: Indicating possible aspiration of residual food or saliva. A cough at rest is indicative of COPD (chronic obstructive pulmonary disease), chronic bronchitis, or other preexisting pulmonary problems or reflux.

Excessive oral secretions: Related to poor sensation, or copious or thick secretions or the inability to effectively manage normally produced oral secretions.

Impaired ability to manage foods of specific sensations or textures: May provide directed clues useful to a more specific diagnosis.

Weight loss, acute or chronic: Indicates inadequate nutrition, or metabolic needs in excess of nutritional intake, for example, undiagnosed cancer, or depression.

Social or behavioral changes related to meals: May provide clues to patient's mental, emotional state, or to degree of debilitation, or to environmental/social factors which may be influencing patient's health and nutrition, such as lack of care or available nutrition.

Family observation of any of above changes.

An interview with a patient's family, friends, and other caregivers, if available, is often very informative. Family and friends may provide information related to observed changes in the patient's eating habits and changes in weight that the patient is not aware of or is unable or unwilling to communicate.

Observations During Meals

A Nursing screening swallow evaluation may be initially performed by the patients nurse. If there is concern regarding dysphagia, further investigations are indicated. Together, the dysphagia team nurse and a speech-language pathologist trained in swallowing work synergistically to offer a complete clinical evaluation. This type of clinical evaluation is discussed in depth in Chapter 8. The assessment reviewed here focuses primarily on the preliminary findings that suggest a patient is dysphagic and requires further diagnostic workup necessitating a bedside evaluation, FEES, and or videofluoroscopy. For this purpose, the nurse observes the patient during one or more mealtimes. A representative sample of the patient's capabilities requires observation at different times of the day, before or after activities or medications. Any changes over time related to fatigue, medication administration, or other factors are noted. Family interviews, or discussions with other caregivers, may be of help in obtaining significant information. The value of information obtained notwithstanding, it is important to remember the limitations of the clinical exam. For example, bedside evaluation alone has been reported to underestimate the frequency of aspiration in patients with neurologic dysfunction (Splaingard et al., 1988). Clinical evaluations must focus on history and physical and signs and symptoms elicited by the exam and interview.

Observations made of the patient during swallow can be of significance and includes the following:

- Change in vocal quality while eating (suggesting presence of material in the larynx on the vocal folds).
- Cough during or after swallow (suggesting possible aspiration) or inability to clear the pharynx or larynx.
- Wet or gurgling sound associated with respiration (suggesting food/liquids in pharynx and an inability to clear the pharynx or larynx).
- Change in ability to take routine medications, that is, pills more difficult, capsules and liquids easier.
- Apparent attempts to compensate for swallowing/food management difficulty, as by multiple swallows of one bolus, manipulating size or consistency of bolus, or by avoidance or preference of particular kinds of foods, or by assuming particular postures, that is, chin-tuck, head turning.
- Fatigue during meal; time needed to complete meal (amount of food/time).
- Increasing frequency of eating attempts with decreasing volumes and weight loss.
- Alteration of normal laminar airflow during auscultation of the larynx.
- Unexplained weight loss.

Chest and Cervical Auscultation

Auscultation of the chest and cervical airway are important techniques in the clinical evaluation of any person suspected of dysphagia and possible aspiration. Normal airflow associated with normal respiration has a characteristic laminar sound that can be detected by placing a stethoscope over various parts of the airway. Large airway sounds differ from small airway sounds because of the density of tissue the air is traveling through to reach the stethoscope, (Bickley, 2009) and each area of the chest has a unique sound dependent on its distance from the large airways and the chest wall.

Laryngeal auscultation may be especially useful in evaluating dysphagic, or possibly dysphagic, patients (Hamlet, Nelson, & Patterson, 1990; Hamlet, Penny, & Formolo, 1994; Selley, Ellis, Flack, Baylis, & Pearce, 1994; Takahashi, Groher, & Michi, 1994; Zenner, Losinski, & Mills, 1995). Placing the stethoscope gently on the lateral aspect of the larynx, and listening to airflow

in normal breathing, during swallowing, or speech, will provide the listener with experience in identifying this sound and differentiating it from other sounds (Figure 7–1). In a dysphagic patient who aspirates during swallow, the quality of sound generated may be altered, as would be expected if fluids and air are mixed. In addition to airflow, some mechanical events associated with swallow have characteristic sounds. Such events may include elevation of the larynx and bolus flow through the pharyngoesophageal segment, although exact correspondences between sounds and events remain to be identified. A listener experienced with the characteristics of these mechanical "event" sounds may be able to differentiate normal and altered sound generation, however. Laryngeal auscultation should focus on the documentation

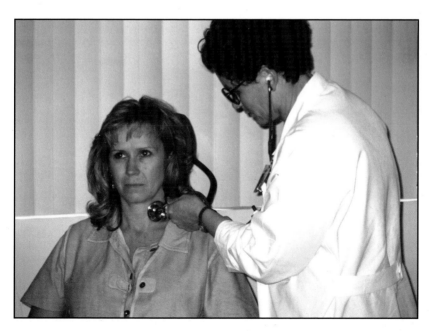

Figure 7–1. Laryngeal auscultation. Proper placement of bell of stethoscope while patient completes swallowing and speech maneuvers.

of laminar versus nonlaminar airflow, **not** on the swallow. Chest auscultation is of particular help in defining daily changes related to aspiration and aspiration pneumonia. Chest radiographs are indicated if pneumonia is suspected on chest auscultation.

NURSING CARE IN DYSPHAGIC PATIENTS

Aspiration Precautions

Aspiration precautions are indicated in many settings such as acute care hospitalized patients, patients in nursing home settings, and home health patients. However, precautions *must* be modified for each individual patient to match his or her type of dysphagia, nutritional needs, and treatment plan. Again, continual diligence is required because many dysphagic patients aspirate without giving any external sign of food or liquid entering the airway (Logeman, 1986). This plan of care must be developed on the basis of objective data. Refer to Table 7–1 (Metheny, 2002).

Inpatient aspiration precautions may include the following:

Oral Feeding:

- Do not allow patient to eat unattended or unobserved.
- If patient is taking an oral diet, follow the diet recommendations and restrictions generated by an objective dysphagia assessment plan. (Coordinate with the physician's orders for consistency, amount, and frequency.)
- Position patient in optimally safe upper body position as recommended, or 90° in a chair with head/neck flexion, if possible. Address head stability during meals.
- Observe for coughing, choking, throat clearing, or struggle during eating.
- Minimize distractions (maintain quiet environment, no television, no talking during eating).
- Continually assess the patient's pulmonary status for fevers, rales, rhonchi, and clinical signs of aspiration.

Enteral Feeding:

- Ensure placement of tube is confirmed by radiograph and monitor for evidence of tube migration, by measurement.
- Observe reflux precautions (proper positioning. limit nocturnal feeds, elevate the head of the bed).
- Check residuals before beginning enteral feeding (Metheny, 2012).
- Improve oral care (Munro, 2004; Niederman & Craven, 2005).

Outpatient aspiration precautions are similar and may include:

Oral Feeding:

- Avoid eating/drinking when alone.
- Minimize distractions (quiet environment, no television, no talking during eating).
- Observe food consistency, amount, and frequency recommendations by the dysphagia team.
- Observe optimally safe upper body position as recommended, or use 90° upper body position with chin tuck. Assess head stability during eating.

- Ensure that family/caregivers are familiar with Heimlich maneuver, CPR, and signs of aspiration.
- Cough, throat clear, "wet" voice, voice changes, struggle associated with eating/drinking (Metheny, 2007).
- Frequently assess for changes in pulmonary status reflective of aspiration (rales, fevers, rhonchi).
- Oral care before and after meals (Munroe, 2004).

Enteral Feeding:

- Monitor tube position for evidence that it has migrated.
- Observe reflux positions.
- Check residuals before feeding (Metheny, 2012). Monitor and document tolerance or intolerance to the enteral feeding regimen.

Feeding Precautions

Observation of Patients with Enteral Nutrition

Individuals whose primary mode of nutrition is by feeding tube (NG, NJ, GT/J) are still susceptible to aspiration from gastroesophageal reflux and improper placement or migration of the enteral tube. As early as 1986 Metheny stated that aspiration pneumonia is unquestionably the most potentially lethal complication of tube feeding (Metheny, 1986). GI reflux may occur with both continuous or bolus feeding and can also occur with gastric secretions alone. Reflux and potential aspiration in patients with gastrostomy tubes can be caused by lower esophageal sphincter (LES) relaxation secondary to gastric distention of the stomach

(Takahashi et al., 1994). These patients require rigorous monitoring because this type of aspiration may be silent and its symptoms are elusive to cursory examination. Initial gastric placement is confirmed by radiograph. Vomiting, coughing, retching, or suctioning can cause the distal tip to migrate upward into the esophagus or downward into the duodenum, or may become coiled in the pharynx (Simmons, 2012). The nurse must be aware of the position of the patient during enteral feeding and medication. Antireflux precautions such as elevating the head of the bed should be integrated into practice.

Coughing following a feeding (especially bolus feeding), with a full stomach, is a strong indication of reflux and potentially aspiration. When feeding is administered lower in the GI tract, via jejunostomy, reflux of gastric acid after feeding may still occur (Coben, Weintraub, DiMarino, & Cohen, 1994; Sands, 1991). The acidity (pH <3) of the gastric secretions is extremely damaging to the larynx and lungs (even more so than the content of tube feeds) and medications designed to modify stomach acidity, such as antacids and H2-blockers, should be considered. Elpern et al. (1987) found that 77% of patients with tubes in place aspirated material at some time during the study period.

Proper position and monitoring of the enteral feeding tube is critical to the correct administration of proper nutrition. Radiographic documentation of tube placement is the standard of care (McClave et al., 2009). If the patient is discharged home with an enteral feeding tube family members should be taught assessment for placement. With a nasogastric tube in place, the nasolabial tip should be protected with a skin barrier, and tape placement must be appropriate to avoid nasal tip necrosis (Figure 7–2). Similarly, gastrostomy and jejunostomy tubes necessitate protection of the anterior abdominal wall, and require skin barriers around the tube insertion site. In the home radiographic determination is also indicated if there is any concern regarding clinical interpretation of the tube placement. In the home, belly auscultation, measurement, instillation of air, and gastric contents checks are used to assess correct placement of enteral tubes. Blue vegetable dye placed in a very small amount of the tube feeding formula of patients with a tracheostomy can be a useful test for reflux and subsequent aspiration. Blue dye is contraindicated for routine enteral feeding assessment (Metheny, 2002). If in the trial blue dye is suctioned from the tracheostomy, the test is considered positive. Glucose monitoring of pulmonary secretions is not a reliable indicator of formulas that have been refluxed into the airway.

When drugs are mixed with enteral products, it is important to assess the mixture for physical and chemical compatibility. In some instances, there is a potential for the drugs and/or enteral products to undergo degradation and inactivation when combined (Cutie, Altman, & Lenkel, 1983). Always consult your Pharmacist for guidance regarding drug and formula interaction and incompatibility. Suctioning through a tracheostomy tube may cause a patient to cough and the increased intrathoracic pressure generated during a cough may cause reflux. Consequently, suctioning should be effective to remove secretions but gentle to prevent the reflexive coughing, particularly if aspiration is suspected during a reflux episode. Following suctioning, a patient may be asked to cough voluntarily, without suction, to further determine if there is refluxed material in the airway, but this is not always a reliable indicator.

In addition to monitoring patients for evidence of aspiration, the nurse caring for the patient with enteral feeding must work closely with the physician and dietitian to assure the patient's tolerance and progression to the feeding regimen. Monitoring fluctuations in weight, protein and albumin levels, and blood chemistry are routine measures. Also observe for alterations in the patient's level of consciousness as these may affect the patient's ability to airway protect their airway. Attention to the patient's physical well-being, of course, must also be accompanied by attention to maintaining the best quality of life possible in the face of what may represent a radical alteration in lifestyle.

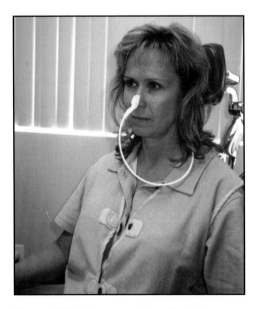

Figure 7–2. The correct method of securing a nasogastric tube to prevent dislodgement and nasal tip/alae necrosis.

Observation of Patients with Artificial Airways

In patients with an artificial airway in place, the disease process as well as the presence of the appliance may influence the patient's ability to swallow. The presence of food (or enteral feeding in the case of a tube-fed patient) in a tracheostomy, or endotracheal secretions, are obvious indicators of aspiration or reflux and aspiration. This observation requires an immediate response from the treatment team to treat an aspiration event. Patients with an artificial airway in place should be immediately suctioned in the event of a witnessed aspiration. The primary cause of pneumonia in patients on ventilators is the ongoing microaspiration around the cuff of the artificial airway (Minei, 2006; Niederman, 2005).

A patient with an artificial airway often intimidates the novice clinician, but it is through understanding that the patient receives appropriate care (Sievers, 2010). Clinicians involved in the care of the person with dysphagia must have an intimate knowledge of the kinds, uses, and complications of artificial airways used in their patient population (Lindholm, 1985). Halum et al. (2011) have investigated the prevalence of tracheotomy tube complications and risk factors associated with their occurrence. This analytical article discusses such care issues as mucous plugs, accidental decannulation, airway stenosis, and bleeding. Health care providers responsible of the care of patients with tracheostomy will find this useful in their practice reviews. The following is an overview of some of the types of tracheostomy tubes used in the acute care setting.

Cuffed tracheostomy tubes (Figure 7–3) are used to seal the airway for positive pressure ventilation and to attempt to prevent aspiration of secretions into the lungs (Lindholm, 1985). Intracuff pressures are established at no more than 20 to 30 mm Hg in order not to exceed end capillary pressures (McGuinnis, Shively, & Patterson, 1971). These tubes are typically used in critical care settings and with patients on positive pressure ventilators or during surgical procedures requiring anesthesia. Patients are infrequently sent home with cuffed tubes. This happens only if they require positive pressure ventilation, such as the patient with end stage amyotrophic lateral sclerosis (ALS). When a patient does not require positive pressure ventilation, and is breathing independently, the cuff is always deflated to avoid pressure and scarring of the tracheal walls (tracheal stenosis). Cuff deflation is the precursor to replacing the cuffed tube with a non-cuffed tube and eventual decannulation.

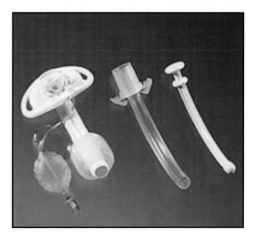

Figure 7–3. Cuffed tracheostomy tube: cuffed tube with pilot balloon; disposable inner cannula; insertion obturator. (Photo courtesy of Mallinckrodt Medical, Inc.)

Uncuffed/cuffless tracheostomy tubes (Figure 7–4) are used to provide an airway when the patient is able to breathe on his or her own but still requires assistance with secretion removal and airway maintenance. These tracheostomy tubes are typically used for tracheostomy patients for long-term airway support. The tube itself may tether the larynx and interfere with its normal elevation during swallow (Johnson, Reilly, & Mallory, 1985). The goal is to use the smallest tube possible that allows the patient to ventilate with maximum tidal volume without restriction.

Fenestrated tubes (Figure 7–5) are tubes that are rarely used for weaning and decannulation, and are generally smaller in size than tubes used for traditional airway maintenance. Their secondary benefit as they are smaller may make for improved speech for selected individuals. When the inner cannula is removed and the tube is capped, the patient is breathing via the fenestra, as well as around the tube (Lindholm, 1985). Fenestrated tubes are not left in place for long periods of times, no more than 3 to 5 days, because of the possibility of invagination of fragile tracheal mucosa into the fenestra, therefore obstructing the patient's airway (Figure 7–6). Prior to decannulation, the patient should have the tube capped for 18 to 24 hours to test tolerance, and then be decannulated early in the morning. This allows for the most hours of intense observation of the patient's accommodation and airway competence immediately following decannulation. (See Figure 7–7 UCD Sievers Decannulation protocol.)

Speech and Swallowing with a Tracheostomy

When medically stable, the patient with a noncuffed tracheostomy should be taught to cover the tube opening and

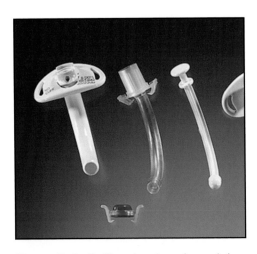

Figure 7-4. Cuffless tracheostomy tube: outer cannula; disposable inner cannula; decannulation cannula; thumb screw inner cannula; insertion obturator. (Photo courtesy of Mallinckrodt Medical, Inc.)

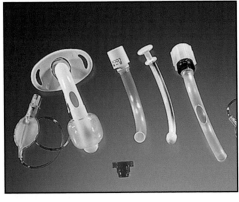

Figure 7-5. Fenestrated tracheostomy tube: outer cannula; decannulation plug (*red*); 35-mm reusable inner cannula; insertion obturator; fenestrated reusable inner cannula with decannulation cap in place. (Photo courtesy of Mallinckrodt Medical, Inc.)

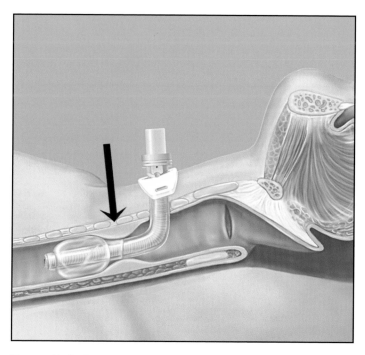

Figure 7–6. Tracheostomy tube with fenestra occluded by granulation tissue growth from the posterior tracheal wall.

talk. The use of finger control speech or the use of a one-way valve speaking system is predicated upon the ability of the patient to successfully use this technique without compromising their ability to clear their secretions. The patient and family should be instructed in the proper method of speech and breathing, that is, inhale through the tracheostomy tube, cover the tube at peak inhalation, and speak on exhalation. It is important to remind the patient to then release the cover and again breathe in through the tube. Once the technique is mastered, patients usually quickly become adept at speaking. The use of the vocal folds for speech is believed to facilitate function of the larynx for swallow. In addition, the patient's ability to communicate orally may be of great help in identifying problems,

discussing needs, and maintaining interactions with significant others and their care givers (Hoit, 2003). Speaking related shortness of breath is characterized by air hunger and physical exertions and the difficulty in coordination with swallowing may be detrimental to their quality of life (Hoit, 2007). Communication while intubated or with a tracheostomy can significantly interfere with issues of quality of life and manipulation of the artificial airway and ventilator may enhance their ability to communicate. Care providers must improve the patient's ability to communicate. Assessment by skilled bedside clinicians can reveal patients' communication potential and facilitate useful augmentative and alternative communication tools and strategies for patients and their families (Broyles, 2012).

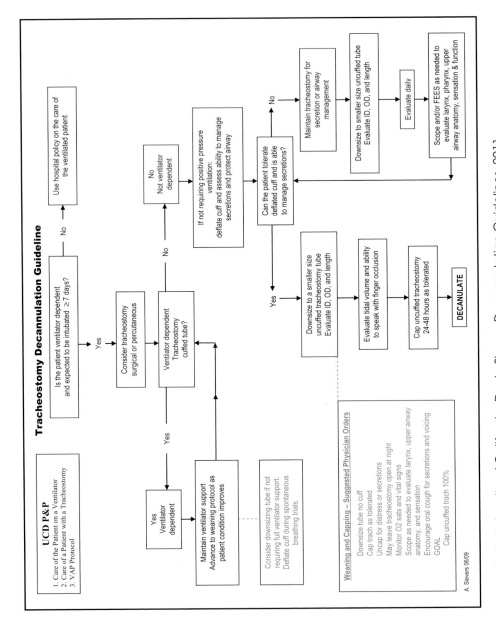

Figure 7-7. University of California, Davis, Sievers Decannulation Guidelines, 2011.

Observation of Patients from Tube to Oral Feeding

Nursing intervention during transition from tube feeding to oral feeding includes assurance of overall adequate nutrition, monitoring of progress, and *slow careful* advancement of the treatment plan. Patients who are in the process of transition from enteral feeding to oral feeding must be carefully followed for possible complications of aspiration, weight loss, intolerance and changes in chemistry panels on routine evaluations. It is cautious to maintain aspiration and reflux precautions throughout this period. Any alteration or acute changes of pulmonary function that may indicate aspiration, necessitates intervention and therapy by the physician managing the patient's care. Patients may initially view a return to oral eating as a huge success, and indeed it is. But, in their enthusiasm, they may also fail to observe necessary precautions. Patients must be monitored to ensure that they, and their families, understand and observe the precautions prescribed.

Observation of Patients on Modified Oral Nutrition

When a treatment plan permits the patient to eat orally, but with modifications or restrictions, the nurse and dysphagia therapist can work together to ensure that the protocol is communicated to and understood by, the patient (to the extent possible), family members, other professionals, and caregivers. This attention to implementation of dietary modifications, compensatory strategies, or other recommendations that comprise the treatment plan continues while the patient is in the hospi-

tal, and may also need to be extended to other environments, for example, when the patient is transferred to another floor, discharged to another facility, or sent home. Use of adaptive devices for feeding must be carefully monitored for safety (Sievers, Leonard, & McKenzie, 1992). Feedback regarding the effectiveness of the plan also needs to be communicated regularly to other members of the dysphagia team, so that plan updates occur as the patient progresses.

Psychosocial Factors

Nurses are extremely influential in teaching patients how to cope with life's illnesses. This is true of the nurse in the acute care hospital, the skilled facility, the rehabilitation hospital, and the home. As part of a dysphagia team, the nurse should address a patient's psychosocial issues with concern, and with accurate information.

Quality of life issues are of great import for people who have a diagnosis of a swallowing disorder, particularly after head and neck cancer resections (Dropkin, 1997; Luckett, 2011). Patients with dysphagia, with or without aspiration, may experience a change in normally established eating habits. Issues related to safe nutrition, eating with friends and family, eating in public, alteration of normal routines, and the need for increased time for feeding may become pressing. The relationship between food and eating to quality of life, perhaps universally, is significant. Television has many advertisements emphasizing food; eating is a major part of holiday or just social activities. But for the dysphagic patient, and others in his or her environment, eating may be a stressful chore, not a pleasure. Coping skills can be sorely challenged during this time. Strategies for coping with the changes and the stressors they induce are a part of the patient education process, and the responsibility of all dysphagia team members who have contact with the patient. Nursing care, in particular, should include attention to these details, and to the resolution of issues that can separate rather than unite a family during a time of illness. The goal is success with nutrition whether it be oral or enteral.

TEAM COLLABORATION

As has been emphasized frequently in this manual, the best approach to the dysphagic patient is a team approach. The integration of many disciplines is needed for complete diagnosis and treatment, and the interaction of these professionals on a regular basis, that is, daily or weekly, ensures that necessary feedback regarding the patient's progress is available to appropriately revise and update the plan as needed. The team approach represents the best care for patients, and allows members of the team to advance their own knowledge through shared experiences, skills, and information.

STUDY QUESTIONS

1. The nurse's role in the treatment of dysphagia includes:
2. What is the optimum bed position recommended in the literature to prevent aspiration in critical patients?
3. How does laryngeal auscultation help you in the evaluation of a patients swallow and airway?

4. How does a complete history help in the evaluation of a patient with a swallowing complaint?
5. What should be the first response if a patient is observed with significant swallowing difficulties?
6. Describe the correct method of securing a nasogastric tube in place.

REFERENCES

American College of Chest Physicians/Society of Critical Care Medicine Consensus Conference: Definitions for sepsis and organ failure and guidelines for the use of innovative therapies in sepsis. (1992). *Critical Care Medicine, 20*(6), 864–874.

Altman, L., & Lenkel, J. B. (1983). Compatibility of enteral products with commonly employed drug additives. *Journal of Parenteral Enteral Nutrition, 7*, 186–191.

August, D., & Teitelbaum, D. (2002). Guidelines for the use of parenteral and enteral nutrition in adult and pediatric patients, ASPEN Board of Directors and The Clinical Guidelines Task Force. *Journal of Parenteral and Enteral Nutrition, 26*(1 Suppl.), S1–96.

Bickley, L., Szilagyi, P., & Hoekelman, R. A. (2009). Interviewing the health history. In B. Bates & R. Hoekelman (Eds.), *A guide to physical examination and history taking.* (4th ed., Chap. 1). Philadelphia, PA: Wolters, Kluwer, Health/Lippincott Williams & Wilkins.

Broyles, L. M., Tate, J. A., & Happ, M. B. (2012) Use of augmentative and alternative communications strategies by family members in the intensive care unit. *American Journal of Critical Care, 21*, e21–e32.

Coben, R., Weintraub, A., DiMarino, A., & Cohen, S. (1994). Gastroesophageal reflux during gastrostomy feeding. *Gastroenterology, 106*, 13–18

Cutie, A. E., Altman, L., & Lenkel, J. B. (1983). Compatibility of enteral products with commonly employed drug additives. *Journal of Parenteral Enteral Nutrition, 7*, 186–191.

Dixon, S. W. (2005). Nutrition care issues in the ambulatory (outpatient) head and neck cancer patient. *Support Line, 27*, 3–10.

Dropkin, M. J. (1997). Coping with disfigurement/dysfunction and length of hospital stay after head and neck cancer surgery. *ORL-Head and Neck Nursing, 15*, 22–26.

Elpern, E. H., Jacobs, E. R., & Bone, R. C. (1987). Incidence of aspiration in tracheally intubated adults. *Heart and Lung, 16*, 527–531.

Esper, D. H., & Harb, W. A. (2005). The cancer cachexia syndrome: A review of metabolic and clinical manifestations. *Nutrition in Clinical Practice, 20*, 369–376.

Halum, S. L., Ting, J. Y., Plowman, E. K., Belafsky, P. C., Harbarger, C. F., Postma, G. N., . . . Merati, A. L. (2012). A multiinstitutional analysis of tracheotomy complications. *Laryngoscope, 122*, 38–45.

Hamlet, S., Patterson, R. J., & Nelson, R. L. (1990). Interpreting the sounds of swallowing: Fluid flow through the cricopharyngeus. *Annals of Otology, Rhinology, and Laryngology, 99*, 749–752.

Hamlet, S., Penney, D. G., & Formolo, J. (1994). Stethoscope acoustics and cervical auscultation of swallowing. *Dysphagia, 9*, 63–68.

Hoit, J. D., Banzett, R. B., Lohmeier, H. L., Hixon, T. J., & Brown, R. (2003). Clinical ventilator adjustments that improve speech. *Chest, 124*, 1512–1521.

Hoit, J. D., Lansing, R. W., & Perona, K. E. (2007). Speaking related dyspnea in healthy adults, *Journal of Speech, Language, and Hearing Research, 50*, 361–374.

Horner, J., & Massey, E. (1998). Silent aspiration following stroke. *Neurology, 38*, 317–319.

Johnson, J., Reilly, J., & Mallory, G. (1985). Decannulation. In E. Myers, S. Stool, & J. Johnson (Eds.), *Tracheostomy* (Chap. 12). New York, NY: Churchill Livingston.

Lindholm, C. (1985). Choice of tracheostomy tube. In E. Myers, S. Stool, & J. Johnson (Eds.), *Tracheostomy* (Chap. 8). New York, NY: Churchill Livingston.

Logemann, J. (1986). Treatment for aspiration related to dysphagia: An overview. *Dysphagia, 1*, 34–38.

Luckett, T., Britton, B., Clover, K., & Rankin, N. M. (2011) Evidence for interventions to improve psychological outcomes in people with head and neck cancer: A systematic review of the literature. *Support Care Cancer, 19*, 871–881.

McClave, S. A., Demeo, M. T., DeLegge, M. H., DiSario, J. A., Heyland, D. K., Maloney, J. P, . . . Zaloga, G. P. (2002). North American Summit of Aspiration in the Critically Ill Patient: Consensus statement. *Journal of Parenteral and Enteral Nutrition, 26*(Suppl. 6), S80–S85.

McClave, S. A., Martindale, R. G., Vanek, V. W., McCarthy, M., Roberts, P., Taylor, B., . . . Cresci, G.: A.S.P.E.N. Board of Directors; American College of Critical Care Medicine; Society of Critical Care Medicine. (2009). Guidelines for the provision and assessment of nutrition support therapy I: The adult critically ill patient. *Journal Parenteral Enteral Nutrition, 33*, 277–316.

McGuinnis, G. E., Shively, J. G., Patterson, R. L., & Magovern, G. J. (1971). An engineering analysis of intratracheal tube cuffs. *Anesthesia and Analgesia, 50*, 557–564.

Metheny, N. A. (2002). Risk factors for aspiration. *Journal of Parenteral and Enteral Nutrition, 26*(Suppl. 6), S26–S33.

Metheny, N. A. (2007, 2011). Preventing aspiration in older adults with dysphagia: Best practices in nursing care to older adults. *ORL-Head and Neck Nursing, 29*, 20–21.

Metheny, N. A., Aud, M. A., & Wunderlich, R. J. (1999). A survey of bedside methods used to detect pulmonary aspiration of enteral formula in intubated tube-fed patients. *American Journal of Critical Care, 8*, 160–169.

Metheny, N. A., Dahms, T. E., Stewart, B. J., Stone, K. S., Edwards, S. J., Defer, J. E., & Clouse, R. E. (2002). Efficacy of dye-stained enteral formula in detecting pulmonary aspiration. *Chest, 121*, 1–6.

Metheny, N. A., Eisenberg, P., & Spies, M. (1986). Aspiration pneumonia in patients fed through nasoenteral tubes. *Heart and Lung, 15*, 256–261.

Metheny, N. P., Mills, A. C., & Stewart, B. J. (2012). Monitoring for intolerance to gastric tube feedings: A national survey. *American Journal Critical Care, 21*, e33–e40.

Minei, J. P., Nathens, A. B., West, M., Harbrecht, B. G., Moore, E. E., Shapiro, M. B., . . . Maier, R. V. (2006). Inflammation and the host response to injury, a large scale collaborative project: Patient-oriented research core—standard operating procedures for clinical care. I. Guidelines for mechanical ventilation of the trauma patient. *Journal of Trauma, (60*(5), 1106–1113.

Munro, C. L., & Grap, M. J. (2004). Oral health and care in the intensive care unit: State of the science. *American Journal of Critical Care, 13*, 65–74.

Niederman, M. S., & Craven, D. E. (2005). Guidelines for the management of adults with hospital acquired ventilator associated and healthcare associated pneumonia. *American Journal of Respiratory Critical Care Medicine, 171*, 388–416.

Sands, J. (1991). Incidence of pulmonary aspiration in intubated patients receiving enteral nutrition through wide- and narrow-bore nasogastric feeding tubes. *Heart and Lung, 20*, 75–80.

Selley, W. G., Ellis, R. E., Flack, F. C., Bayliss, C. R., & Pearce, V. R. (1994). The synchronization of respiration and swallow sounds with videofluoroscopy during swallowing. *Dysphagia, 9*, 162–167.

Sievers, A. E. F. (2010). Caring for the patient with upper airway disorders. In K. S. Osborn, C. E. Wraa, & A. B. Watson (Eds.), *Medical surgical nursing preparation for practice* (Chap. 34). Boston, MA: Pearson.

Sievers, A. R., Leonard, R. J., & McKenzie, S. (1992). The safe use of an adaptive early feeding device for impaired patients. *ORL-Head and Neck Nursing, 10*, 17–19.

Simons, S. R., & Abdallah, L. M. (2012). Bedside assessment of enteral tube placement: Aligning practice with evidence. *American Journal of Nursing, 112*, 40–46.

Splaingard, M. B., Hutchins, L., Sulton, G., & Chaudhuri, G. (1988). Aspiration in rehabilitation patients: videofluoroscopy vs. bedside clinical assessment. *Archives of Physical Medicine and Rehabilitation, 69*, 637–640.

Takahashi, K., Groher, M. E., & Michi, K. (1994a). Methodology for detecting swallowing sounds. *Dysphagia, 9*, 54–62.

Takahashi, K., Groher, M. E., & Michi, K. (1994b). Symmetry and reproducibility of swallowing sounds. *Dysphagia, 9*, 168–173.

Trieger, N. (2004). Oral care in the intensive care unit. *American Journal of Critical Care, 13*, 24–33.

Zenner, P. M., Losinski, D. S., & Mills, R. H. (1995). Using cervical auscultation in the clinical dysphagia examination in long-term care. *Dysphagia, 10*, 27–31.

RECOMMENDED READINGS

Sievers, A. (2008). Dysphagia and swallowing. In L. Harris & M. Huntoon (Eds.), *Core curriculum*. New Smyrna Beach, FL: Society of Otolaryngology-Head and Neck Nurses.

Society of Otorhinolaryngology Head and Neck Nursing Standards of Practice Committee. (1996). *Guidelines for otorhinolaryngology nursing practice*. New Smyrna Beach, FL: Society of Otorhinolaryngology-Head and Neck Nursing.

8

Clinical Swallow Evaluation

Susan J. Goodrich
Alice I. Walker

The "clinical" swallow examination is done, classically, in the "clinic," without medical instrumentation. It involves clinician-driven gathering of information, including a medical and feeding history, clinical examination of oral structures and function, and observational evaluation of patients and their swallowing function.

SWALLOW "SCREEN" VERSUS CLINICAL EVALUATION

"Screening" tests related to dysphagia should be differentiated from standard clinical evaluations. As the term implies, a swallowing "screen" is performed, often at bedside, to determine if a patient is dysphagic and, more particularly, if a patient is aspirating. Primary questions addressed are whether the patient can eat orally, safely, or whether a more comprehensive assessment for dysphagia is indicated. Screens are frequently mandated in hospitals for acute CVA or head injured patients, that is, "at-risk" patient populations. Although

often performed by SLPs, screens may also be undertaken by nursing staff or physicians. A number of screening tools have been described; ones noted here are of interest in that they represent different approaches.

"Water swallow tests," perhaps one of the most frequently used bedside screening approaches, involve giving a patient some amount of water with instruction to drink it as quickly as possible. If coughing or voice change is noted during or after the swallow (assuming the task can be completed), additional monitoring or screening or, possibly, referral for instrumental examination, will be recommended (De Pippo, Holas, Reding, Mandel, & Leser, 1994; Kidd, Lawson, Nesbitt, & MacMahon, 1993; Suiter & Leder, 2008). The Volume-Viscosity Swallow Test (VVST) expands on water swallow tests by requiring the clinician to present 5 to 20-cc amounts of thin-liquid, and pudding-, and nectar-thick materials, respectively, to the patient (Clave, 2008), again monitoring for evidence of aspiration/swallowing difficulty. Other investigators have reported the use of tartaric acid to provoke and assess a patient's cough reflex and laryngeal sensation (Addington, Stephens, & Gilliland, 1999). Martino and colleagues have described both a screening tool and an associated training program for its use (Martino, Silver, Teasell, Bayley, Nicholoson, et al., 2009.) This screen, the Toronto Bedside Swallowing Test (TOR-BSST), incorporates both swallowing tasks and a brief oral-motor assessment in the bedside screen.

Other techniques that are intriguing, but that to date have produced variable and sometimes contradictory results, involve the use of cervical auscultation and pulse oximetry, respectively. The use of cervical auscultation, which involves recording airway or swallowing sounds via stethoscope or perhaps laryngeal microphone, is based on the assumption that sounds associated with impaired swallowing or aspirate in the airway can be uniquely identified (Borr, Hielscher-Fastabend, & Lucking, 2007; Leslie, Finn, Ford, & Wilson, 2004; Zenner, Losinski, & Mills, 1995). Pulse oximetry has been used in an attempt to detect changes in arterial blood oxygenation in response to aspiration, again with mixed results (Colodny, 2000; Zaidi et al., 1995). A recent review of screening tests, however, suggests that a water swallow test combined with pulse oximetry may be of particular value (Rofes, Arreola, Almirall, Cabre, Campins, et al., 2011).

In contrast to "screens," the clinical swallow evaluation consists of a medical and feeding history review, both written (medical records/chart review) and oral (including current method and schedule of feeding), a physical examination of oral-motor anatomy and function, and observation of swallowing. As in any clinical evaluation, the goal is a working hypothesis of the problem. In addition to observations regarding the patient's swallow behaviors, the clinical swallow evaluation should be concerned with the patient's overall health, cognitive status, and physical limitations. It should also assess appropriateness and readiness to undergo more in-depth evaluation, such as endoscopy (Langmore, Schatz, & Olsen, 1988) or fluoroscopy (Logemann, 1983). The information obtained in the clinical evaluation begins the process toward treatment strategy recommendations (Cherney, 1994; Gelb, 1985; Groher, 2009; Steefel, 1981). The remainder of this chapter deals with the comprehensive clinical evaluation.

INDICATIONS

A clinical swallow evaluation is indicated in any patient referred for assessment of a suspected swallowing problem. Referral usually takes place when the patient, the family, caregiver, feeder, and/or the physician express concerns regarding eating or swallowing, when weight loss or nutrition failure occur, and/or when pulmonary history suggests aspiration. Crucial to the assessment process is an understanding of the referral question, so that recommendations may specifically address concerns raised. For example, the question of whether a person may be therapeutically fed small amounts differs greatly from the question of whether a non-oral source of nutrition may be discontinued. Knowing the concerns of the patient, referring health care provider and the caregiver, which may be the same or may differ, will enable the assessor to provide more helpful information.

The clinical swallowing evaluation is a first and critical step toward providing information relevant to both the diagnostic and therapeutic processes. It enables the clinician to describe and elucidate symptomatology, more thoroughly examine the sensory and motor aspects of the oral mechanism, and determine the need and readiness for further diagnostic workup. Clinical assessment of a patient and the patient's presenting complaint is best performed before any diagnostic swallowing procedure, for example, fluoroscopy (dynamic swallow study, or "DSS") or endoscopy ("FEES").

Clinical assessment also allows the examiner to determine optimal timing of further evaluation, if needed. Instrumental exams performed immediately or very soon after a traumatic or crucial event may, of course, produce quite different results from exams performed when the patient's condition is more stable. Careful clinical monitoring of a patient allows for the most efficacious timing of additional exams and, consequently, the most useful information. Indications for clinical exam may also change. For example, if a patient with a diagnosis of head and neck cancer is undergoing radiation therapy, repeat clinical exams may be appropriate at different intervals throughout the therapy, depending on the patient's ongoing swallow function.

LIMITATIONS

The clinical swallowing examination is crucial in any assessment of swallowing function, but it is not all inclusive. It does not allow evaluation of the entire swallowing tract and thus cannot provide complete information regarding oral, pharyngeal, and laryngeal structures and function. Because the pharynx is not visualized, it cannot provide information about timing of the swallow through the pharynx, or pharyngeal strength, or whether residue remains after the swallow. Because the larynx is not visualized, the clinical exam cannot provide definitive information about aspiration (Linden, Kuhlemeier, & Patterson, 1993; Splaingard, Hutchins, Sulton, & Choudhuri, 1988). Clinical evaluation is not intended as a substitute for an instrumental exam; however, it should not be bypassed when DSS or FEES are scheduled, but included as part of the total evaluation. As noted, understanding the patient's history, and careful clinical assessment, combined with the results of any instrumental exams, will facilitate and optimize appropriate treatment decisions.

Limitations of the clinical swallow evaluation may be imposed by other factors. For example, if a patient is for some reason unable to physically cooperate with a full exam, a history may need to be obtained from other sources, for example, chart review, referral source, and a limited physical evaluation performed.

EQUIPMENT

Paper and pencil for recording history and patient information are the foundation of the exam, but most useful are basic supplies such as a small flashlight and a tongue blade. A lateral view diagram of normal anatomy is useful for explaining normal swallowing to the patient. Other supplies may include the following: small laryngeal mirror (for tactile and/or cold stimulation); feeding apparatus such as a spoon and cup, possibly a syringe and catheter, straw, or pipette if observation of other feeding methods is needed; food and liquid such as water, ice chips, thick liquid, puree, cracker, or other similar solid requiring some chewing; emesis basin; washcloth, towel, or paper towels. Suction should be available if problems with airway maintenance needs, for example, tracheotomy tube, are anticipated. Supplies helpful for introducing stimuli without food (and in therapy) include gauze rolls or gauze to wrap around flexible straws, and lemon juice, sugar water, and saline. A "clinical swallowing kit" containing these items may help the clinician be better prepared for the evaluation.

TASKS/EVALUATION

Medical History and Swallowing Complaint

Gathering of a complete and thorough medical and feeding history is critical. Pertinent medical history should be gleaned from the patient's medical chart and gathered by communication with professionals involved in the patient's care, including the referral source. Written medical information may come in the form of the medical chart, progress notes, or referral forms. Sources of information may include the patient, patient's family and medical personnel. A patient's primary diagnosis, general medical status and referral question should be understood and discussed with the patient, the referral source and the patient's physician when necessary and appropriate, as each may have a direct bearing on the reason for referral, decisions regarding further workup, and forthcoming recommendations. The specific concerns of the referrer can then be addressed directly in the assessment report and recommendations. Equally important is the patient's complaint or concerns, as this sometimes differs from the concerns of the referral source. A number of tools have been developed that permit patients to objectively describe their problems, and the impact of swallowing difficulty on their lives (Belafsky, Mouadeb, Rees, Pryor, Postma, & Leonard, 2008; Chen, Frankowski, Bishop-Leone, Hebert, Leyk, Lewin, & Goepfert, 2001).

Gathering of case history should follow the model of the standard history and physical interview, beginning with identifying information and patient complaint. The complaint is then elucidated, citing onset time and type, symptoms, precipitating events, and current manifestations and character (description of the problem[s]). Past medical history should cover multiple systems, including cardiac, pulmonary, gastrointestinal, neurological, otolaryngological, and so forth. Cardiac problems or illnesses of other types should be noted, as their effect on general patient conditioning and fatigue may prove important (Selnes & McKhann, 2005). Airway status should be understood, with consultation with the patient's physician and/or a pulmonologist or otolaryngologist, if warranted. Pulmonary problems should be recorded, including history and types of pneumonia, as well as any disease process that may contribute to pulmonary compromise and reduced tolerance for aspiration. Gastrointestinal information is important, especially a history of gastroesophageal reflux, as problems in this area may directly or indirectly impact laryngeal, pharyngeal, and oral symptoms and problems (Groher, 2009; Koufman, 2002). Neurological problems could impact sensory and/or motor systems for swallowing, and should be documented. Information from otolaryngological, or head and neck, exam, is crucial in understanding known problems of the oral, pharyngeal, and laryngeal anatomy. Report of oral care and dental condition is important, if available (Langmore et al., 1998; Loeb, Becker, Eady, & Walker-Dilks, 2003). If structures of the larynx, including the vocal folds, have been recently evaluated, this information will be important in assessing the patient's airway protection capabilities.

Any other medical problems, hospitalizations, and surgeries should be recorded, including dates of occurrence. Prior voice, speech, or swallowing problems, and intervention given, whether medical, surgical, or radiological, may impact swallowing and thus should be noted. Psychiatric and social history, including independence and availability of support, may impact the diagnostic and/or rehabilitative processes, and should be included, if relevant. A list of medications currently taken is important, as medications may cause xerostomia, drowsiness, or other symptoms relevant to swallowing. Further questions are guided by knowledge of the complaint and history. Information presented in the next few sections represents an abbreviated template of steps and considerations in performing a clinical swallow evaluation.

Swallowing History

Method and Schedule of Feeding or Eating

The current method of nutritional intake is noted, that is, oral with utensils or syringe, or non-oral feeding tubes, such as, nasogastric, gastrostomy, duodenum, or jejunum tubes. Some of these methods may be used in combination, with one supplementing the other (see Chapter 10). Thus, it is important to ask the patient or caregiver which feeding method is used, at what times, and with what substances.

Diet

Note the type, amount, and frequency of food and liquid intake, as well as food preferences. Preferences for certain substances may provide important information about the patient's comfort level managing certain foods. Have the patient's eating habits changed because of his specific complaints? Are particular foods or liquids avoided, or sought? Changes in eating habits over the course of a day should also be documented. For instance, does the patient eat more or less at one time of day than another? Noting time and amount of intake for each type of meal will provide baseline information, and also give clues as to a patient's compensatory strategies for eating. The Functional Oral Intake Scale (FOIS), a seven-point ordinal scale that describes oral intake, may be useful in documenting overall functional change over time (Crary, Carnaby, Mann, & Groher, 2005).

Onset of Problem

The time and date of the onset of swallowing problems, and whether gradual or sudden, should be noted. Were problems concurrent with other medical problems, or did they occur following particular incidents? Were there multiple incidents of problems? Have the problems changed, and in what way, over time?

Description of Problem

Whenever possible, the swallowing problem should be described in detail by the patient. During the interview, it can be important to focus the patient on descriptions of symptoms, rather than the perceived diagnosis. Questions should attempt to elicit symptoms, current manifestations and the character of the swallowing problem.

1. *Context:* When do swallow problems occur? Do they occur at particular times of the day or during particular meals, and when during these meals (beginning, middle, end of meals, or sometime after)? Are these meals at home, outside the home, with others, or when alone? (Are distractions such as talking during swallowing occurring?) Do the same or similar problems occur at other times besides eating?

2. *Cough or choke:* Do coughing and/or choking occur; if so, with what frequency and severity? Is the problem a tickle responded to with a cough or throat clear, or does it produce an uncontrollable cough? Has it interfered with breathing? Do coughing/choking occur during or after swallowing, and/or at other times of the day, for example, when meals are not being taken? Does food "get stuck?" (If so, ask the patient to point to "sticking" point.) Does it eventually go down, or require a liquid wash to clear? Has the patient ever needed the Heimlich maneuver to dislodge material from the airway?

3. *Weight loss:* Has the patient experienced recent weight change, and is it related to a change in eating habits? Note the patient's height and present weight compared to past weight.

4. *Localization and characterization:* Are there any other subjective descriptions of the problem? For example, can the patient point to an area in the mouth, throat, or chest where the problems seem to occur? Does food "pocket" in certain areas? Is there any pain associated with swallowing? Have appetite changes been experienced? Does the patient experience dry mouth?

5. *Social or emotional impact:* How does the patient feel about the swallowing problem? Is it of concern? Have experiences with swallowing been frightening? Does the patient have a certain eating goal? A checklist may also be employed to record the patient's subjective impression of the problem's impact on quality of life. Examples of inventories that provide such information are the M.D. Anderson Dysphagia Inven-

tory (MDADI or ADI) (Chen et al., 2001) and the Eating Assessment Tool (EAT-10) (Belafsky et al., 2008).

Variability

The variable characteristics of the problem should be described, such as:

1. *Foods:* Do problems occur with certain foods or food types (including pills, medications)? Note whether problems occur usually with liquids and/or solids, and the texture and consistency of those foods. This information may be used later in trial swallows. Are some foods easier to swallow than others? More difficult? Are liquids difficult to control? Do particular foods get "stuck"? Are certain liquids or foods avoided due to problems? (Ask about dental care and problems chewing as this is often overlooked as an important factor with solids.)

2. *Temperature:* Is the ease of swallowing affected by the temperature of the food? Are hot or cold foods easier or more difficult to swallow?

3. *Eating time:* How long does it take to eat a meal? Is this usual for the patient? Longer eating times may indicate more problems are occurring during the meal, or that the patient is eating more slowly to compensate for problems. Shorter times may indicate rushed or poor intake, or lack of interest or attention.

4. *Secretions:* How is the patient handling secretions? Are there problems with drooling? Are secretions copious, or conversely, is there a lack of saliva (xerostomia may occur as a consequence of radiation therapy, and dry mouth is a common side effect of some medications.)?

Compensations

What has the patient found helpful in dealing with the swallowing problem? Have any particular strategies been useful in helping the patient compensate? Consider the following:

1. *Rate:* Is the patient altering the rate of eating, slower or faster, to better handle food?

2. *Consistency:* Has the consistency of foods eaten been altered? Are certain foods blended or avoided altogether?

3. *Posture:* Are particular body postures or positions, that is, leaning, tucking the chin, turning the head, helpful to swallowing?

4. *Other:* Have any other tactics proven useful? For example, is food placed in a certain place in the oral cavity to facilitate chewing and/or swallowing? Is a syringe used for food placement, or a straw for drinking? Have the amounts of food attempted on one swallow been altered? Does the patient think coughing or throat-clearing help?

Clinical Examination or Observation

Overall Conditioning, Including Cognition or Alertness/Endurance

The patient's general overall conditioning, level of awareness, alertness, and cooperation should be noted, along with apparent strength and potential for fatigue. Readiness for instrumental studies may also be assessed at this time: A person should be awake, alert, and able to accept food voluntarily.

Body Tone, Size, Posture, or Positioning

The general body tone and specific oral tone are important to note, as well as the patient's typical sitting position during eating, and whether or not postural support is required. For the radiographic study, the patient must be positioned in a reasonably appropriate posture in the radiology suite, so size and upper body postural support needs may be crucial factors. If special chairs, safety straps, or other accommodations are needed for special positioning, these should be considered, especially if further diagnostic testing is necessary.

Airway

Status of the airway should be noted. If the patient is breathing through a tracheostomy tube, the type and status (cuffed or uncuffed) of the tube should be recorded. Note if breathing appears labored or audible in any way before, during, or after the evaluation.

Following Instructions

How well is the patient able to follow directions? Are verbal or gestural cues needed to elicit desired behaviors? Is demonstration needed for imitation? Does a hearing loss or vision problem impact perception, and can compensation be made for this? Is a language translator needed for further assistance for the patient or family?

Self-Feeding Potential

Is the patient able to feed independently, and to what degree? Are special utensils or delivery systems needed?

Direct Physical Evaluation

Oral Phase

1. *Structure:* The jaw, dentition, lips, tongue, buccal cavity, gum, faucal pillars, palate, and velum should all be observed carefully. Tissue condition, including color, configuration, shape, size, symmetry, and any additional findings such as scarring or tethering should be recorded. Observe the presence or absence of tonsil, including size, placement, and condition. Missing teeth, especially molars used in chewing, are important to note.

2. *Sensation:* Sensitivity in and around the oral cavity can be assessed by applying light touch to areas of the lips, tongue, buccal cavity, gums, and so on. Areas of reduced or hypersensitivity should be noted, as well as unilateral differences in responses. This information may have implications for bolus management and trigger of the swallow sequence.

   Note: Facial sensation is controlled by cranial nerve (CN) V (Trigeminal). Sensation for the anterior two thirds of the tongue is provided by the lingual nerve, a branch of CN V. (Taste for the anterior two thirds of the tongue is provided by CN VII [Facial].) Sensation and taste for the posterior one third of the tongue and the pharynx is provided by CN IX (Fuller,

1993). Noting the area of impaired sensation should provide information about particular cranial nerve involvement.

3. *Reflexes and responses/nonvolitional movements:* Assessment of normal oral reflexes in the adult is usually limited to the gag reflex, as other primitive reflexes are usually not present beyond 6 to 8 months of age.

Impairment of reflexes and responses, or presence of primitive or infantile reflexes, such as the bite reflex, may suggest neurological problems (Groher, 2009). Presence or absence of reflexes and responses, and symmetry of movement, are usually noted by tactile stimulation with a tongue blade.

   a. The gag reflex includes a head and jaw extension, rhythmical tongue protrusions, and pharyngeal contractions in response to stimulation at the posterior part of the oral cavity, usually the faucial pillars or base of the tongue.

   b. The transverse tongue response is a lateral movement of the tongue in response to tactile stimulation at the lateral border.

   c. The bite reflex is clamping of the teeth or up and down movement of the jaw in response to stimulation of the gum, molar, or sometimes other dental surfaces.

4. *Volitional movement:* Volitional movements of the oral-motor mechanism should be assessed in terms of strength, rate, accuracy, and range of motion. Again, noting the area of impairment should provide information about particular cranial nerve involvement.

   a. Jaw: Ability to open and close the jaw, relative ease, and amount of movement should be observed. Jaw opening may actually be measured in millimeters to note any significant trismus, and to compare to normative data. Measurements may be compared to normative data to note limitations (interincisal distance in adults should approximate 40 to 50 mm; if below 20 to 25 mm, it may impact introduction of food into oral cavity) (Gelb, 1985). Ask the patient to clench the teeth, while palpating masseter and temporalis muscles for evidence of contractions.

   Note: Muscles of motor control of mastication are controlled by CN V (Trigeminal) (Fuller, 1993).

   b. Lips: Labial closure at rest and during swallowing should be observed to note the patient's ability to maintain lip competence, and to breathe through the nose during eating. Pursing and retraction of the lips should be noted in isolation and in alternating tasks. Note symmetry of smile and showing of teeth.

   Note: Muscles of facial expression are controlled by CN VII (Facial) (Fuller, 1993).

   c. Tongue: Anterior lingual movement may be assessed by having the patient extend, lateralize, elevate, and depress the tip, and by having the patient sweep the tongue from the front to the back of the oral cavity along the roof of the mouth. Note symmetry, strength, range of motion, accuracy of movement, and mark inaccurate, weak movements, or searching behaviors. Posterior lingual movement can be observed by having the patient elevate the back of the tongue, as in producing a /k/ sound. Strength can be assessed by asking the patient to push the tongue against a tongue depressor or into the cheek on both sides. Is the cheek pushed outward by this gesture?

Note: Lingual movement is controlled by CN XII (Hypoglossal) (Fuller, 1993).

d. Velum: Movement of the velum, or soft palate, may be assessed by having the patient open the mouth, and then observing palatal movement during production of a sustained /a/ sound. Amount and vigor of elevation, as well as symmetry, can be noted. Compare to gag movement.

Note: Palatal, pharyngeal, and laryngeal movement are controlled by CN IX (Glossopharyngeal) and CN X (Vagus) (Fuller, 1993).

5. *Oral sensorimotor integrity:* In addition to assessing isolated sensory versus oral-motor skills, the integrity of the two working in concert may be important to explore systematically, as the unique interplay of sensation and movement may have implications for bolus manipulation and the oral stage of swallowing. For example, the light touch sensation of a small bolus may not be enough to allow adequate oral manipulation or to trigger a swallow response. A bolus with greater mass or heavier weight, however,

may stimulate an adequate motor response.

6. *Secretions:* Oral secretions should be observed, including approximate amount and type, and how the patient manages these during the assessment. The patient may be swallowing, or actively or passively expectorating. Inquiry should be made regarding changes in secretion type, amount or management.

7. *Articulation:* Observation of a patient's articulatory behaviors and patterns may offer much information about oral function. For instance, ability to produce an anterior lingua-alveolar stop /t/ may provide information about anterior lingual movement and control, just as production of /k/ may provide information about posterior lingual movement and control. These sounds may be elicited in diadochokinetic tasks to note agility and speed. Articulation in connected speech may give an indication of the timing and precision of movement of articulatory structures.

8. *Resonance:* Observe resonance during speech for problems with oral-nasal coupling. Be alert to problems with velar function that could impact bolus containment and pressure generation.

Pharyngeal and Laryngeal Evaluation

1. *Vocal quality or changes:* Note changes in vocal quality from the norm, such as hoarseness or breathiness. This could possibly indicate a problem with laryngeal anatomy or function, which may relate to problems with closure to protect the airway. If otolaryngology consultation

has not been obtained, problems in this area may indicate a need for such.

2. *Pitch control or range:* The patient should be asked (or this behavior should be elicited through demonstration) to glide up and down his or her pitch range to assess laryngeal agility. This may provide some information about laryngeal control and elevation.

3. *Breathing:* Note any problems with breathing, including stridor or audible breath sounds at rest, which may alert the clinician to respiratory compromise. Note weak vocal intensity or the reported phenomenon of "running out of air" or becoming short of breath, with or without speech.

4. *Volitional cough or throat clear:* Assess the patient's ability to cough or throat-clear on command by simply asking the patient to cough and clear the throat. The behavior may also be demonstrated to obtain an imitative response. Your goal is to assess the ability to volitionally expectorate aspirated material.

5. *Saliva swallow and laryngeal management:* During the clinical examination, before assessing a liquid or food swallow, the examiner should listen carefully to the patient's voice to note any lack of clarity, "wetness," and so on. Note whether the patient coughs or clears the throat during the interview. The patient may be asked to initiate a "dry" swallow of saliva present, and cough and throat-clear, with voice quality noted afterward.

6. *Liquid and/or food swallow:* Liquid and/or food swallow during clinical evaluation should only be at-tempted under safe circumstances. Ideally, suction should be available in case problems are encountered with either aspiration or food retrieval. A small bolus can be given to determine management, ability to swallow, and clinical signs of aspiration. However, the patient should not be given any substance that may compromise his or her health. First, note the patient's ability to contain the bolus within the oral cavity. Oral manipulation of the bolus is better observed with purees or solids. Timing and effortfulness of the swallow may be grossly observed, as well as the presence or absence of cough or throat-clear following the attempt. The patient's voice should then be attended to for lack of clarity, "wetness," and so on.

Example form for clinical evaluation is included in Appendix 8–A at the end of this chapter.

IMPRESSIONS AND RECOMMENDATIONS

A summary of the clinical findings should contain information relevant to the swallowing problem and provide an impression of factors that may impact and, in fact, dictate further intervention. If the clinical assessment reveals only oral problems or cognitive/behavioral problems, recommendations and therapy usually can be planned without further studies. Even a cursory clinical and history is necessary to pair with the FEES information in order to address the specific dysphagia question at hand.

If there are indications of problems at the pharyngeal or laryngeal stages of swallowing, further studies may be recommended, for example, a dynamic swallowing study or FEES may be indicated to assess function as well as provide information about the safety of continuing oral feeding and/or to determine more specific techniques to manage the swallowing problem. Most obviously, if a person demonstrates coughing or choking during eating, further studies of the swallowing mechanism would be indicated. If inability to maintain nutrition or hydration by mouth has resulted in weight loss or compromised health, further studies may be warranted. If pulmonary health has suffered, imaging of the swallow may provide illumination. And if known problems exist, imaging or direct visualization may guide the development of strategies to improve swallow safety and/or efficiency.

The specific findings of the clinical evaluation will facilitate procedural considerations during the imaging studies. If a patient has posturing or movement limitations, mechanical adjustments may be anticipated and changed. If certain substances are tolerated differently during swallow, by observation or report, they may be used following administration of the standard protocol.

The clinical swallow evaluation may also provide baseline information about swallowing function, making it easier to track and compare a patient's swallowing ability over time. If the patient is not ready for a further workup initially, some aspects of the evaluation may be repeated over time to determine readiness for further workup at a later date.

In summary and reiteration, the clinical swallowing evaluation is a first and crucial step toward providing critical information relevant to both the diagnostic and therapeutic processes. It describes and elucidates symptomatology and the dysphagia question, more thoroughly examines the sensory and motor aspects of the oral mechanism, begins the process toward strategies and intervention and helps determine the need and readiness for further diagnostic workup.

STUDY QUESTIONS

1. What is the likely difference between a "bedside" and "clinical" evaluation?
2. Why are history and physical evaluations considered necessary before further imaging studies, such as videofluroscopic evaluation?
3. What are some reasons you may not recommend further studies after your clinical evaluation?
4. What are the clinical signs and symptoms of silent aspiration?
5. What are the symptoms of left cranial nerve XII damage and what oral problems would you expect to find during your evaluation?
6. Describe the clinical impact of xerostomia, that is, what might be the effect on eating and swallowing?

REFERENCES

Addington, W. R., Stephens, R. E., & Gilliland, K. A. (1999). Assessing the laryngeal cough reflex and the risk of pneumonia after stroke: An interhospital comparison. *Stroke, 6,* 1203–1217.

Belafsky, P. C., Mouadeb, D. A., Rees, C. J., Pryor, J. S., Postma, G. N., & Leonard, R. J. (2008). The validity and reliability of the eating assessment tool (EAT-10). *Annals of Otology, Rhinology, and Laryngology, 117*, 919–924.

Borr, C., Hielscher-Fastabend, M., & Lücking, A. (2007). Reliability and validity of cervical auscultation. *Dysphagia, 22*, 225–234.

Chen, A. Y., Frankowski, R., Bishop-Leone, J., Hebert, T., Leyk, S., Lewin, J., & Goepfert, H. (2001). The development and validation of a dysphagia-specific quality-of-life questionnaire for patients with head and neck cancer. *Archives of Otolaryngology-Head and Neck Surgery, 127*(7), 870–876.

Cherney, L. R. (1994). *Clinical management of dysphagia in adults and children*. Gaithersberg, MD: Aspen.

Clavé, P., Arreola,V., Romea, M., Medina, L., Palomera, E., & Serra-Prat, M. (2008). Accuracy of the volume-viscosity swallow test for clinical screening of oropharyngeal dysphagia and aspiration. *Clinical Nutrition, 27*, 806–815.

Colodny, N. (2000). Comparison of dysphagics and nondysphagics on pulse oximetry during oral feeding. *Dysphagia, 15*, 68–73.

Crary, M. A., Carnaby Mann, G. D., & Groher, M. E. (2005). Initial psychometric assessment of a functional oral intake scale for dysphagia in stroke patients. *Archives of Physical Medicine Rehabilitation, 86*, 1516–1520.

DePippo, K. L., Holas, M. A., Reding, M. J., Mandel, F. S., & Lesser, M. S. (1994). Dysphagia therapy following stroke: A controlled trial. *Neurology, 44*, 1655–1660.

Fuller, G. (1993). *Neurological examination made easy*. New York, NY: Churchill Livingstone.

Gelb, H. (1985). Patient evaluation. In H. Gelb (Ed.), *Clinical management of head, neck and TMJ pain and dysfunction* (Chap. 3). Philadelphia, PA: W. B. Saunders.

Groher, M. E., & Crary, M. A. (2009). *Dysphagia: Clinical management in adults and children*. Maryland Heights, MO: Mosby.

Kidd, D., Lawson, J., Nesbitt, R., & MacMahon, J. (1993). Aspiration in acute stroke: A clinical study with videofluoroscopy. *QJM: An International Journal of Medicine, 86*, 825–829.

Koufman, J. A. (2002). Laryngopharyngeal reflux is different from classic gastroesophageal reflux disease. *Ear Nose and Throat Journal, 81*(9 Suppl. 2), 7.

Langmore, S., Schatz, K., & Olsen, N. (1988) Fibreoptic endoscopic examination of swallowing safety: A new procedure. *Dysphagia, 2*, 216–219.

Langmore, S. E., Terpenning, M. S., Schork, A., Chen, Y., Murray, J. T., Lopatin, D., & Loesche, W. J. (1998). Predictors of aspiration pneumonia: How important is dysphagia? *Dysphagia, 13*, 69–81.

Leslie, P., Drinnan, M. J., Finn, P., Ford, G. A., & Wilson, J. A. (2004). Reliability and validity of cervical auscultation: A controlled comparison using fluoroscopy. *Dysphagia, 19*, 231–240.

Linden, P., Kuhlemeier, K. V., & Patterson, C. (1993). The probability of correctly predicting subglottic penetration from clinical observations. *Dysphagia, 8*, 170–179.

Loeb, M. B., Becker, M., Eady, A., & Walker-Dilks, C. (2003). Interventions to prevent aspiration pneumonia in older adults: A systematic review. *Journal of the American Geriatric Society, 51*, 1018–1022.

Logemann, J. A. (1983). *Evaluation and treatment of swallowing disorders*. Boston, MA: College-Hill.

Martino, R., Silver, F., Teasell, R., Bayley, M., Nicholson, G., Streiner, D. L., & Diamant, N. E. (2009). The Toronto bedside swallowing screening test (TOR-BSST): Development and validation of a dysphagia screening tool for patients with stroke. *Stroke, 40*, 555–561.

Rofes, L., Arreola, V., Almirall, J., Cabré, M., Campins, L., García-Peris, P., . . . Clave, P. (2011). Diagnosis and management of oropharyngeal dysphagia and its nutritional and respiratory complications in the elderly. *Gastroenterology Research and Practice*. Epub, 2010, Aug. 3.

Selnes, O. A., & McKhann, G. M. (2005). Neurocognitive complications after coronary artery bypass surgery. *Annals of Neurology, 57,* 615–621.

Splaingard, M. L., Hutchins, B., Sulton, L. D., & Chaudhuri, G. (1988). Aspiration in rehabilitation patients: Videofluoroscopy vs. bedside clinical assessment. *Archives of Physical Medicine and Rehabilitation, 69,* 637–640.

Steefel, J. S. (1981). *Dysphagia rehabilitation for adults.* Springfield, IL: Charles C. Thomas.

Suiter, D. M., & Leder, S. B. (2008). Clinical utility of the 3-oz water swallow test. *Dysphagia.* Epub, 2007, Dec. 4.

Zaidi , N. H., Smith, H. A., King, S. C., Park, C., O'Neill, P. A., & Connolly, M. J. (2004). Oxygen desaturation on swallowing as a potential marker of aspiration in acute stroke. *Age Ageing, 24,* 267–270.

Zenner, P. M., Losinski, D. S., & Mills, R. H. (1995). Using cervical auscultation in the clinical dysphagia examination in long-term care. *Dysphagia, 10,* 27–31.

Clinical Swallow Evaluation Form

UNIVERSITY OF CALIFORNIA, DAVIS MEDICAL CENTER
SACRAMENTO, CALIFORNIA

OPD PROGRESS RECORD

VOICE, SPEECH AND SWALLOWING CENTER   **OTOLARYNGOLOGY CLINIC**

PT. NAME: **UCD ID#:**

BIRTHDATE: **DATE OF VISIT:**

Diagnosis: **Referral:**

Concern on referral:

Related Medical Hx/results of testing:
Cardiac:
GI:
Pulmonary:
Neurological:
ENT:
Other:
Dental:
Medications:
Speech/Voice:
Services:
Social/Family:

Feeding Hx:
Method:
Schedule:
Onset:
Variability: secretions: foods:
                        temperature: time of day/meal:
Cough/choke: context: frequency/severity:
Compensations: rate:
                        consistencies (prep, alternate, avoid):
                        posture:
Weight: present: usual: time/loss:

Clinical Observations:
Airway: trach: cuffed/uncuffed:
                        voluntary cough: breath-hold:

continues

127

continued

	labial	lingual	palatal	mandibular	dental
Oral exam: structure:					
tone:					
movement:					
sense:					
reflexes:					
secretions:					

Speech: articulation:

voice: resonance:

intelligibility:

Swallow:	substance/delivery system	cough/choke	voice	other
liquid:				
puree/pudding:				
cracker/solid:				

9

Pediatric Clinical Feeding Assessment

Janet Pitcher
Margie Crandall
Susan J. Goodrich

Pediatric feeding problems have been recognized in the literature for the past 35 to 40 years (Illingworth, 1969; Logan & Bosma, 1967). Although no comprehensive definition of pediatric feeding problems has been widely accepted, infants and children experiencing feeding difficulties may demonstrate a refusal to eat orally, have difficulty with the act of feeding, or be unable to sustain oral feedings to maintain adequate caloric intake. Feeding problems have been defined by both etiology and function, including categories of food refusal, food selectivity by type or texture, oral-motor delays, or dysphagia (Babbit, Hoch, & Coe, 1994; Field, Garland, & Williams, 2003). In fact, some authors have proposed, and more studies are indicating, that most feeding problems have underlying organic causes (Manikam & Perman, 2000).

Clinically, the health care provider may note that the infant/child is failing to thrive, has impaired oral feeding skills, is potentially aspirating, and/or has difficulty transitioning from enteral to oral feedings. Despite the lack of a universally accepted definition of pediatric feeding problems, numerous articles have identified groups of children who are at risk for feeding problems (Arvedson & Brodsky, 1994; Bier, Ferguson, Cho, Oh, & Vohr, 1993; Case-Smith, Cooper, & Scala, 1989; Herbst, 1981; Imhoff & Wigginton, 1991; Luiselli, 1994; Mercado-Deane et al., 2001; Morris & Klein, 2000; Mueller, 1972; Palmer, Crawley, & Blanco, 1993; Reilly & Skuse, 1992; Reilly, Skuse, Mathisen, & Dieter, 1995; Samour & King, 2005; Stevenson & Allaire, 1991).

Although etiologies of pediatric feeding problems are not a specific focus of this chapter, it is essential that any physical reason for feeding problems be addressed prior to or in conjunction with any behavioral therapeutic intervention. These may include neurological or gastroenterological diseases or dysfunction, structural anomalies, and cardiac compromise (Imhoff & Wiggington, 1991). Table 9–1 lists commonly associated etiologies.

Feeding difficulties can be a problem in infants with gastroesophageal reflux (GER) (Falconer, 2010). Hymen (1994), in addition to offering GER as " . . . one reason why baby won't eat," also suggests a possible contributing mechanism is visceral hyperalgesia, "a neuropathic condition in which prior experience changes sensory nerves so that previously innocuous stimuli are perceived as painful." Thus, children may perceive feeding and swallowing as painful in the absence of tissue damage.

A more recent addition to medical knowledge found to be a factor in some pediatric feeding disorders is the existence of an inflammatory disease found in the digestive tract on biopsy, known

Table 9–1. Common Etiologies Associated with Feeding Problems

- Neurological dysfunction
- Gastrointestinal diseases/dysfunction
- Cardio-respiratory compromise
- Sensory deprivation
- Structural anomalies
- Social-behavioral maladaptation

Source: Adapted from "Identifying feeding and swallowing in infants and young children." By S. Imhoff and V. Wigginton, 1991, *Clinical Communication Disorders, 1,* 59–67.

as eosinophilic esophagitis (EoE). Food allergy is an associated finding in most patients (Orenstein et.al., 2001). EoE has been confused with, but now begun to be distinguished from, esophageal inflammation due to gastroesophageal reflux (Orenstein et al., 2001), which may also contribute to feeding problems (Hyman, 1994). In a large review of upper endoscopies of 743 patients less than 21 years of age, Sorser and colleagues (in press) recently found that 44, or 5.8% showed significant EoE.

Recent studies have found EoE to manifest itself, or present differently, in different patient populations (Ferreira et al., 2008; Levine et al., 2012; Orenstein et al., 2001; Rodrigues et al., 2001; Sorser et al., in press). In Orenstein et al.'s (2001) review, children presenting with vomiting and feeding disorders were younger, and children presenting with heartburn and dysphagia, older. Rodrigues and colleagues (2001) found clinical expression to be in feeding disorders and vomiting or abdominal pain in children, dysphagia and esophageal food impaction in teenagers and adults. Ferriera et al. (2008) found children less than four years of age presented with feeding disorder and failure-to-thrive, children ages 5 to 8 years with abdominal pain and symptoms associated with reflux (heartburn and/or vomiting), and children over 8 years with abdominal pain, dysphagia, and occasional food impaction. The possibility of EoE presenting as a pediatric feeding problem thus suggests this be included in a possible diagnostic differential, and prompts clinical assessment to include questions regarding food allergies.

Treatment for EoE at this time consists of dietary management and anti-inflammatory pharmacotherapy (Ferreira et al., 2008; Levine et al., 2012; Orenstein et al., 2001; Rodrigues et al., 2001). Orenstein and colleagues (2001) suggest proton-pump inhibitor (PPI) treatment may be useful in maintenance control of symptoms despite persistent eosinophilic inflammation found on esophageal biopsy. Levine and others (2012) suggest a diagnosis of EoE be considered when symptoms of gastroesophageal reflux do not respond to conventional treatment. Medical management would be in the purview of the treating physician, but in the case of EoE, as well as other medical problems such as gastroesophageal reflux, the pediatric feeding clinician may play a role in differential diagnostic assessment and referral to appropriate specialists, as well as managing feeding behaviors related to the medical diagnosis.

More information is now available to provide a basis for assessing feeding problems in children (Arvedson & Brodsky, 1994; Einarsson-Backes, Deitz, Price, Glass, & Hays, 1994; Field et al., 1982; Frappier, Marino, & Shishmanian, 1987; Gisel, 1994; Herbst, 1981; Imhoff & Wigginton, 1991; Measel & Anderson, 1979; Meier & Anderson, 1987; Mueller, 1972; Palmer, Crawley, & Blanco, 1993; Reilly & Skuse, 1992; Reilly et al., 1995; Rogers & Arvedson, 2005; Skuse, Stevenson, Reilly, App, & Mathisen, 1995; Stevenson & Allaire, 1991). Evidence suggests that inadequate nutritional intake is associated with behavioral, developmental, and cognitive impairments (Luiselli, 1994; Oates, Peacock, & Forrest, 1985; Sanders, Patel, LeGrice, & Shepherd, 1993; Singer & Fagan, 1984), and that critical, sensitive periods of feeding development may be influenced by delay of oral feeding or stimu-

lation (Beratis, Kolb, Sperling, & Stein, 1981; Illingworth & Lister, 1964). Therefore, a feeding assessment that provides a framework for early intervention is critical when there is a question whether a child has feeding difficulties.

A clinical feeding assessment is a comprehensive, systematic biopsychosocial approach to the evaluation of a child with feeding difficulties. The assessment can help professionals identify potential or actual feeding problems, including possible etiologies, and develop appropriate interventions. The diagnostic use and value of instrumental procedures including the dynamic swallow study in infants and children is not discussed here (see Chapter 14), but may complement the clinical feeding assessment presented.

A comprehensive feeding assessment includes the medical history, feeding history, developmental history, anatomy and physiology, diet, and psychosocial environment, including a caregiver interview. Assessment involves not only review of a patient's medical chart and direct patient examination, as in the adult patient, but should include a review of the child's educational and therapeutic records. Additionally, in this population, one must consider the complex nature of parent-child interactions and their influence on feeding and swallowing behaviors.

The pediatric feeding assessment is best approached by a multidisciplinary team (Manikam & Perman, 2000). Team members may include the following: physicians, including specialty physicians such as pediatric otolaryngologists, pediatric gastroenterologists, developmental pediatricians, pediatric neurologists, pediatric pulmonologists, pediatric radiologists if radiographic testing is included in the assessment, and pediatric psychiatrists; nurses, including clinical nurse specialists in feeding, neurology, gastroenterology, pulmonology, and so forth; speech pathologists and occupational therapists with specialties in dysphagia; nutritionist/dieticians; behavioral psychologists; and social workers.

PEDIATRIC FEEDING ASSESSMENT

The feeding assessment consists of five parts:

1. Data Collection (obtained before evaluating the child)
2. Nutritional Screening, Feeding History, and Developmental Milestones (obtained from parent or caregiver interview)
3. Physical Assessment
4. Oral Sensory-Motor and Feeding Skills Assessment
5. Psychosocial Interactional Assessment.

Data Collection

Data collection is done before the evaluation of the child. Data collection includes a review of the infant or child's:

■ Medical history
■ Growth chart
■ Current clinical nutritional status.

Medical History

The medical history review includes evaluating the perinatal and neonatal history, medical diagnosis, previous hospitalizations, and significant ill-

nesses, focusing on organic precursors or causes of feeding problems. The perinatal and neonatal history may provide information detailing any fetal distress, the infant's response during delivery, prematurity, any significant congenital anomalies, and any major illness during the first few months of life. Congenital anomalies, central nervous system insults, or chronic illnesses may affect the child's ability to eat orally. For example, respiratory problems may make it difficult for the infant to breathe comfortably during feeding, cardiac problems may contribute to fatigue during feeding sessions, and/or gastroesophageal reflux may cause association of feeding with discomfort. Neurological problems may prevent the development of normal oral-motor skills as well as interfere with the pharyngeal swallow. Previous hospitalizations and significant illnesses can influence or disrupt the child's developmental skills, including feeding skills. As stated earlier, all or any of these findings can be associated with the infant or child's refusal to eat, oral-motor organization, and/or ability to sustain adequate oral intake. All should be noted when taking a medical history, as well as current health status and medications taken.

Growth Chart

It is critical to review the growth chart to determine the child's nutritional status. Prolonged inadequate caloric intake results in an infant or child nutritionally failing to thrive. A child is defined as having failure to thrive when: (1) the weight-to-length ratio is <5% for age and gender, or body mass index (BMI) for children beginning at age 2 years, (2) the weight is <5% for age and gender, or (3) the weight percentage has decreased two standard deviations or more below the norm. In the United States, growth charts were developed by the National Center for Health Statistics in collaboration with the Centers for Disease Control, based on data from national probability samples. The 2000 CDC growth charts represent the revised version of the 1977 NCHS growth charts. These growth charts now have body mass index for-age charts. They are available through the CDC at http://www.cdc.gov/growthcharts. However, other growth charts for some specific patient populations, such as Down syndrome and premature infants, are available. Examples of growth charts are provided in Appendix 9, A through F.

The causes of failure to thrive may be organic (physical cause), nonorganic (psychosocial), or a combination of both. However, not all growth patterns are strictly related to nutrition. The child's medical condition may influence individual patterns of growth. For example, genetic or intrauterine insults (i.e., fetal alcohol syndrome) may result in growth retardation, with the infant's weight, height, weight for height ratio, and head circumference being less than the fifth percentile for age and gender.

Current Clinical Nutritional Status

A review of the current clinical nutritional status should include laboratory tests and possibly anthropometrics. Laboratory tests can help define nutritional deficiencies. The most readily available screening tests are the complete blood count and a chemistry panel. A complete blood count may reveal concerns such as iron-deficiency anemia or altered immune status. The chemistry panel may reveal electrolyte abnormalities (i.e., sodium and chloride) and protein deficiency (i.e., a low albumin and total protein). Anthropometrics measures triceps skinfold thickness and mid-arm circumference as a serial indicator of body fat and muscle mass (American Academy of Pediatrics, 1985). Anthropometrics may be a preferred measurement of nutritional status compared to growth charts when the infant or child's age is unclear.

NUTRITIONAL SCREENING, FEEDING HISTORY, AND DEVELOPMENTAL MILESTONES

This information is usually elicited from the parent or caregiver. Feeding history should include past methods and patterns of feeding from birth onward, including transitions to new foods/textures. It is useful to know when the feeding problem began, what medical and social circumstances existed at the time, and the course of progression. The current feeding status needs to include the parent's perception of the feeding problem or difficulty and a thorough description of the child's mealtimes, including the method and schedule of feeding. Information gathered should include type of food, amounts, textures, temperatures, duration of feeding, physical environment including seating and posture, family members usually present, the child's behavior, and any interventions attempted. A 24-hour dietary recall of the child's feeding routine and schedule is helpful to assess individual nutritional patterns. A review of the child's developmental progress with the parent or caregiver helps them to understand what general skills the child has that relate to the child's ability to eat. Normal feeding skills will be discussed later under oral sensory-motor and feeding skills.

PHYSICAL ASSESSMENT

An assessment of the child's general physical appearance and findings will provide information about the child's nutritional status. When performing this assessment, one must consider the infant or child's:

- Behavior
- Development
- Physical appearance.

Behavior

When observing the behavioral state, observe how the child acts. Is the child alert, active, irritable, or apathetic? The alert and rested child provides the most realistic information about feeding behaviors. Irritability and apathy are commonly seen with malnutrition.

Observe also the child's apparent response to food presentation and attitude toward eating: is the child hungry, cautious, anxious, relaxed? Is this behavior in direct response to food presentation or to any other stimulus during the feeding?

Development

The developmental assessment involves observing the child's fine and gross motor skills and muscle tone. Is the

child performing tasks at the expected age, or is the child showing some developmental delays? Many children who are developmentally delayed exhibit some alteration in muscle tone, either hypertonia, hypotonia, or mixed tone. Both the child's motor skills and muscle tone influence his or her ability to eat.

Physical Appearance

The physical appearance involves assessing the child's:

- Skin
- Hair
- Eyes
- Mouth and oral cavity.

Skin. First, check the skin for color, bruises, rashes, and turgor. A pale color may indicate iron-deficiency anemia. Bruising may be due to vitamin K deficiency. Essential fatty acids, zinc, or vitamin deficiencies are known to cause skin rashes. When inadequate fluid intake accompanies poor caloric intake, the skin will be dry. Loose skin covering the decreased subcutaneous fat indicates both a calorie and protein inadequacy (marasmus). Excessive fluid retention resulting in edema may be due to insufficient protein intake (kwashiorkor) or electrolyte imbalances.

Hair. Check hair for texture, color, and distribution. Hair that is brittle, pale blond colored, and sparsely distributed is seen with protein malnutrition.

Eyes. Check eyes for hydration status and infection. Xerophthalmia, or dryness, may be due to vitamin A deficiency. Malnutrition can affect the immune system and cause conjunctivitis (Kleiman & Warman, 1994).

Mouth and Oral Cavity. The physical appearance of the mouth and oral cavity portion are checked as part of the oral reflexes and feeding skills evaluation, which is discussed next. Incorporating this aspect of the physical assessment with the evaluation of oral reflexes and feeding skills will diminish additional infant stress and crying associated with oral inspection.

ORAL SENSORY-MOTOR AND FEEDING SKILLS ASSESSMENT

The infant or child's oral sensory-motor and feeding skills determine the types of foods safely handled. During the first 3 years of life, dramatic oral-motor and developmental feeding skill changes have profound effects on the types of food, textures, and feeding methods the infant or child can safely control. Table 9–2 details pediatric feeding skills development.

The approach recommended for assessing oral sensory-motor and feeding skills is to progress from the least frightening or threatening (external touching of the face and mouth) to the most threatening (internal inspection of the mouth).

Some oral reflexes are common to all ages, but the most rapid oral reflex and feeding skill changes occur in infancy. Therefore, the oral reflexes and feeding skills assessments will be divided into three infant developmental stages covering the first year of life:

- Birth to 4 months
- 5 to 7 months
- 8 to 12 months.

It is important to note that, although infants are referred to in this section, the clinician may find similar primitive reflexes still present in an older child with neurological deficits. Reflexes that are common to all age groups will be explained once, during the assessment of the oral reflexes and feeding skills of the infant from birth to 4 months.

Birth to 4 Months

Developmental feeding skills are affected by the infant's gestational age. For example, preterm infants frequently demonstrate generalized hypotonia and immature development of their suck/swallow/breathing, thus affecting their feeding efficiency. However, somewhere around 33 to 34 weeks gestation, the healthy growing premature infant's oral-motor maturation allows for suck/swallow/breathing coordination and the introduction of oral feedings (Casaer, Delieger, Decock, & Eggermont, 1982; Wolff, 1968). (See Table 9–2, Pediatric Feeding Skills Development; Preterm Infant.)

For term infants and premature infants whose postnatal age is corrected considering their prematurity the following reflexes and responses exist:

- Rooting reflex
- Suck reflex
- Bite reflex
- Gag reflex
- Tongue protrusion reflex
- Swallow reflex
- Lip and jaw closure
- Tongue mobility.

Table 9–2. Pediatric Feeding Skills Development

Age	Positional Stability	Reflexes	Feeding Skills	Types of Food
Preterm infants (34 to 36 wks)	Lower tone More extension Reduced buccal pads Reduced cup shape of tongue	Gag reflex develops usually around 32 weeks gestation Suck reflex functionally mature at 32 to 34 weeks Rooting reflex elicited at 32 weeks	Coordinated suck/swallow/breathing at 34 to 37 weeks Feeding readiness: gags with gavage tube insertion, competently swallows oral secretions, demonstrates rhythmic nonnutritive suck	Breast milk or formula
Newborn to 3 months (full-term)	Buccal pads present Lip closure Cup-shaped tongue facilitates transfer of liquid to pharynx Oral and pharyngeal structural mobility support both respiration and feeding Limited neck stability	Gag reflex Rooting reflex Tongue protrusion reflex Biting reflex Suck/swallow reflex	Rhythmic sucking pattern (average 1 suck burst/second for nutritive sucking, 2 sucks/sec for nonnutritive suck) Oral-pharyngeal area is shared for feeding and breathing Hand to mouth activity Hand reaching toward bottle	Breast milk or formula
4 to 6 months	Increasing stability of neck and shoulders Lower lip positions around spoon Tongue fills less space in oral cavity allowing for greater mobility and posterior positional shift	Transitional period—primitive reflexes are disappearing except for gag reflex	Beginning of up-and-down chewing (munching) Lateral tongue movement Lip closure around spoon begins Both hands to hold bottle Cup drinking introduced	Breast milk or formula May begin to introduce solid foods with spoon

Age	Positional Stability	Reflexes	Feeding Skills	Types of Food
7 to 9 months	Teeth eruption (central and lateral incisors) Upper lip more mobility to stabilize spoon feeding	Gag reflex similar to adult	More mature lip movement, mobility, and stabilization Tongue lateralization present Rotary (diagonal) chewing begins Assisting with spoon Beginning to drink from cup held by caregiver	Breast milk or formula Finger foods Crackers, toast Soft fruits and vegetables Strained foods
10 to 12 months	Molar eruption Corners of lips and cheek are drawn inward during chewing. The cheeks are used to control and move food	Gag reflex	Continued maturation of feeding skills Holding bottle or cup Liquid loss from mouth with cup drinking may be noted Pincer grasp Self-feeding by grasping spoon with whole hand Holds cup with two hands Has 4 to 5 consecutive swallows	Breast milk or formula Soft table foods
13 to 18 months	External jaw stabilization begins Full eruption of incisors and molars increases the vertical diameter of oral cavity	Gag reflex	Up-and-down jaw movement stops Rotary chewing becomes more mature Increasing control of liquid during cup drinking Bites down on rim of cup	Whole cow's milk Solid foods Chopped foods

continues

Table 9–2. *continued*

Age	Positional Stability	Reflexes	Feeding Skills	Types of Food
13 to 18 months *continued*			Uses long sequence of drinking at one time Begins to develop controlled bite Chews with lips closed	
19 to 24 months		Gag reflex	No longer uses bite to stabilize cup for cup drinking Child cleans lip with tongue May begin to transfer food from one side of mouth to other side Rotary chewing is mature Begin to suck with a straw Skills are refined for independent feeding	Chopped, fine food to regular Firmer meats for chewing can be introduced
25 to 36 months	Anatomic changes continue to place demands on oral sensorymotor agility, and adaptation: continued eruption of molars, inferior-anterior growth of the mandible, and descent of the hyoid and larynx with the hypopharynx. Changes continue through puberty.	Gag reflex is elicited from the posterior third of the tongue (as in adults) and by adulthood can be under some voluntary control.	Skills continue refinement (child develops finer control) as sensory-motor experience continues to shape central representation of feeding. Speech skills and head/neck postural stability develop in parallel with feeding maturation. Electromyography suggests mastication coordination is fully mature at 3 to 6 years.	Regular table food. Concerns re judgment and distractibility may limit foods offered.

When assessing these movements, start with the rooting reflex. Elicit the reflex by gently stroking the infant's cheek. The infant will turn his or her head toward the touch with mouth open. The rooting reflex disappears between 3 and 5 months.

The suck reflex is easily assessed following the rooting reflex. Alert the infant to your finger insertion by progressive touch from cheek to lip, then into the mouth. Gently insert finger with pad side up toward the hard palate. During the sucking reflex, the tongue extends over the gums or lip, with a motion moving from tongue tip to the back of the tongue. A pulling pressure is felt with the inserted finger being pulled to feel the soft palate. The sucking reflex disappears at approximately 6 months.

When assessing the rooting or suck reflexes, oral hypersensitivity may be noted. For example, the infant may demonstrate agitation, facial grimace, arching, and gagging even with gentle touching of the face. Oral hypersensitivity is defined as an aversion to touch or to eating food by mouth and/or food refusal of certain food types or textures. It may occur in children who have experienced prolonged periods of restricted eating or drinking, children who have experienced discomfort associated with feeding or even medical intervention, or children who have impaired oral sensory-motor feeding skills.

When assessing the mouth and oral cavity look at the structure and movement of the mouth and oral cavity, including:

- Gum and mucous membranes
- Palate
- Dentition

- Airway status, including jaw size and presence of tonsils
- Tongue.

The gums are checked for hyperplasia (i.e., excessive growth of gum tissue) because of possible side effects of anti-convulsants. Both the gums and mucous membranes are observed for bleeding, sores, and hydration status. The palate is checked for architecture and cleft deformities. If teeth are present, they should be observed for number, caries, grinding, and occlusion. During the oral assessment, the bite reflex is assessed. The bite reflex is demonstrated during infancy by an up-and-down movement of the jaw. Pressure on the anterior and lateral aspects of the gums elicits this response. It usually disappears between 3 and 5 months.

Next assess the gag reflex. The gag reflex is present at birth and throughout our lives. It is elicited by placing a tongue blade on the anterior one third of the tongue and gently "walking back" until the tongue "humps" or elevates. This is one of the signs indicating the child can protect the airway during swallowing. An absent or diminished gag reflex may lead to aspiration. At this point, it is usually necessary to soothe and quiet the infant before proceeding.

Once the infant is quiet, assess the protrusion reflex. The tongue protrusion reflex is present during the first 4 months. This immature tongue movement pushes solid food out of the mouth when it is placed on the anterior part of the tongue. It can be assessed by placing a small quantity of food on the tongue and observing the tongue movement. The tongue protrusion reflex is one of the reasons why infants should not be fed solid foods for the first 4 to 6 months of life.

The swallow reflex can be observed or felt by the upward and forward movement of the cricoid cartilage during the introduction of liquids or solids. Listen for sound change including "wet"-sounding breathing or voice, as well as cough/choke. Coughing or choking may occur with an inadequate swallow, but is not always present during a clinical exam, even if the pharyngeal swallow is incompetent. If an incompetent pharyngeal swallow is suspected, or the child is at risk for pulmonary compromise, pharyngeal imaging may need to be considered (see criteria for Dynamic Swallow Study [Chapters 14–17]).

Lip and jaw closure and tongue mobility are necessary for eating and swallowing. They can be assessed when observing a feeding or with infants when assessing the suck. Inadequate lip or jaw closure makes eating and swallowing difficult because of an inability to create adequate seal around the bottle, resulting in insufficient negative intraoral pressures. Impaired tongue mobility affects both intraoral pressure and oral transfer of a food bolus before swallow.

5 to 7 Months

This is a transitional time for the maturing infant. The infant is:

- Losing the primitive reflexes for rooting, sucking, biting, and tongue protrusion
- Gaining voluntary oral control by alerting with mouth opening at the sight of food, elevating the tongue, and beginning to manipulate food orally
- Starting to initiate self-feeding behaviors.

Again assess the structure and movement of the mouth and oral cavity, including:

- Rooting reflex (disappearing at age 3–5 months)
- Suck reflex (disappearing at approximately age 6 months)
- Tongue movements (protrusion reflex disappearing at age 4 months)
- Bite reflex (disappearing at 3–5 months)
- Gag reflex (lifelong).

Besides assessing for previous physical findings, whenever possible, observe for maturing tongue movements. They include tongue elevation (tongue pushes back and touches palate) and lateral (side to side) movements.

To assess voluntary oral control, offer solid pureed food. When the food is first offered, voluntary alerting and mouth opening to accept food are seen in an infant at this stage. The infant may become very active and excited at the sight of food. It may be important to schedule the feeding assessment near or at a regularly scheduled mealtime to assess the infant's genuine response to food at a time normally fed.

If tongue elevation is not noted during the oral assessment, it can be assessed by offering food with a spoon. Tongue elevation clears food from the roof of the mouth and is necessary for the infant to eat and swallow pureed foods. Tongue elevation will be seen when the infant loses the protrusion reflex and gains the ability to manipulate and swallow pureed foods given by spoon. The swallow reflex may be assessed at this time (the same assessment previously described for the younger infant).

Food manipulation or munching involve jaw movements and tongue lateralization, (the ability of the tongue to move side to side). Jaw movements mash the food. Tongue lateralization enables the food to be moved to and from the gums and teeth for swallowing. The beginning stages of food manipulation or chewing start at 5 months of age with voluntary up-and-down jaw movements ("vertical munch"). Tongue lateralization begins at 6 to 7 months of age. The up-and-down jaw movements are followed by lateral jaw movements (and later by mature rotary movements: "rotary grind"). During this initial stage, up-and-down and lateral jaw movement, with tongue lateralization, are normal. Food manipulation can be evaluated by observing the infant's control of food. Jaw movements and tongue lateralization need to be noted. Tongue lateralization, if not observed during oral cavity assessment, can be judged by placing a small quantity of food on the gums, teeth, or in the lateral oral cavity and observing the infant's ability to mash or manipulate the food and then move it to the tongue for swallowing. Inadequate food manipulation or lack of tongue lateralization makes eating textured food difficult or impossible.

Self-feeding is observed during mealtime when food is offered. Self-feeding at this stage is demonstrated by:

- Increasing midline stability to sit independently and begin to hold a bottle or cup.

- The palmar grasp (the infant's ability to pick up large pieces of food between the thumb and palm.)
- Gross motor skills, including voluntary shoulder adduction and abduction, and elbow flexion with supination and pronation.

8 to 12 Months

During this stage there is a continued maturing of feeding skills. The important aspects of the feeding assessment are:

- Primitive reflexes disappear
- Food manipulation or chewing skills continue to develop
- Self-feeding skills continue to develop.

First assess the mouth and oral cavity, including both structure and function, as mentioned previously. Teeth may be present, most notably, deciduous, or primary central incisors. Lateral incisors may be present or erupting. Voluntary tongue movements may be observed. Assess the gag reflex.

Next, offer the infant food and observe for:

- Voluntary oral control
- Voluntary alerting
- Tongue elevation
- Food manipulation or chewing.

The up-and-down and lateral chewing now progresses to the beginning of a mature rotary-type movement. The infant's increasing number of teeth will enable him or her to handle more food textures and larger pieces of food, though true tearing of food may coincide more with eruption of the lateral canines at 16 to 23 months of age, and rotary chewing usually coincides more with eruption of the first molars, from 13 to 19 months of age. The swallow reflex is assessed while the infant is eating.

Self-feeding skills in this age group are demonstrated by:

- Midline stability to sit alone in the chair and to hold a bottle or cup.
- Maturing gross motor control enables easier cup holding with less spillage and smoother control of food from hand to mouth.
- Fine motor skills to self-feed progress from palmer to pincer grasp. The pincer grasp allows the infant to pick up food between his thumb and finger, enabling self-feeding with utensils and the ability to self-feed bite-size pieces of food.
- Independent eating is increasingly occurring as development progresses.

Feeding skills acquired during the first year of life are further refined during the toddler years. These are primarily chewing and further development of fine motor skills and control. See Table 9–2, Pediatric Feeding Skills Development.

PSYCHOSOCIAL INTERACTIONAL FEEDING ASSESSMENT

The relationship and interaction between the infant and parent or caregiver are extremely important. This interaction may have profound effects on the child's nutrition and feeding. For example, parents may be confused and not offer food to their infant if the infant does not provide clear hunger cues (i.e., agitation, crying, and mouth opening). In contrast, the infant who does provide clear cues may not be offered food if caregivers are insensitive to the cues. Therefore the quality of the interaction between the parent or caregiver and infant may have a significant impact on the amount of food ingested, even if the infant has normal feeding skills. An interactional assessment tool such, as Parent-Child Feeding Scale (NCASTAVENUW, 2006), provides information about the relationship between the parent and child during the feeding. This information focuses on the parent's sensitivity to the infant's cues, distress, social-emotional and cognitive growth fostering behavior, as well as the infant's clarity of cues and responsiveness to the parent.

In addition to observing interaction patterns, it is critical to note the behavior of the child before, during, and after the mealtime experience. The infant or child's cues of pleasure or distress are fundamental to determining how and where the feeding process is interrupted.

INTERVENTIONS FOR PEDIATRIC FEEDING DIFFICULTIES

Intervention for pediatric feeding disorders, of course, will depend on etiology and information found in the clinical assessment. Once physical causes or contributors to the problem have been addressed, the focus becomes normalizing feeding.

Comrie and Helm (1997) advocate a team approach to the child with feeding problems, stating the individual needs and cues of the child must be read, respected, and responded to, and families must be an integral part of the intervention. The individual infant or child's assessed feeding abilities determine the starting point and plan of interventions. Manikam and Perman (2000) advocate focus on antecedent manipulation (modifying and adapting the environment and caregiver behaviors) rather than relying on management of consequences. Dietician Ellyn Satter (2000) advocates a division of responsibility in successful feeding or eating, with parents being responsible for the what, when, and where of feeding, and children being responsible for how much and whether they eat. This way, the caregiver controls antecedents, yet the child is encouraged and allowed to explore eating at their own comfort and skill level. Common areas of intervention include positioning, control of environmental stimulation, appropriate feeding utensils, appropriate consistencies of food based on the assessed feeding skills level (see Table 9–2), and respect for the infant or child's behavioral cues of acceptance and refusal of food, all based on supporting the natural development of feeding skills.

Refusal to accept oral feedings may be due to a variety of reasons, including organic causes, sensory issues, motor difficulties, and fear due to real or perceived threat of aspiration. Manikam and Perman (2000) have suggested that feeding problems be viewed as on a continuum between organic and psychosocial factors. Therefore, force-feedings are discouraged. The purpose of a feeding evaluation is to determine "why" a child is not feeding appropriately, leading to interventions designed to support a normal developmental feeding sequence, allowing feeding to become both safe and pleasurable.

Infants and children who have feeding difficulties frequently require supplemental nutrition support, such as nasogastric or gastrostomy feedings. Supplemental feedings provide adequate nutrition whereas oral sensory-motor therapy is focused on maintaining and developing the infant or child's feeding skills. Specific stimulation treatments for children with oral-motor impairments are controversial and efficacy is not yet definitively proven. Research, however, is ongoing, and in some instances encouraging (Lamm, DeFelice, & Cargan, 2005).

Interventions relating to feeding difficulties require significant time and investment by family and health care professionals. In addition, infants or children with feeding difficulties may plateau at various oral sensory-motor feeding skill developmental levels. Therefore, some infants or children may require long-term supplemental nutrition to sustain them. In cases where it is unsafe for the infant or child to eat (i.e., because of aspiration risk), the goal of therapy is usually good oral hygiene and dental care, and helping to maximize quality of life through safe patient nutritional intake and pleasurable family interaction.

CONCLUSION

Various pediatric feeding problems have been identified for over 40 years. One approach to a comprehensive pediatric feeding assessment has been provided, based on normal feeding skills of children from birth to 3 years. This approach provides the practitioner with knowledge to identify potential or actual problems a child may have with eating.

From problem identification, appropriate supportive interventions can be provided to caregivers to help make eating a safe and pleasant experience for their child. Because feeding is a major component of the caregiver's role, information and interventions to help them in providing nutrition to the child will diminish family stress and support their role as caregivers.

STUDY QUESTIONS

1. Who might be members of a Pediatric Swallowing Team, and what contributions might each make?
2. How might an infant's cardiac problems impact his or her feeding or eating?
3. What are the technical criteria for a diagnosis of "failure to thrive"?
4. What information about the child's feeding method, schedule, or behavior is important to elicit from the family or caregivers when taking a *feeding* history?
5. What is the difference between using antecedent manipulation versus focus on consequences to manage feeding behaviors? What might be advantages and disadvantages of each method?

REFERENCES

American Academy of Pediatrics, Committee on Nutrition. (1985). In G. B. Forbes & C. W. Woodruff (Eds.), *Pediatric nutrition handbook* (2nd ed.). Elk Grove Village, IL: Author.

Arvedson, J. C., & Brodsky, L. (Eds.) (1994). *Pediatric swallowing and feeding: Assessment and management*. San Diego, CA: Singular.

Babbit, R. L., Hoch, T. A., & Coe, D. A. (1994). Behavioral feeding disorders. In D. N. Tuchman & R. Walters (Eds.), *Pediatric feeding and swallowing disorders: Pathophysiology, diagnosis and treatment* (pp. 77–96). San Diego, CA: Singular.

Beratis, S., Kolb, R., Sperling, E., & Stein, R. (1981). Development of child with long-lasting deprivation of oral feeding. *American Academy of Child Psychiatry, 20*, 53–64.

Bier, J. B., Ferguson, A., Cho, C., Oh, W., & Vohr, B. R. (1993). The oral motor development of low-birth-weight infants who underwent orotracheal intubation during the neonatal period. *American Journal of Diseases of Children, 147*, 858–862.

Casaer, D., Daniels, H., Devlieger, H., Decock, P., & Eggermont, E. (1982). Feeding behavior in preterm neonates. *Early Human Development, 7*, 331–346.

Case-Smith, J., Cooper, P., & Scala, V. (1989). Feeding efficiency of premature neonates. *American Journal of Occupational Therapy, 43*, 245–250.

Centers for Disease Control and Prevention, National Center for Health Statistics. CDC growth charts: United States. Available from: http://www.cdc.gov/ growthcharts/ May 30, 2000.

Comrie, J., & Helm, J. (1997). Common feeding problems in the intensive care nursery: Maturation, organization, evaluation, and management strategies. *Seminars in Speech and Language, 18*, 239–260.

Einarsson-Backes, L., Deitz, J., Price, R., Glass, R., & Hays, R. (1994). The effect of oral support on sucking efficiency in preterm infants. *American Journal of Occupational Therapy, 48*, 490–498.

Falconer, J. (2010). Gastro-oesophageal reflux and gastrooesophageal reflux disease in infants and children. *Family Health Care, 20*, 175–177.

Ferreira, C. T., Vieira, M. C., Vieira, S. M., Silva, G. S., Yamamoto, D. R., & Silveira, T. R. (2008). Eosinophilic esophagitis in 29 pediatric patients. *Archives of Gastroenterology, 45*, 141–146.

Field, D., Garland, M., & Williams, K. (2003). Correlates of specific childhood feeding problems. *Journal of Paediatrics and Child Health, 39*, 299–304.

Field, T., Ignatoff, E., Stringer, S., Brennan, J., Greenberg, R., Widmayer, S., & Anderson, G. C. (1982). Nonnutritive sucking during tube feedings: Effects on preterm neonates in an intensive care unit. *Pediatrics, 70*, 381–385.

Frappier, P., Marino, B., & Shishmanian, E. (1987). Nursing assessment of infant feeding problems. *Journal of Pediatric Nursing, 2*, 37–44.

Gisel, E. G. (1994). Oral-motor skills following sensorimotor intervention in the moderately eating-impaired child with cerebral palsy. *Dysphagia, 9*, 180–192.

Herbst, J. (1981). Development of sucking and swallowing. In E. Lebenthal (Ed.), *Textbook of gastroenterology and nutrition in infancy* (pp. 97–107). New York, NY: Raven.

Hymen, P. E. (1994). Gastroesophageal reflux: One reason why baby won't eat. *Journal of Pediatrics, 125*, S103–S109.

Illingworth, R. (1969). Sucking and swallowing difficulties in infancy: Diagnostic problem of dysphagia. *Archives of Disorders in Children, 44*, 655–665

Illingworth, R., & Lister, J. (1964). The critical or sensitive period, with special reference to certain feeding preterms in infants and children. *Journal of Pediatrics, 65*, 839–848.

Imhoff, S., & Wigginton, V. (1991). Identifying feeding and swallowing problems in infants and young children. *Clinical Communication Disorders, 1*, 59–67.

Kleiman, R., & Warman, K. (1994). Nutrition in liver disease. In S. Baker, R. Baker, & A. Davis (Eds.), *Pediatric enteral nutrition* (Chap. 17). New York, NY: Chapman and Hall.

Lamm, N., DeFelice, A. M., & Cargan, A. (2005). Effect of tactile stimulation on lingual motor function in pediatric lingual dysphagia. *Dysphagia, 20*, 311–324.

Levine, J., Lai, J., Edelman, M., & Schuval, S. J. (2012). Conservative long-term treatment of children with eosinophilic esophagitis. *Annals of Allergy Asthma and Immunology, 108*, 363–366.

Logan, W., & Bosma, J. (1967). Oral and pharyngeal dysphagia in infancy. *Pediatric Clinics of North America, 14*, 47–61.

Luiselli, J. K. (1994). Oral feeding treatment of children with chronic food refusal and multiple developmental disabilities. *American Association of Mental Retardation, 98*, 646–655.

Manikam, R., & Perman, J. A. (2000). Pediatric feeding disorders. *Journal of Clinical Gastroenterology, 30*, 34–46.

Measel, C., & Anderson, G. (1979). Nonnutritive sucking during tube feeding: Effect on clinical course in premature infants. *Journal of Obstetrics, Gynecology and Neonatal Nursing, 8*, 265–272.

Meier, P., & Anderson, G. (1987). Responses of small preterm infants to bottle and breast-feeding. *Maternal and Child Health Nursing, 12*, 97–105.

Mercado-Deane, M., Burton, E., Harlow, S., Glover, A., Deane, D., Guill, M., & Hudson, V. (2001). Swallowing dysfunction in infants less than 1 year of age. *Pediatric Radiology, 31*, 423–428.

Morris, S., & Klein, M. (2000). *Pre-feeding skills.* Tucson, AZ: Therapy Skill Builders.

Mueller, H. (1972). Facilitating feeding and prespeech. In P. Pearson & C. Williams (Eds.), *Physical therapy services in the developmental disabilities* (pp. 283–310), Springfield, IL: Charles C. Thomas.

NCAST-AVENUW. (2006). Parent Child Interaction (PCI) Program. Retrieved from http://www.ncast.org/index.cfm?fuseaction=category.display&category_id=24

Oates, R., Peacock, A., & Forrest, D. (1985). Long-term effects of nonorganic failure to thrive. *Pediatrics, 75*, 36–40.

Orenstein, S. R., Shalaby, T. M., Di Lorenzo, C., Putnam, P. E., Sigurdsson, L., Mousa, H., & Kocoshis, S. A. (2001). The spectrum of pediatric eosinophilic esophagitis beyond infancy: A clinical series of 30 children. *American Journal of Gastroenterology, 96*, 22–90.

Palmer, M., Crawley, K., & Blanco, I. (1993). Neonatal oral-motor assessment scale:

A reliability study. *Journal of Perinatology*, *13*, 28–35.

Reilly, S., & Skuse, D. (1992). Characteristics and management of feeding problems of young children with cerebral palsy. *Developmental Medicine in Child Neurology*, *34*, 379–388.

Reilly, S., Skuse, D., Mathisen, B., & Dieter, W. (1995). The objective rating of oral-motor functions during feeding. *Dysphagia*, *10*, 177–191.

Rodrigues, A. L., Palha, A. M., & Lopes, A. I. (2011). Eosinophilic esophagitis: Clinical expression at pediatric age. *Acta Med Portugual*, *6*, 1065–1074.

Rogers, B., & Arvedson, J. (2005). Assessment of infant oral sensorimotor and swallowing function. *Mental Retardation and Developmental Disabilities Research Reviews*, *11*(1), 74–82.

Samour, P. Q., & King, K. (2005). *Handbook of pediatric nutrition* (3rd ed.). Sudbury, MA. Jones & Bartlett.

Sanders, M., Patel, R., LeGrice, B., & Shepherd, R. (1993). Children with persistent feeding difficulties: An observational analysis of the feeding interactions of problem and non-problem eaters. *Health Psychology*, *12*, 64–73.

Satter, E. (2000). *Child of mine: Feeding with love and good sense*. Palo Alto, CA: Bull.

Singer, L., & Fagan, J. (1984). Cognitive development in failure-to-thrive infant: A three-year longitudinal study. *Journal of Pediatric Psychology*, *9*, 363–383.

Skuse, D., Stevenson, J., Reilly, S., App, B., & Mathisen, B. (1995). Schedule for oral-motor assessment (SOMA): Methods of validation. *Dysphagia*, *10*, 192–202.

Sorser, S. A., Barawi, M., Hagglund, K., Almojaned, M., & Lyons, H. (in press). Eosinophilic esophagitis in children and adolescents: Epidemiology, clinical presentation and seasonal variation. *Journal of Gastroenterology*.

Stevenson, R., & Allaire, J. (1991). The development of normal feeding and swallowing. *Pediatric Clinics of North America*, *38*, 1439–1452.

Wolff, P. (1968). The serial organization of sucking in the young infant. *Pediatrics*, *42*, 943–956.

APPENDIX 9–A

Growth Chart

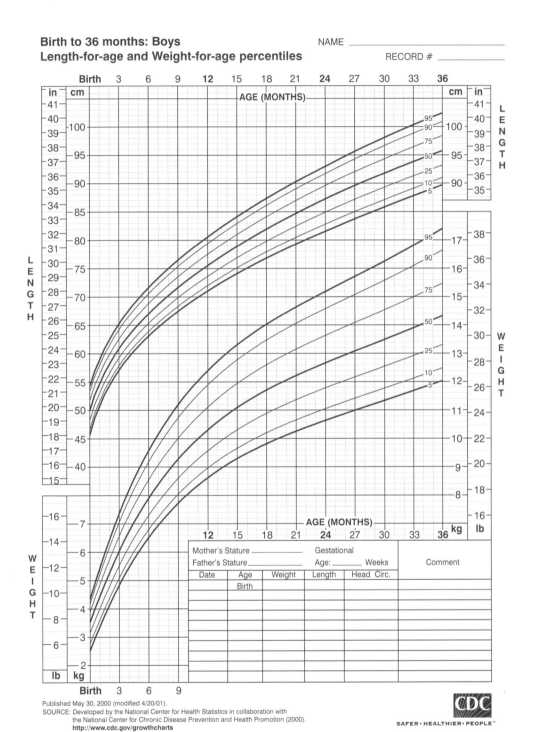

Birth to 36 months: Boys
Length-for-age and Weight-for-age percentiles

NAME _____

RECORD # _____

Published May 30, 2000 (modified 4/20/01).
SOURCE: Developed by the National Center for Health Statistics in collaboration with
the National Center for Chronic Disease Prevention and Health Promotion (2000).
http://www.cdc.gov/growthcharts

APPENDIX 9–B

Growth Chart

Birth to 36 months: Girls
Length-for-age and Weight-for-age percentiles

NAME _____

RECORD # _____

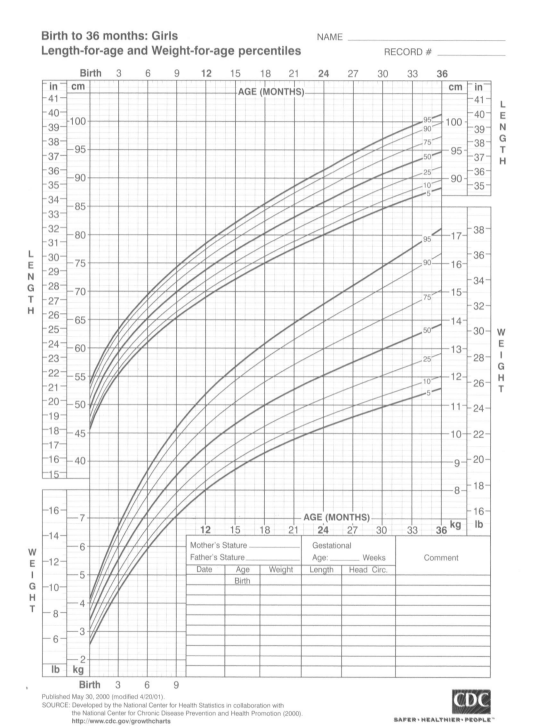

Published May 30, 2000 (modified 4/20/01).
SOURCE: Developed by the National Center for Health Statistics in collaboration with
the National Center for Chronic Disease Prevention and Health Promotion (2000).
http://www.cdc.gov/growthcharts

CDC
SAFER · HEALTHIER · PEOPLE™

148

APPENDIX 9–C

Growth Chart

2 to 20 years: Boys
Stature-for-age and Weight-for-age percentiles

NAME _____

RECORD # _____

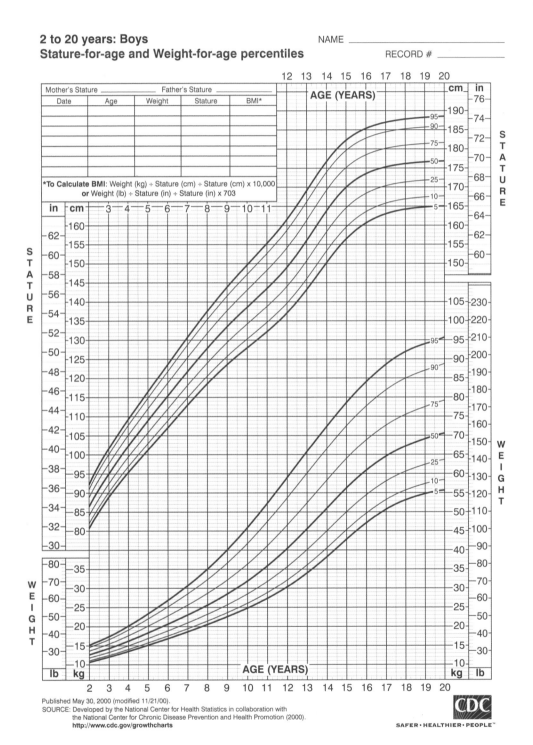

Published May 30, 2000 (modified 11/21/00).
SOURCE: Developed by the National Center for Health Statistics in collaboration with
the National Center for Chronic Disease Prevention and Health Promotion (2000).
http://www.cdc.gov/growthcharts

APPENDIX 9–D

Growth Chart

2 to 20 years: Boys
Body mass index-for-age percentiles

NAME _____

RECORD # _____

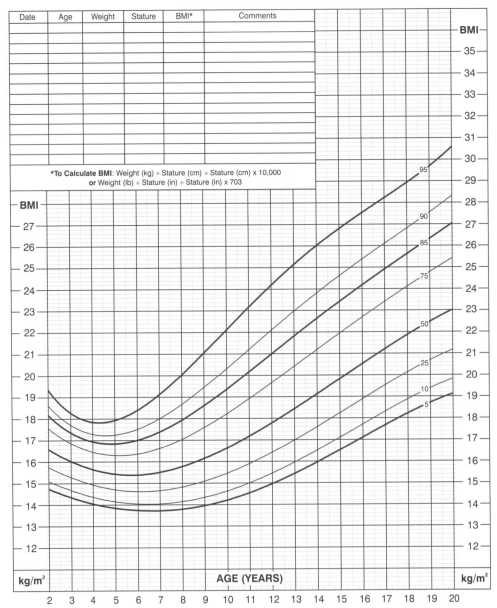

*To Calculate BMI: Weight (kg) ÷ Stature (cm) ÷ Stature (cm) x 10,000
or Weight (lb) ÷ Stature (in) ÷ Stature (in) x 703

Published May 30, 2000 (modified 10/16/00).

SOURCE: Developed by the National Center for Health Statistics in collaboration with
the National Center for Chronic Disease Prevention and Health Promotion (2000).
http://www.cdc.gov/growthcharts

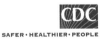

APPENDIX 9–E

Growth Chart

2 to 20 years: Girls
Body mass index-for-age percentiles

NAME _____

RECORD # _____

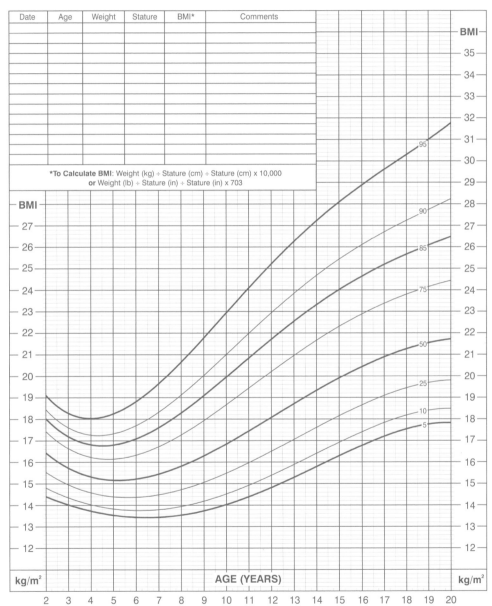

Date	Age	Weight	Stature	BMI*	Comments

*To Calculate BMI: Weight (kg) ÷ Stature (cm) ÷ Stature (cm) x 10,000
or Weight (lb) ÷ Stature (in) ÷ Stature (in) x 703

Published May 30, 2000 (modified 10/16/00).
SOURCE: Developed by the National Center for Health Statistics in collaboration with
the National Center for Chronic Disease Prevention and Health Promotion (2000).
http://www.cdc.gov/growthcharts

SAFER · HEALTHIER · PEOPLE

APPENDIX 9–F

Growth Chart

2 to 20 years: Girls
Stature-for-age and Weight-for-age percentiles

NAME _____

RECORD # _____

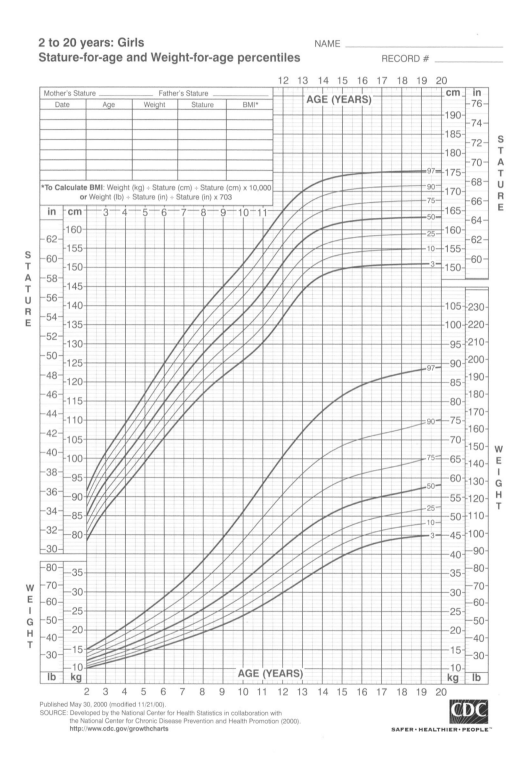

CDC
SAFER · HEALTHIER · PEOPLE™

10

Nutritional Concerns and Assessment in Dysphagia

Beverly Lorens

Successful management of dietary needs in dysphagic patients requires the efforts of all involved caregivers. The particular responsibility of the dietitian is to assess a patient's nutrition and hydration needs, and then to translate these needs into a diet that meets restrictions imposed by the team. These restraints may be unrestricted oral feeding, oral feeding with compensatory safeguards or facilitators, enteral (nonoral) feeding, or combined enteral and oral feeding. As these needs change, the dietitian should be involved to make the transition as effective as possible. Another important responsibility of the dietitian is to make the diet prescribed as appealing and palatable to a patient as possible. Implicit in this obligation is the recognition that eating is not an isolated act of nutrient provision, but is also associated with strong social, cultural, religious, and other influences in patients' lives. To the extent possible, these influences must also be considered in evaluating and treating the dysphagic patient.

Both screening and comprehensive nutritional evaluations require consideration of a patient's *anthropometric characteristics, dietary intake, relevant clinical* and *physical findings,* and *socioeconomic considerations*. Comprehensive assessment will elaborate each of these areas, for example, dietary intake will be assessed in terms of calories, protein, vitamins, minerals, and fluid, and evaluated for adequacy based on the patient's individual needs (Huyck, 1990; Nutrition Assessment, 1992; Nutritional Screening Initiative, 1994; Webber & Splett, 1995).

INDICATIONS

Nutritional assessment should be considered when a patient's means of feeding has been altered, when such a change is anticipated, or when there are concerns about the amount and/ or nutrition or hydration value of a patient's diet (Wood, 2005).

Patient Populations at Risk for Nutritional Compromise

Populations considered here are those most likely to benefit from a team evaluation, for example, a patient for whom there is a possibility of safe oral feeding and whose mentation level is judged adequate for at least a minimal level of cooperation with team objectives. The dysphagia may be a result of traumatic accident, surgical or medical event, neuromuscular progressive disease process, or developmental anomaly. Although some patients may be relatively stable in terms of their swallowing ability, others may reflect great variability over time. Many recent-event stroke patients, head trauma patients, and head and neck surgical patients will progress in swallowing during the period of therapeutic intervention. Over time, partial or even full recovery of function may be realized (Goguen et al., 2006). Patients with progressive neurogenic conditions, such as Parkinson's syndrome, demyelinating disease, Huntington's chorea, amyotrophic lateral sclerosis, or multiple sclerosis, may experience periods of stability but, in general, will decline consistent with their disease. Age groupings of patients have additional significance. For example, one can generally expect the CVA (cerebral vascular accident) population to be older, and the head trauma population to be younger. Such differences not only have implications for dietary needs, but also may influence a patient's eligibility for funding

sources that support nutritional needs. Funding resources need to be evaluated early to provide for implementation or exploration of alternatives. Innovative adjustments in formula choice or method of enteral feeding can provide cost savings for the unfunded person.

Other distinctions in patient groups have implications for the timing and frequency of dietary monitoring and/ or intervention. In some populations, changes in eating status are *anticipated*, and dietary needs can be addressed before the expected event (Fietkau, Iro, Sailer, & Sauer, 1991; Raykher et al., 2007; Senft, Fietkau, Iro, Sailor, & Sauer, 1993). One example of such a change is the intermittent interruption of nutrition because of treatment-related nausea, where the goal may be to maximize nutrition or hydration during nontreatment periods. Additional examples of an expected change are the compromised nutritional intake in the head and neck cancer patient undergoing radiotherapy (Ahmed, Samant, & Vieira, 2005; Fietkau et al., 1991; Senft et al., 1993), or an extended NPO (nothing per oral) status in a postoperative patient (Koehler & Buhl, 1991). In other populations, the need for nutritional assistance is *acute and unanticipated*. Patients who are apparently well and then experience a sudden insult, that is, CVA or trauma, are examples of this kind of population (Nyswonger & Helmchen, 1992). Other patients may be maintaining adequate nutrition or hydration but have few reserves to cope with new or unexpected problems that compromise their nutritional well being. In such cases, changes in nutrition or hydration status are *not entirely unanticipated*. Careful monitoring to ensure prompt intervention is necessary. For example, a patient with a degenerative disease who has been doing well for a long period of time may begin to fail. Or a patient recovering from surgery may leave the hospital doing well, but experience difficulty later in the postoperative period.

"Red Flags" for Formal Dietitian Consult

Significant changes in *weight trends* and *hydration* status in a patient signal the need for a comprehensive nutritional evaluation. Guidelines for determining the severity of unintentional weight loss are presented in Table 10–1.

In general, a person losing 10 to 20% of his or her usual weight may sustain moderate impairment, whereas a loss of greater than 20% of usual weight indicates severe impairment (Phinney, 1995). In both situations, thorough elaboration of the cause of weight loss will be required.

Red flags for suboptimal hydration include rapid weight loss (a 48-hour weight loss of 4 pounds can mean a negative fluid balance of 2 liters), complaint of thirst, skin turgor changes, decreased urination, change in blood chemistry, such as a rising blood urea nitrogen level [BUN] in the absence of other renal indicators, and an increased serum sodium level (hypernatremia). Patients with thin liquid dysphagia may be at particular risk for alterations in hydration status. They will have difficulty augmenting fluid intake to compensate for increased fluid losses because of secondary illness and are also more vulnerable to other fluid depleting conditions such as fever, diarrhea, or increased perspiration related to heat or physical exertion.

NUTRITIONAL ASSESSMENT

As noted, careful monitoring of patients' nutritional status can and should be undertaken by members of the dysphagia team and other caregivers. However, expedient referral to the dietitian is indicated when there is any question regarding the patient's ability to safely maintain adequate nutrition

Table 10-1. Evaluation of Weight Change

Time	Significant Weight Loss (% of Change)	Severe Weight Loss (% of Change)
1 week	1–2	>2
1 month	5	>5
3 months	7.5	>7.5
6 months	10	>10

Source: Blackburn, G. L., Bistrian, B. R., Maini, B. S., Schlamm, H. T., & Smith, M. F. (1977). Nutritional and metabolic assessment of the hospitalized patient. *Journal of Parenteral and Enteral Nutrition, 1,* 15.

or hydration via the current means of food intake. Typically, another member of the team has nutritionally screened dysphagic patients and this has triggered a referral to the dietitian for a more comprehensive assessment. Components of the dietitian's examination include the following.

Anthropometric Data

(Krystofiak & Mueller, 2007; Nutritional Assessment, 1992; Pesce-Hammond & Wessel, 2005)

As indicated, a primary cue for dietary referral is weight change. Appropriate weight range is impacted by gender, age, height, and frame. The patient's usual weight, any change in this amount, over what period of time, and whether any change was intentional must be determined (see Table 10–1). If weight loss is too rapid, and in particular if it is associated with inadequate protein intake, it may adversely impact the body's immune function. The ability to resist disease and infection is compromised (Linn, Robinson, & Klimas, 1988). The patient's energy level and ability to

participate in the prescribed rehabilitation program may also be affected. Presented in Table 10–2 are guidelines for interpreting nutritional status based on percent of ideal body weight (IBW) and percent of usual body weight (UBW).

Laboratory Data

(Krystofiak & Mueller, 2007; Nutritional Assessment, 1992; Pesce-Hammond & Wessel, 2005)

Visceral protein status is frequently screened by obtaining a *serum albumin* value (from a blood sample, usually requested as part of a Comprehensive Medical Panel). A value of less than 3.2 (Zeman, 1991, pp. 56, 77) to 3.5 (Nutrition Screening Initiative, 1994, p. 19) is suggestive of the patient being at nutritional risk. Different laboratories may have different normal ranges and some adjust normal range based on age. Prealbumin can provide a more sensitive indicator of current protein status. However, pre-albumin may be lowered in the presence of metabolic stressors, inflammation, or infection, irrespective of nutritional state, and is referred to as

Table 10-2. Evaluation of Nutritional Status Based on a Percentage of Weight

	% of Ideal Body Weight	% of Usual Body Weight
Mild malnutrition	80–90%	85–95%
Moderate malnutrition	70–79%	75–84%
Severe malnutrition	0–69%	0–74%

Source: Koehler, J., & Buhl, K. (1991). Percutaneous endoscopic gastrostomy for postoperative rehabilitation after maxillofacial tumor surgery. *International Journal of Oral and Maxillofacial Surgery, 20,* 38–39.

a "negative acute phase protein." Therefore, a low pre-albumin value may not, by itself, reflect compromised protein or nutrition status. C-reactive protein (CRP), a positive acute phase protein, can be used as an indicator of stress or inflammation (Pesce-Hammond & Wessell, 2005, p. 19). If CRP is within normal limits, then the pre-albumin can more confidently be accepted to reflect actual protein status.

Laboratory blood chemistry values that are both commonly available and useful for evaluating hydration status are *serum sodium* and *blood urea nitrogen*. Elevated values are typical in the dehydrated patient. Additionally, albumin will be elevated in dehydration. One needs to remain mindful that hypoalbuminemia may be masked by mild to moderate dehydration causing hemoconcentration and a falsely elevated albumin value. In dehydration, low urine output will occur as the body seeks to conserve fluid (Zeman, 1991, p. 71). A useful caveat is never look at individual blood results by isolated values, rather, view them together as in a composite picture.

Nutrition History

(Krystofiak & Mueller, 2007; Nutritional Assessment, 1992, pp. 75–77; Nutrition and Your Health, 1995; Pesce-Hammond & Wessell, 2005)

Between the time of referral and the time the patient is evaluated, it is extremely helpful to have obtained a *food diary record* (i.e., a 3-day history up to a 7-day history of dietary intake). The patient or caregiver is instructed to record the time food or drink is consumed, the amount consumed, and a description of the food and how it was prepared, that is, steamed, fried, broiled (Appendix 10–A). The amount of food should be described using standardized measurements. For example, a "glass" of juice might be 4, 8, 12, or even 16 ounces, depending on the size of container and how full it was filled *and* if all was consumed. The patient is also asked to note if this is a typical meal pattern and, if not, how it differs from the usual. Any nutrient label information concerning calories and protein per serving size should also be included in the report. It is important to appreciate that merely recording one's dietary intake may alter the usual pattern of intake.

Additional measures obtained by the dietitian are a recent (last 24 hours) food intake record as recalled by the patient (referred to as a *24-hour recall*), and a *food frequency list,* which describes how often the patient has had different types of foods over a recent time period.

The history of food intake provided by the patient or caregiver, and the translation of this information in terms of nutrient content are, at best, only approximate. The patient's ability to recall type and quantity of dietary intake may be flawed. In addition, our understanding of the nutrient content of foods and the patient's individual nutrient requirements is not absolute. These limitations notwithstanding, it is still important to make the best interpretation possible from the available information. From all measures considered, the dietitian will compare the patient's dietary intake to standard referents of dietary requirements. For example, the United States Department of Agriculture (USDA) MyPyramid food guidance system (Appendix 10–B) recommendations for daily dietary requirements include:

- 5 to 10 servings of grains, emphasizing whole grains and higher fiber choices
- 1½ to 2½ cups of fruit, eating more in the fresh and natural form
- 2 to 4 cups of vegetables, emphasis on variety and color
- 3 cups from the milk group that also includes fortified soymilk, cheese, yogurt, and tofu
- 5 to 7 ounce equivalents from the meat and bean group (includes poultry, meats, eggs, and nuts)
- 5 to 10 teaspoons from oils (vegetable)
- 130 to 500 calories from discretionary calories group that includes sweets, solid fats, and higher calorie forms of food.

It should also be underscored that establishment of nutritional needs is *an estimate* and, as such, simply provides a place to begin. Subsequent monitoring of weight, laboratory values, and the patient's global sense of well-being will assist in fine tuning the nutrition goals.

The USDA has issued a "Plate Method" for guiding nutrition intake. This is a graphic illustration that illustrates amounts of space, on a plate (with cup and side dish), that should be devoted to particular types and textures of foods, for example, fruits, grains, vegetables, protein, and drink. This author finds the MyPyramid a more useful guide with the dysphagic population. Textural modification can result in a meal that presents far from the standard plate, cup, and side dish. More significantly, the focus with the former approach is on including all food groups, when the textures of some groups may not lend themselves readily to dysphagic patients.

Clinical and Physical Findings

Assessment of the patient's oral peripheral structures is addressed at length in other chapters, and will not be reviewed here. Typically, the dysphagia therapist has completed this evaluation before a dietitian consult. It is important to stress that oral cavity structures and their functional integrity impact both how and what type of nutrition a patient may be able to manage. For example, the patient's ability to chew to a ground or puree texture will influence the texture(s) of food that can be offered.

Also important to the nutritional evaluation is the patient's level of physical activity. If activity is minimal, the patient's energy need and number of calories required will be low, necessitating the selection of nutrient dense food. "Nutrient dense" means that food with calorie content needs also to provide a significant balance of protein, vitamins, and minerals, with so-called "empty" calories kept to a minimum. The goal is to ensure nutritional adequacy of protein, vitamins, and minerals without excess weight gain from excess calories that would further impact mobility.

Concurrent chronic conditions, such as diabetes, coronary artery disease, renal, and pulmonary impairment that may have pre-existing diet management in place, must also be noted. Pre-existing therapeutic diet modifications may be counterproductive to adequate nutrition or hydration in a patient with newly developed dysphagia. A cardiac patient's low-fat diet may be inappropriate if the patient is unable to consume adequate calories while adhering to the low-fat regimen. The initial priority is to maintain weight. Once this is achieved, a patient may begin incorporating lower fat food choices if the low fat diet is still indicated. Diabetic diets have undergone significant changes since 1994. The emphasis is on individualizing the diet based on the medical nutrition needs and the results of self-monitoring of blood glucose. Patients may need guidance in adjusting their prior "diabetic" diet within the new constraints of their dysphagia. Additionally, increased reliance on pharmaceutical intervention may be indicated if conditions such as hyperlipidemia or hyperglycemia are not adequately controlled. Chronic medication use, with particular attention to food–drug interactions, must also be evaluated.

Mental health status, and in particular, recent changes in this status, must also be considered. Alterations in cognitive skills, ability to attend, or to speak will affect communication and social interaction. This can have implications for a patient's compliance with treatment objectives. Such changes may also trigger depression or a diminished sense of well being, with resultant decreased appetite and failure to maintain weight.

The social environment a patient is in, or will enter upon leaving the hospital or care facility, is screened as a part of the nutritional evaluation. In particular, adequate funds to purchase food, as well as a living situation that allows food preparation, are important factors to assess. The dysphagic patient will have a greater diet variety if the means

to acquire appropriate foods and then prepare them to proper texture and viscosity are available. Also important to the assessment are observations regarding the patient's level of isolation, dependence on others for food procurement or preparation, current or former occupation, cultural background, and other factors that may influence food choices or eating.

NUTRITIONAL GOALS IN TREATMENT PLANNING

Establishing Energy, Protein, and Fluid

For purposes of this chapter, the primary nutritional goal for a dysphagic patient is to approximate nutrition needs that will allow achievement or maintenance of healthy body weight. Patients should be monitored closely and the dietitian again consulted if desired outcomes of weight maintenance, gain, or loss are not obtained.

Energy
(American Society of Parenteral and Enteral Nutrition, 1993; Hopkins, 1993; Nutritional Assessment, 1992; Recommended Dietary Allowances, 1989, pp. 24–38; Wooley & Frankenfield, 2007)

Adults. Daily energy requirements for adults are based on a calculated reference (ideal) weight for height in kilograms (Table 10–3). A maintenance base is 25 to 35 kcal per kg reference weight per day. Additional allowance must be made for increased activity or metabolic stress. The obese patient may lose

Table 10–3. Calculating Reference Weight (Ideal Body Weight)

Adult Male (Hamwi Method)*	106 lbs for first 5 feet; 6 lbs for each inch over 5 feet *Example:* 5'9" Reference weight = 160 lb = 72.7 kg
Adult Female (Hamwi Method)*	100 lbs for first 5 feet; 5 lbs for each inch over 5 feet *Example:* 5'4" Reference weight = 120 lb = 54.5 kg
Children	Consult standardized Growth Curves. Some modified growth curves are available for specific conditions, i.e., Downs syndrome

Source: Gottschlich, M., Matarese, L., & Shronts, E. (Eds.). (1993). *Nutrition support dietetics core curriculum* (2nd ed.). Silver Spring, MD: American Society for Parenteral and Enteral Nutrition.

weight using his or her "ideal" weight in the calculation and require adjustment of energy goal if weight loss is unacceptable.

Children. Daily energy requirements for children must be individualized to age group and weight, activity, spasticity, and also for catch-up growth. Recommended dietary allowances are established for healthy children. These are used as a base that can be modified for an individual child in a specific situation.

Protein
(Hopkins, 1993, pp. 58–63; Nutritional Assessment, 1992; Recommended Dietary Allowances, 1989, pp. 52–77; Shaw, Wildbore, & Wolfe, 1987; Young, Kearns, & Schoepfel, 2007)

Adults. 0.8 gram protein per kilogram reference weight is the recommended daily dietary intake for an adult. This level is increased or decreased depending on specific disease consideration, level of nutritional debilitation, and metabolic stress, for example, related to fever or sepsis. For anabolism or during

periods of stress, the value is typically increased to between 1.0 and 1.5 grams protein per kilogram reference weight. In burn and trauma patients, protein may be increased to 2.0 g protein per kg.

Children. Appropriate daily protein levels for children are highly variable depending on age and metabolic stressors. Infants' and children needs range from 2.2 to 1.0 g per kg with the value decreasing to the adult level of 0.8 protein per kg at age 15 years for females and age 19 years for males (Recommended Dietary Allowances, 1989).

Fluid
(Hopkins, 1992, p. 63; Nutritional Assessment, 1992; Recommended Dietary Allowances, 1989, pp. 247–250)

Adults. There are many accepted formulas to determine appropriate fluid levels for adults. A general guideline is 1 ml fluid per kcal. Another method uses a range: 25 to 40 ml per kg reference weight per day. Fluid needs decrease with age. Influences on fluid requirements include amount of total body surface area, illness, activity level, and temperature of the environment. Fluid needs are, in part, proportional to body surface area. The obese person would have increased needs over the person within their ideal weight range.

Children. For the first 10 kg of body weight, add 100 ml/kg per day; for the second 10 kg of body weight, add 50 ml per kg per day; for each additional kilogram, add 20 mL per kg per day.

Vitamins and Minerals

(Clark, 2007, pp. 129–159; Hopkins, 1993, pp. 42–51; Nutritional Assessment, 1992; Recommended Dietary Allowances, 1989; Standing Committee on the Scientific Evaluation of Dietary Reference Intakes, Food and Nutrition Board, Institute of Medicine, 1997 and 1998)

Adequacy of the overall diet needs to be assessed for the provision of sufficient vitamins and minerals within the calorie density consumed. In an adult eating orally, a multiple vitamin/mineral supplement is generally indicated if nutritional energy needs are less than 1,500 kcals per day. (ADA Reports, 2005; Fairfield & Fletcher, 2002; Fletcher & Fairfield, 2002).

TRANSLATING ENERGY-PROTEIN-FLUID NEEDS INTO A TREATMENT PLAN

Once the target values for calories, protein, and fluid have been established, the route of nutrient ingestion must be considered. The dysphagia team has typically discussed the available alternatives and decided the best option for the patient. Conventional oral eating, facilitated by strategies as needed, is the most desirable. Oral intake combined with enteral tube feeding may also be recommended. This combination may be used when fatigue or some other limitation may impact the patient's ability to rely totally on oral feeding. Other patients will require enteral feeding for all their nutrition. Whatever method is prescribed, constant re-evaluation is needed to determine if the current option is working or remains appropriate. During these periods, the dietitian provides the team and the physician managing the patient's care with a quantitative analysis of food consumption by reviewing food diaries kept by the patient or caregiver.

Oral Feeding

If oral feeding is recommended for the patient, the dysphagia therapist will determine what restrictions must be applied to ensure safe oral feeding. The dietitian will help identify foods that both appeal to the patient and meet the safety requirements imposed. In short, the dietitian will translate the team's prescription into everyday foods that the patient can consume in sufficient quantities to meet nutrition or hydration needs.

Textures range over a continuum from pourable liquids with varying viscosities to gel consistencies, to slippery puree foods that deform from shape with gravity, to stiffer purees that hold their shape, to combinations of puree and ground texture, to fine chop. Potentially, texture will be unrestricted, but the length of time required to eat may require selection of nutrient dense foods. The normal adult swallower enjoys the full range of the texture or viscosity continuum from the least to most viscous. The dysphagic patient may find the tolerable viscosity range restricted, that is, shifted to the low or high end, or compressed from both extremes. The texture continuum in relation to transit ability and airway protection is presented in Table 10–4.

An exercise found useful in our setting was to have members of the dysphagia team meet in the central kitchen. A smorgasbord of food was sampled from our patient tray line. Team members jointly developed a matrix classification of what foods would be considered thick or thin liquids, allowed on puree or ground diet. This process significantly strengthened the complementary relationship the dysphagia therapist and dietitian share in treating the dysphagic patient. The dysphagia therapists gained insights regarding how limited a meal may become given multiple restrictions, and the dietitians gained, among other things, an understanding of how thin a "thick liquid" may be and how broad a range would be acceptable for other characterizations of food used by the therapists. Also emerging from this experience was an appreciation for the *range* of viscosity included in the categories "thick liquid" and "puree" and for the difficulty involved in correlating findings regarding viscosities sampled on the dynamic swallow study with the subjective determination of a tolerable range of viscosities made during the bedside evaluation. Information presented in Appendix 10–C represents the result of the group collaboration.

It should be noted that the categories of textures presented are not ironclad. Individualizing dietary restriction to the patient's specific impairment provides maximum variety.

Subsequently, the National Dysphagia Diet: Standardization for Optimal Care (National Dysphagia Diet Task Force, 2002) was published as a start toward providing a level of consistency in terminology used to describe dysphagia diets and textures, and viscosity standards of liquids.

Our Food and Nutrition Department has adopted the National Dysphagia Diet groupings while retaining some in-between diet texture stages (McCallum, 2003). We also use descriptive titles for the diet instead of a numerical reference. We do not want to suggest that one has to start at Level 1 and progress through a series of advancing textures. We have two modified texture diet series. The first one provides texture changes for those without aspiration risk or cognitive impairment. Typically they are patients that can make modification to the food item to consume it more easily and safely. The patient also enjoys more food variety. In contrast to dysphagia diets, rice and bread are included. The second is the Dysphagia Series. The National Dysphagia Diet has Level 1: Dyphagia Pureed; Level 2: Dysphagia Mechanically Altered Characteristics; and Level 3: Dysphagia Advanced. In addition we have inserted "Dyphagia Puree with Ground Meat" between Levels 1 and 2. This level allows oatmeal, fruited yogurt, scrambled egg, and finely ground meat with a side dish of gravy so the patient or caregiver can further moisten the meat or mashed potatoes to needed amounts. All other foods are pureed (see Table 10–4).

Table 10-4. Texture or Viscosity Continuum

TEXTURE OR VISCOSITY CONTINUUM

Places stress on agility of airway closure oral for swallow but facilitates bolus transfer ⟷ Relieves demands on agility of airway closure and facilitates bolus transfer ⟷ Places stress on oral preparation and and pharyngeal transfer competence

	Thin Liquids	Thick Liquids	Slippery Puree	Puree	Foods Requiring Mastication in order of ascending difficulty
EXAMPLE	(assumed to be at body temperature) apple juice, cranberry juice, non-, lowfat, and whole milk, fruit ice, sherbet, jello, soft drinks	(assumed to be at body temperature) tomato juice, nectar, apple juice with thickener, Instant Breakfast, ≥1.5 cal/cc commercial supplement	(assumed to be at body temperature) pudding, custard, puree fruit, puree vegetables (not starches)	Mashed potatoes, puree scrambled eggs, puree meat	ground meat, regular scrambled eggs, canned fruit, soft cooked carrots, beets, bread
					chopped meat, sandwiches (tuna, egg, bologna)
					unrestricted diet
PROPERTIES	Easily deformed, moves very readily in response to gravity and compression.	Less easily deformed than thin liquids, moves fairly readily in response to gravity or compression.	Less easily deformed so may obstruct a narrow passage. Slides in response to gravity or compression.	Less easily deformed, thus can obstruct a narrow passage. Transferred mostly by compression.	As the bolus becomes more viscous, it is less and less easily deformed, less likely to move in response to gravity, more reliant on dental and lingual competence for mastication and transit, sensory competence and judgment of bolus characteristics, adequate salivation, and healthy mucosa.

continues

163

Table 10–4. *continued*

	Thin Liquids	Thick Liquids	Slippery Puree	Puree	Foods Requiring Mastication in order of ascending difficulty
TRANSIT	Thin liquids are most likely to move through the upper digestive tract quickly and completely.	Variably likely (depending on the degree of thickness) to move through the digestive tract easily without falling into the airway and to pass fairly well through narrow sites such as strictures.	Slippery purees are more likely to stop at obstacles such as webs and strictures, but may be less likely to "stick."	Purees are likely to stop at obstacles and may not slide easily along dry mucosa. Purees will not move through the pharynx without adequate compression/ constriction. Complete transit requires adequate salivary and mucosal health.	Adequate oral and pharyngeal patency and strength of constriction/compression is requisite for safe swallow of high viscosity foods once mastication has transformed the solid into a puree. Adequate transfer requires adequate salivary and mucosal health.
AIRWAY	Agility of laryngeal airway closure for swallow is a prerequisite for ingestion of thin liquids.	Swallow of thick liquids requires less laryngeal agility because thick liquids are less easily deformed and move more slowly (speed varies with thickness) in response to gravity or compression.	Slippery purees require less laryngeal agility but more competent oral and pharyngeal constriction. If the bolus is not adequately transferred, residue may fall into the airway after the swallow. The properties of purees present a greater risk of obstructing the airway than liquids.	Because they do not move readily in response to gravity, purees are less likely to fall into the airway quickly. However, if oral and pharyngeal clearing is incomplete due to poor constriction or xerostomia, pharyngeal residue presents a risk to the airway after the swallow has been completed. The properties of purees present a greater risk of obstructing the airway than liquids.	Adequate airway protection during swallow of solids is reliant on adequately complete oral and pharyngeal transit. The airway can be obstructed if penetrated by solid bolus residue, even if mastication is fairly adequate. The properties of solids present a greater risk of obstructing the airway than liquids.

	Thin Liquids	Thick Liquids	Slippery Puree	Puree	Foods Requiring Mastication in order of ascending difficulty
PATIENTS	Patients with prolonged or incomplete oral, pharyngeal, or esophageal transit due to poor muscular constriction or to narrowing, (e.g., stricture) but who are alert and enjoy good laryngeal function are most likely to achieve adequate intake with liquid consistencies.	Patients with prolonged or incomplete oral, pharyngeal, or esophageal transit due to poor muscular constriction or to narrowing (e.g., stricture) are most likely to achieve adequate intake with liquid consistencies. Patients with mild cognitive deficits or who show poor oral bolus control or impaired initiation of swallow gestures may require thickened liquids.	Patients who are slow to initiate swallow gestures, including airway closure, but who are able to apply some compression to accomplish oral and pharyngeal bolus transfer would tolerate slippery purees.	Patients who are able to apply adequate pressures to transfer the bolus through the oral and pharyngeal cavities completely will tolerate puree consistencies.	The goal of mastication is to produce a "swallow safe" bolus, probably one approximating a puree. The ability to tolerate degrees of viscosity in the solid range is dependent on lingual agility and ROM, judgment re: bolus readiness, salivary flow, and dentition.

Source: From Susan McKenzie, M.S., and Beverly Lorens, R.D., M.S.

Special Concerns

As previously addressed, the patient with a thin liquid dysphagia may have difficulty maintaining adequate hydration. All fluid intake must be contained in some gradient of thicker liquid to gel-form food. It is helpful that pureed fruit, vegetables, and meat contain a high percent of their weight as water. However, without some form of thick to thickened liquids, a patient will likely consume inadequate fluid. A variety of commercial thickeners are available either by direct order or from local pharmacies. Some common household foods also work well for thickening. Examples of commercial and household products available for this purpose are listed in Appendix 10–D.

If patients are able to consume sufficient fluid in the form of puree foods, gels, and thick liquids, they may find that their total calorie intake is higher than needed. Potentially, most of their fluid will contain calories, in contrast to an individual without thin liquid dysphagia who can consume water for thirst.

Another area of concern is the successful patient who, having mastered weight maintenance with dysphagia to dry foods, has begun to gain excessive weight. This may be a result of the preparation of foods in more sauce or gravy dishes, which increase the moisture and slipperiness of the foods, but also increase the calories. Positive results can be obtained by reducing the caloric value of the food preparation.

Nonoral Feeding Alternatives

Total Parenteral Nutrition

When oral feeding is not an option for a patient, other avenues of food intake

must be considered. One such alternative is total parenteral nutrition (TPN). TPN is able to provide total nutrition using a large flow capacity vein, in contrast to peripheral parenteral nutrition (PPN), that accesses a vein that a simple IV would enter. (PPN cannot usually meet full nutrition needs related to the concentration of nutrients in a low flow, smaller, peripheral vein.) Advances in enteral feeding formulas and feeding tubes have made TPN less popular than in the past. TPN is costly, invasive, represents an infection risk, and bypasses the gut, enhancing potential for bacterial translocation (the integrity of the gut is decreased with lack of exposure to nutrients and bacteria normally retained in the gut can pass to the bloodstream) (Borzotta et al., 1994; Kudsk, 1994; Kudsk et al., 1994; Minard & Kudsk, 1994; Moore & Moore, 1991). However, TPN must be used when the gut is nonfunctional because of prolonged ileus, or short bowel syndrome, or where there is contraindication to placing a feeding tube for whatever reason. Additionally, there are patients who will not leave the feeding tube in place. This is more likely in a patient with a nasogastric tube before conversion to a gastrostomy or jejunostomy feeding tube (jejunostomy tubes enter the intestine in the second section of the small intestine, as much as 12 or more inches beyond the stomach).

Enteral Feeding

A patient's degree of dysphagia may require the placement of a feeding tube if nutrition is to be supplied in a safe and sufficient volume. Access sites of feeding tubes are typically the nose, the stomach, or the jejunum (Figure 10–1). An enteral feeding tube placed nasally may have the tip of the tube located in

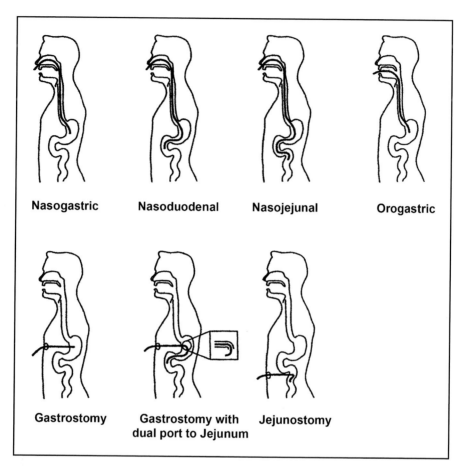

Figure 10-1. Types and access sites of feeding tubes.

the stomach (NG), duodenum (ND), or jejunum (NJ). Tubes placed either by percutaneous endoscopic gastrostomy (PEG) method, radiographically, or surgical gastrostomy may have single or dual lumen tubes, accessing the stomach (GT), or stomach and duodenum (GD) or jejunum (GJ or PEJ, i.e., percutaneous endoscopic jejunostomy). A dual lumen tube has a tube within a tube allowing access to two sites, for example, stomach and duodenum, whereas a single lumen tube delivers to only one site. Lastly, the jejunal feeding tube has both its access and end port in the jejunum (JT). Our otolaryngology surgical team places, at the time of surgery,

a nasogastric, 14 to 18 French silicone sump tube (Figure 10–2) that, if needed (to drain secretions, gas), can be used for gastric decompression (removal of liquid gastric secretions or gas before a post-anesthesia treated patient's stomach begins to regulate and empty contents) and then for feeding once stomach is emptying contents normally. The tube's relatively small diameter and pliability make it a reasonably comfortable tube for extended periods of postsurgical feeding. Additionally, the silicone material does not become rigid over time. This tube can stay in for 30 days if necessary. Non-silicon sump tubes ideally remain in less than a week.

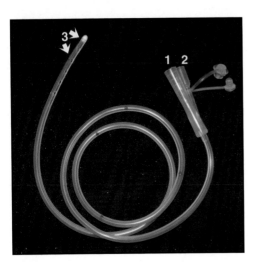

Figure 10-2. Kendall™ Argyle™ silicone Salem Sump™ tube, 16 Fr., 48" length (Tyco/Healthcare). Dual Lumen. Y-connector with: (1) suction drainage lumen/feeding port, (2) suction vent lumen, and (3) closed end tip with multiple exit ports.

Multiple factors are considered concurrently in the decision of what type of feeding tube access will best serve the needs of the patient. These include the following:

- Anticipated duration of enteral feeding (and likelihood of return to oral intake).
- Ability to protect the airway, degree of aspiration risk, and pulmonary reserve to withstand aspiration (delivery sites vary in terms of possible airway risk from reflux).
- Presence of impaired gastric emptying may preclude feeding into the stomach (i.e., gastroparesis).
- Types of enteral feeding formula available (i.e., commercial ready-to-feed, name-brand or store brand, or homemade).
- Availability of feeding pump for continuous feeding (gravity drip bolus or syringe bolus recommended only into the stomach).
- Cosmetic considerations (a nasogastric tube is visible, whereas a GT or JT may be concealed behind clothing).
- Patient compliance with location (i.e., an agitated patient can more easily remove a nasogastric tube than a gastrostomy tube that can be concealed behind a dressing or abdominal binder when not in use).
- Availability and condition of organ to be an access site.
- Selection of feeding schedule (*continuous* or *intermittent* feeds can be delivered into stomach, duodenum, or jejunum but only bolus (gravity or syringe) feeds should be administered into the stomach).

Nasogastric (NG) feeding is generally selected when the duration of time on tube feeding will be relatively short (may be months), there is an intact gag reflex with normal emptying of the stomach and no evidence of uncontrolled esophageal reflux. Particular advantages of the NG tube are its relatively noninvasive placement and cost effectiveness (Figures 10–3 and 10–4).

Nasoduodenal (ND) tubes are appropriate for short-term feeding when gastroesophageal reflux is expected, when there is an increased aspiration risk, or decreased rate of stomach emptying. A continuous feeding rate is employed and commercial formulas are used primarily because these feeding tubes are often smaller in diameter and more prone to plugging. Homemade feedings may not be homogeneous. Also, if they are low enough viscosity to flow, they may be too dilute to deliver an adequate quantity of nutrition (Figure 10–5).

The *nasojejunal* (NJ) feeding route requires a longer tube (43 inches compared to 36 inches for other tubes). It also requires radiographic confirmation of placement and may need to be placed endoscopically. Its primary advantage is that its extended placement into the GI tract minimizes dislodgment back into the stomach and feeding can begin shortly after injury as feeding into the small intestine does not depend on a stomach to be emptying its contents (see Figure 10–5).

Gastrostomy (GT) placement is appropriate if nasoenteric route is unavailable, long-term feeding is required, or swallowing dysfunction is permanent. Location of tip placement in stomach, duodenum, or jejunum would follow the same decision tree used with a nasoenterically placed tube. A prime advantage of gastrostomy is cosmetic as the feeding tube is not outwardly visible (Figures 10–6 and 10–7).

Some dual lumen GTs have a narrow lumen line that serves the duodenum or jejunum (Figure 10–7. This has the advantage of being able to access both the stomach and intestine. Some medications are better absorbed in the stomach. If long-term jejunal feeding is the goal and stomach access is not required, placement directly as a JT may be preferred. Tube length will be shorter, possibly less inclined to clogging. As with the PEG, a PEJ can be placed endoscopically and is therefore

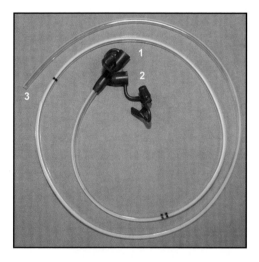

Figure 10–3. Kendall™ Kangaroo™, 12 Fr., 36" length, unweighted (Tyco/Healthcare). Y-connector with: (1) feeding port, (2) irrigation/medication port, and (3) open end tip with exit ports in tubing.

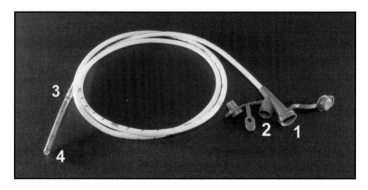

Figure 10–4. Kendall™ Entriflex™ Dual Port Feeding Tube without Sylet 12 Fr., 36" length (Tyco/Healthcare). Y-connector with: (1) feeding port, (2) irrigation/medication port, (3) exit ports, and (4) weighted tip.

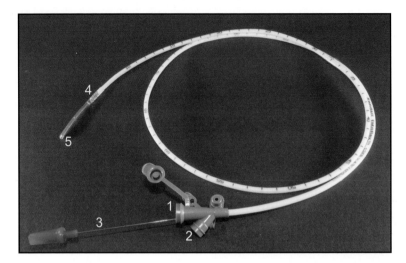

Figure 10–5. Kendall™ Entriflex™ Dual Port Feeding Tube with FLOW THROUGH™ Stylet, 12 Fr., 43" length (Tyco/Healthcare). Y-connector with: (1) feeding port, (2) irrigation/medication port, (3) stylet, (4) exit ports, and (5) weighted tip.

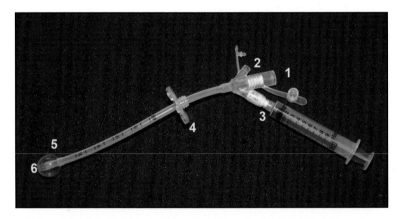

Figure 10–6. Kimberly-Clark™ MIC™ Gastrostomy feeding tube, 20 Fr., 7 to 10-mL balloon (Ballard Medical Products). (1) Feeding port, (2) irrigation/medication port, (3) balloon valve port, (4) external retention disk, (5) balloon, and (6) open tip exit port.

less costly than a surgical jejunostomy. A JT is indicated in the patient with extensive gastroesophageal surgery or disease. (A caveat is that bypassing the duodenum also bypasses the nutrient absorption sites of this part of the intes-tine that may have longer term conse-quences for nutrition status.)

Rustom, Jebreel, Tayyab, England, and Stafford (2006) reviewed 78 head and neck cancer patients for compli-cation rates between three methods

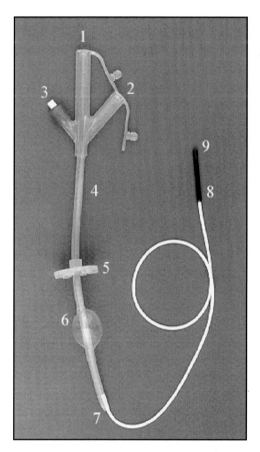

Figure 10–7. MIC™ Gastro Enteric Feeding Tube, 20 Fr. (Medical Innovations, a Division of Ballard Medical Products). (1) Gastric port, (2) jejunal port, (3) balloon valve, (4) dual lumen tube, (5) Secur-Lok® ring, (6) balloon, (7) tapered gastric exit port, (8) multiple exit ports, and (9) weighted tip.

after the surgical resection of tumor and the dragging of the retention bumper of the PEG tube through the neosurgical site is contraindicated. Additionally, Douglas, Koh, and Laramore (2000) reviewed the literature and found six cases of PEG site metastases occurring in patients with head and neck cancer. A later review sites 29 cases of PEG site metastasis (Mincheff, 2005).

A summary of advantages and disadvantages of each feeding tube is presented in Table 10–5. The dietitian is a key resource in assisting selection of the enteral formula appropriate for each, with consideration given to suitability, availability, tolerance, and cost. Some patients may need to *make* their own tube feeding in lieu of one of the multitude of commercially made formulas. The dietitian is invaluable in such situations. Generally, the cost of formula will be lowest if one retains the ability to feed into the stomach. The stomach acts as a reservoir and hypertonic solutions can be fed; whereas, jejunal feeding usually requires an isotonic formula and a feeding pump. As previously noted, the stomach also allows for an intermittent bolus feeding schedule, which may allow the patient more freedom and more of a feeling of normalcy by engaging in feeding at meal periods.

Medications delivered via the feeding tube must be liquid or crushed and sustainable in a slurry. A bolus of water before and after the medication administration will prevent interaction between the medication and feeding that may result in clumping of the feeding which could clog the tube. No sustained release medications can be fed through the feeding tube as crushing will ruin the sustained release property.

of gastrostomy tube insertion: PEG, radiologically inserted gastrostomy (RIG), and surgically inserted gastrostomy (open or laparoscopic). The PEG group had fewer complications and has become their first choice for head and neck cancer patients. At our facility, the RIG method is more commonly used in our head and neck cancer patients. Consideration for this method is that the gastrostomy is more often placed

Table 10-5. Advantages and Disadvantages of Feeding Tubes

Access Site	Advantages	Disadvantages
Nasogastric	• Minimally invasive, easy placement • Suitable for short-term use • Transitional to bolus feeding • Radiographic confirmation not necessarily required	• Cosmetic—feeding tube visible unless patient self-inserts FT each feeding • Risk of sinusitis • Lack of intact gag reflex may indicate increased aspiration risk • Stomach must be uninvolved with primary disease
Nasoduodenal	• Minimally invasive • Suitable for short-term use • Reduced risk of pulmonary aspiration • Useful in conditions of gastroparesis or impaired stomach emptying • Useful if esophageal reflux present • Allows for feeding when bowel sounds are diminished or absent	• Requires radiographic confirmation of placement • Cosmetic—feeding tube is visible • Requires 43" length feeding tube • May not remain placed in duodenum due to tube migration • Typically, smaller diameter tube than NG, more prone to plugging if not properly maintained • Bolus feeding contraindicated • Risk of sinusitis
Nasojejunal	• Same advantages as nasoduodenal • Placement of tip further down GI tract minimizes dislocation to stomach • 60" length tubes available offering even greater placement security	• Similar disadvantages as nasoduodenal except placement of tip more secure
Cervical Esophagostomy	• Improved cosmetic appeal as end of tube more easily concealed • Ease of feeding over gastrostomy as do not need to undress • More suitable for long-term feeding	• Although more suitable for long-term feeding, the lower esophageal sphincter is stented open and same concerns for gastric and esophageal reflux with possible pulmonary aspiration are present as with the NG feeding tube

Table 10–5. *continued*

Access Site	Advantages	Disadvantages
Gastrostomy	• Suitable for long-term feeding • Cosmetically more appealing than a nasally place tube • Minimizes risk of tube migration and aspiration due to voluntary or accidental dislocation of nasoenteric tube by patient • Percutaneous placement available (PEG) • Some GT have large bore tubes which minimizes occlusion from medications and high viscosity formulas • Most suitable of all tubes for use of homemade formula, provided tip is placed in stomach and it is a large bore tube • Bolus feeding option available if tip of tube in stomach	• Potential risk of pulmonary aspiration • Lack of intact gag reflex and/or presence of esophageal reflux may indicate increased risk of aspiration • Insertion site care needed • Potential skin excoriation at stoma site from leakage of gastric secretions • Potential fistula at insertion site after GT removal • If GT feeding tip port is placed in duodenum, usually a smaller bore tube is used and it is subject to more occlusion risk
Jejunostomy	• Suitable for long-term feeding • Minimizes risk of aspiration • Positive gag reflex need not be present • Useful if esophageal reflux is present • Does not depend on functioning stomach • Percutaneous placement (PEJ) available • Minimal risk of dislodgment	• Typically smaller bore tube than a GT and risk of occlusion from medication or viscous formula • Stoma care needed • Potential skin excoriation at stoma site from leakage of gastric secretions • Bolus feeding not an option • Potential fistula at stoma site after JT removal

Source: Adapted from Gottschlich, M., Matarese, L., & Shronts, E. (Eds.). (1993). *Nutrition support dietetics core curriculum* (2nd ed.). Silver Spring, MD: American Society for Parenteral and Enteral Nutrition

TEAM APPROACH

As stated frequently throughout this text, the benefit of a team approach to dysphagic patients is the opportunity it provides for synergism. The dovetailing of the skills and experience of each individual professional in the assessment and treatment of the patient is an enormous advantage, for both the patient and team members. Members of our team have a healthy regard for the individual skills and backgrounds represented by each participant, and this translates to a broad, comprehensive approach to patient management. The team approach also provides opportunities to reinforce the message of other team members or of the collective "team," while individual specialists deliver their own expertise. The patient benefits from multiple exposure to variations of the same treatment theme and hopefully begins to incorporate successful adaptations for his or her individual condition.

STUDY QUESTIONS

1. What is the dietitian's role in the treatment of dysphagia?
   a. Nutritional management
   b. Oral and tube feeding recommendations
   c. Weight management
   d. All of the above
   e. a and c
2. What would be some of the indications to place a gastrostomy feeding tube?
   a. Progressive neurologic condition with feeding difficulties leading to compromise of nutrition
   b. Head injured patient who is expected to need tube feeding for 2 to 3 months who keeps pulling and removing nasogastric tube
   c. Patient who is expected to regain safe and effective swallow function in 2 to 3 weeks and dislikes how she or he looks with a feeding tube
   d. All of the above
   e. a and b
   f. b and c
3. When evaluating whether percent of weight change is significant or severe, both the length of time over which a person's weight has changed and the amount of weight change is considered. *True or False.*
4. Specific guidelines define whether a patient's percent of ideal body weight characterizes them as having mild, moderate, or severe malnutrition. *True or False.*
5. The following elements compose a nutritional assessment:
   a. Anthropometric data
   b. Laboratory data
   c. Nutrition history
   d. Clinical and physical finding
   e. Financial analysis
   f. All of the above
   g. a, b, c, and d.
6. There is clear agreement among dysphagia professionals concerning which food fluids are thin, nectar-like, or honey-like and how to describe textural diets. *True or False.*

REFERENCES

ADA Reports. (2005). Position of the American Dietetic Association: Fortification and nutritional supplements. *Journal of American Dietetic Association, 105,* 1300–1311.

Ahmed, K. A., Samant, S., & Vieira, F. (2005). Gastrostomy tubes in patients with advanced head and neck cancer. *Laryngoscope, 115,* 44–47.

American Society of Parenteral and Enteral Nutrition Board of Directors. Nutrition support for adults with specific diseases and conditions: critical care. (1993). *Journal of Parenteral and Enteral Nutrition, 17*(Suppl.), 20SA–21SA.

Blackburn, G. L., Bistrian, B. R., Maini, B. S., Schlamm, H. T., & Smith, M. F. (1977). Nutritional and metabolic assessment of the hospitalized patient. *Journal of Parenteral and Enteral Nutrition, 1,* 15.

Borzotta A., Pennings J., Papasadero B., Paxton, J., Mardesic, S., & Borsotta, R., Parrott, A., & Bledsoe, F. (1994). Enteral versus parenteral nutrition after severe closed head injury. *Journal of Trauma, 37,* 459–468.

Clark, S. (2007). Vitamins and trace elements. In M. Gottschlich (Ed.), *The A.S.P.E.N. nutrition support core curriculum, a case-based approach—the adult patient* (pp. 129–159). Silver Spring, MD: American Society for Parenteral & Enteral Nutrition.

Douglas, J. G., Koh, W., & Laramore, G. E. (2000). Metastasis to a percutaneous gastrostomy site from head and neck cancer, radiobiologic considerations. *Head and Neck, 22,* 826–830.

Fairfield, K., & Fletcher, R. (2002). Vitamins for chronic disease prevention in adults—scientific review. *Journal of the American Medical Association, 287,* 3116–3126.

Fletcher, R., & Fairfield, K. (2002). Vitamins for chronic disease prevention in adults—clinical applications. *Journal of the American Medical Association, 287,* 3127–3129.

Fietkau, R., Iro, H., Sailer, D., & Sauer, R. (1991). Percutaneous endoscopically guided gastrostomy in patients with head and neck cancer. *Recent Results in Cancer Research, 121,* 209–282.

Goguen, L., Posner, M., Norris, C., Tishler, R., Wirth, L., Annino, D., . . . Haddad, R. (2006). Dysphagia after sequential chemoradiation therapy for advanced head and neck cancer. *Otolaryngology-Head and Neck Surgery, 134,* 916–922.

Gottschlich, M., Matarese, L., & Shronts, E. (Eds.). (1993). *Nutrition support dietetics core curriculum* (2nd ed.). Silver Spring, MD: American Society for Parenteral and Enteral Nutrition.

Hopkins, B. (1993). Assessment of nutritional status. In M. Gottschlich, L. Matarese, & E. Shronts (Eds.), *Nutrition support dietetics core curriculum* (2nd ed., pp. 15–70). Silver Spring, MD: American Society for Parenteral and Enteral Nutrition.

Huyck, N. I. (1990). Screening: A method to prioritize patient care. *Hospital Food and Nutrition Focus, 6,* 1–3.

Koehler, J., & Buhl, K. (1991). Percutaneous endoscopic gastrostomy for postoperative rehabilitation after maxillofacial tumor surgery. *International Journal of Oral and Maxillofacial Surgery, 20,* 38–39.

Krystofiak Russel, M., & Mueller, C. (2007). Nutrition Screening and Assessment. In M. Gottschlich (Ed.), *The A.S.P.E.N. nutrition support core curriculum, a case-based approach—the adult patient* (pp. 163–186). Silver Spring, MD: American Society for Parenteral and Enteral Nutrition.

Kudsk, K. A. (1994). Gut mucosal nutritional support: Enteral nutrition as primary therapy after multiple system trauma. *Gut, 1*(Suppl.), S52–S54.

Kudsk, K. A., Minard, G., Wojtysiak S. L, Croce, M., Fabian, T., & Brown, R. O. (1994). Visceral protein response to enteral versus parenteral nutrition and sepsis in patients with trauma. *Surgery, 116,* 516–523.

Linn, B. S., Robinson, D. S., & Klimas, N. G. (1988). Effects of age and nutritional status on surgical outcomes in head and neck cancer. *Annals of Surgery, 207,* 267–273.

McCallum, S. (2003). The National Dysphagia Diet: Implementation at a regional rehabilitation center and hospital system. *Journal of the American Dietetic Association, 103,* 381–384.

Minard, G., & Kudsk, K. A. (1994). Effect of route of feeding on the incidence of septic complications in critically ill patients. *Seminars in Respiratory Infections, 9,* 228–231.

Mincheff, T. (2005). Metastatic spread to a percutaneous gastrostomy site from head and neck cancer: Case report and literature review. *Journal of the Society of Laparoendoscopic Surgeons, 9,* 466–471.

Moore, E. E., & Moore, F. A. (1991). Immediate enteral nutrition following multisystem trauma: A decade perspective. *Journal of the American College of Nutrition, 10,* 633–648.

National Dysphagia Diet Task Force. (2002). *National Dysphagia Diet: Standardization for Optimal Care.* Chicago, IL: American Dietetic Association.

Nutrition and Your Health: Dietary Guidelines for Americans (4th ed.). (1995). Washington, DC: US Dept of Agriculture, US Dept of Health and Human Services.

Nutritional Assessment. (1992). In American Dietetic Association, *Handbook of clinical dietetics* (2nd ed., Chap. 1). New Haven, CT: Yale University Press.

Nutrition Screening Initiative. (1994). *Incorporating nutrition screening and interventions into medical practice.* Washington, DC: Author.

Nyswonger, G. D., & Helmchen, R. H. (1992). Early enteral nutrition and length of stay in stroke patients. *Journal of Neuroscience Nursing, 24,* 220–223.

Pesce-Hammond, K., & Wessel, J. (2005). Nutrition assessment and decision making. In R. Merritt (Ed.), *The A.S.P.E.N. nutriton support practice manual* (2nd ed., pp. 3–26). Silver Spring, MD: American Society for Parenteral and Enteral Nutrition.

Phinney, S. D. (1995). Advances in diagnosing malnutrition in hospitalized patients. *Nutrition in clinical practice.* Conference Syllabus. Sponsored by UC Davis Division of Clinical Nutrition and Metabolism, Department of Internal Medicine and the Office of Continuing Medical Education April 8, 1995.

Raykher, A., Russo, L., Schattner, M., Schwartz, L., Scott, B., & Shike, M. (2007). Enteral nutrition support of head and neck cancer patients—invited review. *Nutrition in Clinical Practice, 22,* 68–73.

Recommended dietary allowances / Subcommittee on the Tenth Edition of the RDAs, Food and Nutrition Board, Commission on Life Sciences, National Research Council (10th ed.) (1989). Washington, DC: National Academy.

Rombeau, J. L., Caldwell, M. D., Forlaw, L., & Guenter, P. A. (Eds.). (1989). *Atlas of nutritional support techniques.* Boston, MA: Little, Brown.

Rustom, I., Jebreel, A., Tayyab, M., England, R., & Stafford, N. (2006). Percutaneous endoscopic, radiological and surgical gastrostomy tubes: A comparison study in head and neck cancer patients. *Journal of Laryngology and Otology, 120,* 463–466.

Senft, M., Fietkau, R., Iro, H., Sailer, D., & Sauer, R. (1993). The influence of supportive nutritional therapy via percutaneous endoscopically guided gastrostomy on the quality of life of cancer patients. *Supportive Care in Cancer, 1,* 272–275.

Shaw, J. H. F., Wildbore, M., & Wolfe, R. R. (1987). Whole body protein kinetics in severely septic patients: The response to glucose infusion and total parenteral nutrition. *Annals of Surgery, 205,* 288–294.

Standing Committee on the Scientific Evaluation of Dietary Reference Intakes, Food and Nutrition Board, Institute of Medicine. (1997 and 1998). *Dietary reference intakes.* Washington, DC: National Academy Press.

Webber, C. B., & Splett, P. L. (1995). Nutrition risk factors in a home health population. *Home Health Care Services Quarterly, 15,* 97–110.

Wood, K. (2005). Audit of nutritional guidelines for head and neck cancer patients undergoing radiotherapy. *Journal of Human Nutrition and Diet, 18,* 343–351.

Wooley, J., & Frankenfield, D. (2007). Energy. In M. Gottschlich (Ed.), *The A.S.P.E.N. nutrition support core curriculum, a case-based approach—the adult patient* (pp. 19–32). Silver Spring, MD: American Society for Parenteral and Enteral Nutrition.

Young, S., Kearns, L., & Schoepfel, S. (2007). Protein. In M. Gottschlich (Ed.), *The A.S.P.E.N. nutrition support core curriculum, a case-based approach—the adult patient* (pp. 71–87). Silver Spring, MD: American Society for Parenteral and Enteral Nutrition.

Zeman, F. J. (1991). *Clinical nutrition and dietetics* (2nd ed.). New York, NY: Macmillan.

APPENDIX 10-A

Recording Food Intakes

Patient Name _____ DOB _____
UCD MR# _____
Telephone _____
Clinic/Service _____
Ht. _____ Wt. _____

Directions for Recording Your Food Intake:

It is essential that food intake records be filled out as accurately and completely as possible. Each day list all of the foods and beverages you have eaten for any meal and snack. Along with the type of food eaten, record the amount of food and how it was prepared. For example, was it fried? baked? Were bacon drippings or butter added?

Record portion sizes or the amount of food eaten as follows:

tablespoon – Tbsp. Cup – C
teaspoon – tsp. slice – sl.
ounce – oz.

The more details you include, the better we can analyze the diet. For combination dishes and sandwiches, list ingredients: 2 sl. wheat bread, 1 oz. cheese, 1 tsp. mustard.

Carry your daily record with you and fill out the record after you have eaten. Please include times food was eaten.

Equivalent Measures

3 teaspoons = 1 tablespoon
16 tablespoons = 1 cup
1 ounce = 2 tablespoons
8 ounces = 1 cup
16 ounces = 1 pound
32 fluid ounces = 1 quart

SAMPLE PAGE

Date _Tuesday, 4/20_

Vitamin/Mineral Supplements: _50 mg. Vitamin C_

Time	Food/Drink	Amount	Method of Preparation
8:00	eggs	1	soft cooked
	orange juice	1/2 C.	
	toast	1/2 sl.	plain
10:00	vanilla wafers	6	
12:00	turkey sandwich	1	
	whole wheat bread	2 sl.	with 1 tsp. mayonnaise
	turkey	2 sl.	
	low fat milk	4 oz.	
3:00	fresh apple	1/2	(medium size)
5:30	baked fish	1	3 inches x 1/2 inch thick
	mashed potatoes	1/2 C.	made with low fat milk
	spinach	1/2 C.	
	low fat milk	6 oz.	
	salad, tossed	1 C.	w/1 Tbsp. french dressing
8:00	frozen yogurt	1/2 C.	

APPENDIX 10–B

USDA My Pyramid Food Guidance System

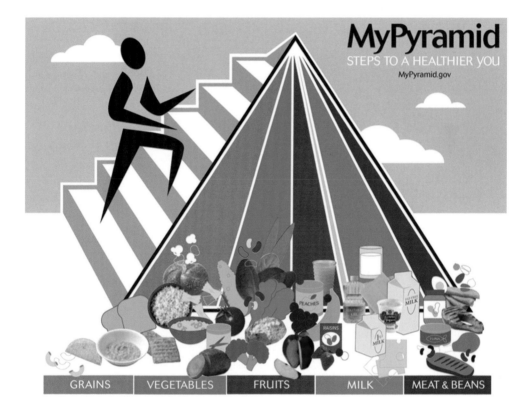

continues

Appendix 10-B. *continued*

GRAINS	VEGETABLES	FRUITS	MILK	MEAT & BEANS
Make half your grains whole	Vary your veggies	Focus on fruits	Get your calcium-rich foods	Go lean with protein
Eat at least 3 oz. of whole-grain cereals, breads, crackers, rice, or pasta every day 1 oz. is about 1 slice of bread, about 1 cup of breakfast cereal, or 1/2 cup of cooked rice, cereal, or pasta	Eat more dark-green veggies like broccoli, spinach, and other dark leafy greens Eat more orange vegetables like carrots and sweetpotatoes Eat more dry beans and peas like pinto beans, kidney beans, and lentils	Eat a variety of fruit Choose fresh, frozen, canned, or dried fruit Go easy on fruit juices	Go low-fat or fat-free when you choose milk, yogurt, and other milk products If you don't or can't consume milk, choose lactose-free products or other calcium sources such as fortified foods and beverages	Choose low-fat or lean meats and poultry Bake it, broil it, or grill it Vary your protein routine — choose more fish, beans, peas, nuts, and seeds

For a 2,000-calorie diet, you need the amounts below from each food group. To find the amounts that are right for you, go to MyPyramid.gov.

GRAINS	VEGETABLES	FRUITS	MILK	MEAT & BEANS
Eat 6 oz. every day	Eat 2½ cups every day	Eat 2 cups every day	Get 3 cups every day; for kids aged 2 to 8, it's 2	Eat 5½ oz. every day

Find your balance between food and physical activity

- Be sure to stay within your daily calorie needs.
- Be physically active for at least 30 minutes most days of the week.
- About 60 minutes a day of physical activity may be needed to prevent weight gain.
- For sustaining weight loss, at least 60 to 90 minutes a day of physical activity may be required.
- Children and teenagers should be physically active for 60 minutes every day, or most days.

Know the limits on fats, sugars, and salt (sodium)

- Make most of your fat sources from fish, nuts, and vegetable oils.
- Limit solid fats like butter, stick margarine, shortening, and lard, as well as foods that contain these.
- Check the Nutrition Facts label to keep saturated fats, *trans* fats, and sodium low.
- Choose food and beverages low in added sugars. Added sugars contribute calories with few, if any, nutrients.

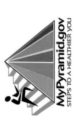

MyPyramid.gov
STEPS TO A HEALTHIER YOU

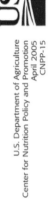

U.S. Department of Agriculture
Center for Nutrition Policy and Promotion
April 2005
CNPP-15

USDA is an equal opportunity provider and employer.

APPENDIX 10–C

Food Texture Continuum Matrix

Thin Liquid ↔	Thick Liquid ↔	Slippery Puree ↔	Puree ↔	Puree Foods + Ground Meat ↔	Soft Foods + Ground Meat ↔	Soft Foods + Chopped Meat
water	NECTAR-LIKE	thin cream of wheat	cooked cream of wheat	cooked oatmeal regular	eggs, all types	*cereal dry
coffee, tea	4 oz. juice + ~1 Tbsp commercial thickener	baby puree meat	pureed scrambled eggs	scrambled eggs	ham, ground	bacon
broth					sausage, ground	sausage
juice:	Commercially made nectar-like:	custard	pregelled, slurried breads on French toast	ham, ground sausage, ground Canadian bacon, ground	Canadian bacon, ground	biscuit
apple		pudding			pancakes	bread
cranberry					muffins	crackers
grape	juices	pureed fruit				toast
orange	milk		entrée meat, pureed	pregelled, slurried breads or French toast	roast beef, ground	waffle
tomato juice	water				roast pork, ground	chicken, chopped
nectar			mashed potatoes, yams	entrée meat, ground		fish
soft drinks			mashed winter squash		meatloaf	hamburger patty
milk:				mashed potatoes, yams	Salisbury steak	hot dog
nonfat			pureed cooked vegetables	mashed winter squash	stew, pieces <1/2 inch	roasts, chopped
lowfat						
whole			soups, blended smooth		noodles	rice
chocolate				pureed cooked vegetables	potatoes	sandwiches:
buttermilk					pasta entrees	tuna, egg, bologna, chicken salad, cheese

continues

Thin Liquid ↔	Thick Liquid ↔	Slippery Puree ↔	Puree ↔	Puree Foods + Ground Meat ↔	Soft Foods + Ground Meat ↔	Soft Foods + Chopped Meat ↔
Instant Breakfast	HONEY-LIKE	pureed cooked vegetables (no potatoes, yams)	pudding	soups, blended smooth	soups	cooked vegetables: broccoli, cauliflower, green beans
commercial supplement	Generally, 4 oz. thin liquids + ~2 Tbsp commercial thickener		custard	pudding	canned beets	
fruit ice			yogurt, smooth (no fruit pieces)	custard	soft cooked vegetables: carrot coins, peas, spinach, zucchini	tomato, fresh sliced
sherbet			pureed fruit	yogurt with fruit pieces		
ice cream				pureed fruit		green lettuce salad
Jello				cottage cheese, small curd	canned fruit, no pineapple	fruit, fresh: banana, melon (cut up), orange (sectioned), pear
					fruit, fresh: banana, strawberries, kiwi	
					cake	graham crackers
					pie, bottom crust only	vanilla wafers
						cookies, no nuts

Thickeners

Patients who need to restrict liquids to a thicker consistency will find that the use of either commercial thickening products or the addition of certain foods and products found in the kitchen cupboard at home will allow them to increase the variety of liquids and foods that they are able to eat.

The amount of thickener added will allow thickening from nectar-like to honey-like, or to an even stiffer spoon-thick consistency. Thickeners can be used to stiffen a pureed food item that may be too thin. Some products work better in hot liquids. Others are supplemented with vitamins and minerals. It is important to compare the amount of product needed to achieve the desired consistency—some products have greater thickening power and, as a result, require less product. Manufactures recommend different amounts of their product to obtain a nectar-like, honey-like, or spoon-thick consistency. The amount of product needed also may differ depending on the temperature, acidity (pH) and amount of sugars and other solids present in solution. Individual product web sites provide information on product use and recipes. Some of the newer gel based thickeners have less alteration in taste and clarity of the liquid being thickened, which for some individuals, improves acceptability and effectiveness.

Following is a list of some search term suggestions, some Web sites, though by no means meant to imply endorsement or a complete list. New products are being developed. Some products are intended (usually gels or powders) to be added to existing fluids at hand to thicken to desired viscosity. Other products can be purchased in a ready-to-consume container with a stated viscosity of nectar-like or honey-like. Currently, there is little standardization between company products and to what viscosity is obtained by following package directions using one of the powder or gel products added to foods at home. Additionally, the viscosity will be altered in the individuals mouth based, in part, by dilution with saliva, length of time it is retained in the mouth, if it is mixed with other food in the mouth. Material in the cup may not maintain the same characteristics as it moves through an individual patient's oral-pharyngeal structures!

Prices vary depending on where purchased and amount ordered. Some companies provide mail order shipping directly to the consumer. Hospital based speech departments may be able to order through their Food Service Department thereby accessing commercial venders. The local drug store usually stocks a thickening product. If not found on the shelves, or behind the counter, the pharmacy can order it.

Some suggested Web-based search terms: "Thickeners-dysphagia" and "therapeutic liquid thickeners." "Precision Foods Thick It," "Thick-It," "Hormel labs–Thick & Easy" (product more likely found in Food Service operations than commercial retail); "Bernard Foods Thixx thickeners."

continues

Some Web sites, not intended to be all inclusive or endorsed:

> **http://www.nestlenutrition.com/us** or **http://www.nestlehealthscience.us**
> Go to "Product & Applications" then " Modified Consistencies/Dysphagia"
> Multiple products available from commercial, "ready-to-drink" thickened
> products to gel-based and powder thickener. Product names include:
> Resource brand of thickened juices, milk, water; "ThickenUp®" (modified
> corn starch), and "ThickenUp®Clear, (non-starch based thickening powder).
> Also: **http://www.nestlenutritionstore.com** Select category: "Swallowing
> difficulties"

> **http://www.SimplyThick.com** (gel–gum based product)

> **http://www.ThickItRetal.com** (powder based product and gum based
> AquaCareH2O™s). Made by Precision.

> **http://www.HormelHealthLabs.com** Order from: **http://www.HomeCare
> Nutrition.com** (Products: Thick and Easy® (powder) and Thick & Easy®Clear
> Instant Food & Beverage Thickener, as well as other specialized food
> products for altered texture needs.)

KITCHEN CUPBOARD RESOURCES:

> Dehydrated potato flakes
>
> Baby instant rice cereal
>
> Pureed vegetables and fruits
>
> Dehydrated baby food
>
> Bread crumbs
>
> Unflavored gelatin—powder needs to be put into solution by heating in liquid,
> then cooled.

Keep in Mind!

> The goal for every patient is a nutritional plan that optimizes recommendations
> from an experienced dysphagia clinician regarding what foods are most likely
> to be appropriate, given the details of impairment. Ideally, the nutrition plan
> should include foods that meet texture and viscosity restrictions, are nutrition-
> ally adequate and, to the extent possible, are acceptable to the patient.

Appendices 10–Db (Thick Liquids) and 10–Dc (Trouble Eating) include examples
of patient education materials developed by dietitians at University California,
Davis Health System.

UCDAVIS
HEALTH SYSTEM

Thick Liquids

Who needs thick liquids?

If you have difficulty swallowing (dysphagia), thin liquids such as water, coffee, and milk may not be safe to drink. Liquids thickened to **nectar consistency** may help you to eat and drink more safely. Examples of nectar thick consistencies are apricot or mango nectar, maple syrup, eggnog, or heavy whipping cream.

What drinks can I have?

May Be Tolerated	**Will Need To Be Thickened**
Tomato juice	Water
<u>Cold</u> Ensure Plus®	Coffee, tea
Fruit nectars	Milk
Yogurt drinks	Regular Ensure®
Buttermilk	Room temperature Ensure Plus®
Smoothies, milkshakes	Jell-O®
Eggnog	Pediasure®
Thick gravy	Thin soups, broth
Thick creamed soups (strained)	Sports drinks
Resource® thickened products	Soda, juice

- Do not eat anything that melts (ice, popsicles, ice cream, sherbet, or Jell-O®).
- Avoid juicy fruits such as oranges, watermelon, or grapes.

How to thicken your drinks:

Commercial Thickeners Find these items at your local pharmacy, drug store, or online	**Household Items**
Thick-it® Thicken Up® by Nestle Nutrition Thick & Easy® by Hormel Health Labs Thixx® Simply Thick®	Add cornstarch, instant potato flakes, mashed potato, or baby foods (meat, vegetable, rice cereal) to thicken soups Add pureed fruit to fruit juices Use pudding or custard mix to make a milkshake Use yogurt or pureed fruit to make a smoothie

Clinical Dietitians & Dietetic Interns, Food & Nutrition Services, UC Davis Medical Center (9/10)
© 2010 The Regents of the University of California. All Rights Reserved.

continues

Tips for thickening liquids:

- **Follow directions.**
  Instructions on your commercial thickener may vary with different products and liquids. In general, add 1 Tablespoon thickener to 4 ounces liquid and stir. Wait 5 minutes before adding more thickener, as it may take some time for liquids to thicken. Too much or too little thickener can make it difficult to swallow.

- **Drink plenty of thickened fluids.**
  People who need thickened liquids often do not get enough fluid each day and can become dehydrated. Ask your Doctor or Dietitian about your fluid needs. In general, aim for 8 cups of fluids each day.

- **Are straws okay?**
  Straws may make it harder to swallow. Your speech therapist will tell you if it is safe for you to use a straw when drinking.

- **Making ice cubes.**
  Using regular ice cubes will thin your beverages as the ice melts. If you want to put ice in your drinks, make your own ice with thickened water. Thicken water using the directions on your commercial thickener and freeze using ice cube trays.

Recipes:

Mint Chocolate Shake
½ cup mint flavored ice cream
½ cup chocolate pudding
½ cup cold chocolate Ensure Plus®

Peanut Butter Drink
½ cup cold vanilla Ensure Plus®
3 Tablespoons creamy peanut butter
3 Tablespoons chocolate syrup

Fruit Smoothie
½ banana
¼ cup peaches
¼ cup strawberries
½ cup orange juice

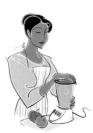

Vanilla Milk
¼ cup milk or vanilla soy milk
½ cup vanilla pudding

Resources:
Visit these websites for more information about your thickener:

- Nestle Nutrition Resource® Thickened Drinks: www.nestlenutritionstore.com
- Simply Thick® Thickened Drinks: www.simplythick.com
- Thick & Easy®: www.hormelhealthlabs.com
- Thick-It® Thickened Drinks: www.thickitretail.com

Clinical Dietitians & Dietetic Interns, Food & Nutrition Services, UC Davis Medical Center (9/10)
© 2010 The Regents of the University of California. All Rights Reserved.

UCDAVIS
HEALTH SYSTEM

When You Have Trouble Eating...

Eating a balanced diet may be difficult if you have:

- Trouble chewing your food due to mouth pain, dental problems, or other issues.
- Trouble swallowing, which can cause coughing, choking, or longer time to finish a meal.
- Shortness of breath or other breathing issues.
- Poor appetite.
- Higher calorie needs for weight gain or to prevent weight loss.
- Other _____

Tips to include all of the food groups and increase calories:

Grains (6 servings)	Hot cereal (cream of wheat, oatmeal, grits) or cold cereal with butter, Half and Half, honey, and/or sugar Toast with butter, jelly, cream cheese, honey, or peanut butter Milk toast (*soak toast in hot milk, and add sugar, cinnamon, melted butter*) Pancakes or French toast with extra butter and syrup Mashed potatoes with extra butter, cream cheese, heavy cream, sour cream, or cheese Pasta with butter, oil, or cream sauce Rice with butter or oil Potato soup Bread pudding
Meat & Other Proteins (5-6 oz)	Canned fish (tuna, salmon),Vienna sausage, canned or soft meats in sauce Meat, tuna, or cheese casserole Stew, chili, lentil soup, split pea soup, or other soups with meat or beans Lentils, canned or refried beans with cheese Tofu or other soy products (*add to soups, casseroles, sauces, etc*) Eggs (such as soft-boiled, poached, or scrambled with cheese, bacon, or avocado)
Vegetables (2 cups)	Fresh, canned, or cooked vegetables with melted cheese, butter, mayonnaise, or salad dressing Tomato or vegetable juice Homemade or canned vegetable soups Pureed yams, pureed winter squash
Fruits (2 cups)	100% fruit juice or fruit nectar Fresh, canned, or stewed fruits (*can add whipped cream*) Pureed fruits (such as applesauce) Fruit smoothies
Milk & Dairy (2 cups or more)	Milk, Lactaid® milk, flavored milk , soymilk (*choose 2% or whole milk to increase calories*) Hot chocolate made with milk Milk shakes or smoothies made with ice cream, frozen yogurt, or whole milk (*can add peanut butter or flavored syrup*) Yogurt, pudding, custard, ice cream Cream soups (such as chicken, mushroom, or asparagus) Cheeses (such as cream cheese, Laughing Cow® cheese, soft cheeses like Brie, or melted cheese dishes) Cottage cheese (*can add fruits, honey, or flavored syrup*)
To increase calories:	Add avocado, butter, mayonnaise, sour cream, cheese, cream cheese, salad dressing, olive oil, canola oil, Half and Half, whipped cream, honey, sugar, flavored syrup, peanut butter

If you still are not able to eat enough...

Add a nutrition supplement such as Carnation Instant Breakfast®, Ensure®, Ensure Plus®, Boost®, Slim Fast®, or store brand equivalents. Ask a pharmacy clerk to help you select or order the product you want.

Clinical Dietitians, Food & Nutrition Services, UC Davis Medical Center (4/09)

continues

Other Tips:

- If you have pain, be sure to tell your Doctor. There may be medications to help with the pain. If your pain is controlled, you will likely eat more.

- If solid food is hard to chew or swallow:
  - Foods can be put in a food processor or blender – let the machine do your chewing! Add broth, gravy, or other liquids to add moisture when blending.
  - Add Instant Breakfast to milk, Lactaid® milk, or soymilk.
  - Increase calories in your Instant Breakfast drink by adding ice cream to make a milkshake.
  - Store-bought nutrition supplements (Ensure Plus®, Boost®, Slim Fast®) are useful if you do not tolerate milk (look for generic brands, which cost less).

- Soups are a favorite. Choose higher calorie soups such as split pea, lentil, chili, clam chowder, or creamed soups made with milk. Cream-based soups are usually higher in calories than broth-based soups.
  - To add more protein to soups or other foods, mix in whey protein powder or powdered milk. Start by adding 1-2 Tbsp and increase according to taste.

- Breakfast foods can be eaten at any time of the day. Eggs are easy to chew and high in protein. Eggs can be prepared in different ways to give variety. Try eggs in French toast, quiche, or bread pudding.

- Eat more frequently. You should eat even if your appetite is poor.
  - Aim for 6-8 small meals (snack-sized), instead of 3 regular meals.
    - A snack can be a carton of yogurt, cottage cheese and fruit, an ice cream sandwich, or a nutrition supplement (such as Ensure®).

- Take a complete multivitamin supplement everyday. If it is hard to swallow a pill, try a children's *chewable* vitamin. If this is hard to chew, crush the multivitamin and eat with applesauce or pudding, or choose a liquid vitamin. Make sure your multivitamin has zinc and iron.

- If you are constipated, you may not eat as much. Constipation can be caused by pain pills, not enough water or fiber, or less physical activity. Talk with your Doctor about medication for constipation, or talk with your Dietitian for ideas to prevent constipation.

NOTES:

Clinical Dietitians, Food & Nutrition Services, UC Davis Medical Center (4/09)

11

Endoscopy in Assessing and Treating Dysphagia

Rebecca Leonard

Endoscopy is a valuable tool in both the assessment and treatment of dysphagic patients. The intent of this chapter is to describe both uses of the instrument in our clinic. Media clips of evaluations and treatment sessions incorporating endoscopy are included in files on the DVD accompanying this text. They can be found in the materials folder for Chapter 11.

procedure is now popularly referred to as "FEES." It has also been referred to as a videoendoscopic evaluation of dysphagia (VEED) (Bastian, 1991). In 1993, Aviv, Martin, Keen, Debell, and Blitzer described flexible endoscopy with sensory testing, referred to as "FEEST." The goal of the latter is to assess laryngeal sensation, but it may also involve an endoscopic assessment of swallowing.

FLEXIBLE ENDOSCOPY AS AN ASSESSMENT TOOL

Flexible endoscopic evaluation of swallowing safety (FEESS) was first described by Langmore, Schatz, and Olsen in 1988, and has been elaborated on frequently in the intervening period by these and other authors (Hyodo, Nishikubo, & Hirose, 2010; Kidder, Langmore, & Martin, 1994; Langmore, 2003; Langmore & McCullough, 1997; Langmore, Schatz, & Olsen, 1991; Suiter & Moorhead, 2007). The original "FEESS"

Preliminary Considerations (Equipment, supplies, patient preparation)

New technologies have greatly enhanced image quality associated with currently available flexible endoscopes. Contemporary videoscopes referred to as "chip in the tip" scopes include the camera chip in the scope's tip, that is, in very close proximity to structures visualized. These scopes offer superb image quality, but are quite expensive and may not be available in every setting. With older scope technology, the camera is attached to the scope's eyepiece, and structures are filmed through the fiber-optic bundle that directs light through the scope into the airway. Structures of interest are thus further away from the camera, and the light source is more limited. In some cases, this can impact observations possible. Faced with this situation, for example, when subtle silent aspiration is suspected, we have sometimes attempted imaging with a rigid oral endoscope (typically used in stroboscopic imaging of the larynx). Although this scope, inserted orally, is not in place during swallow, it can provide a large, very bright view of the larynx and other structures post-swallow. Using this strategy, we have identified small amounts of bolus material on the vocal folds, or even in the subglottic airway, that were not observed with the flexible scope. In short, quality of the study will vary depending on quality of the particular instrument used.

Bolus materials used in the evaluation vary according to clinician preferences, but typically reflect a range of consistencies and textures. Butler, Stuart, Case, Rees, Vitolins, et al. (2011) recently reported, in normal elderly subjects, significantly different scores on the Penetration Aspiration Scale (PAS) according to both liquid type (water vs. milk) and volume, with higher (poorer) scores noted for milk than for skim milk and water, and for larger, as compared to smaller, bolus sizes. Individual dysphagic patients may demonstrate not only variability, but serious limitations, in their management of various bolus types. Supplies that allow the clinician to vary bolus type, and also volume, and to do so in a uniform manner, are important considerations. Multiple options for introducing foods/liquids,

that is, spoon, cup, straw, should also be anticipated. All supplies need to be easily accessed, in particular, when only one clinician is available to perform the study. A FEES "kit" that contains bolus materials likely to accommodate the patient's needs, as well as other requirements of the exam, is useful.

A particular advantage of endoscopy is that it can be performed at bedside or in the clinic, ideally with the patient seated in an upright position. Although not trivial, particularly for inpatients, being able to keep the back straight while bending forward slightly from the waist is helpful. An anesthetic may also optimize the procedure. A topical anesthetic agent (lidocaine, 4%), usually combined with neosynephrine (0.25%) can be introduced to one nasal passage, the most open if there is a difference from left to right. A gel form of the anesthetic can be applied to the tip of the scope which is then inserted slowly into the nostril and held in a stable position until it takes effect. Alternatively, the anesthetic can be delivered in spray form. The topical anesthetic agent may allow the patient to accommodate the procedure more comfortably; however, if it interferes with sensation, study results may be confounded. Some clinicians have, in fact, refrained from using an anesthetic agent because of this concern. In a double-blind crossover study, Johnson, Belafsky, and Postma (2003) reported no differences in laryngopharyngeal sensory testing in patients who underwent multiple exams with different anesthetic agents and a saline sham, respectively. These authors used two sprays in each nostril, and each spray was 1 second in duration. As noted, we typically apply the agent used to only one nostril. If no anesthetic is used (this is most often our practice, and it is generally tolerated well by patients), a small amount of lubricating jelly on the scope may allow more comfortable insertion. The tip of the scope can be dipped into an antifogging agent, as well.

If there is a particular question about velar function, or about the degree of closure of the velopharyngeal port during swallow, the scope may be inserted between the inferior and middle turbinates to ensure a viewing position that will enable simultaneous visualization of the velum, and lateral and posterior pharyngeal walls. For observation of other structures during swallow, the scope is inserted along the floor of the nose. Observation of oropharyngeal structures is completed with the tip of the scope in the oropharynx, typically at or just below where the inferior soft palate would be at rest during quiet breathing (mouth closed), with the tongue base, piriform sinuses, posterior pharyngeal wall, posterior cricoid area, and laryngeal structures in view. Laryngeal structures are better viewed with the scope tip lower, at about the epiglottis, with the full length of the true vocal folds visible. With the scope appropriately placed, the patient is asked to engage in tasks directed to evaluating the integrity of swallowing structures, and the safety or efficiency of swallowing. Recording the evaluation permits not only the examiner but others present, including the patient, to view the study.

Indications for FEES

Evaluation of swallowing function with FEES does not provide the same information as a dynamic videofluoroscopic study (DSS) of swallow; rather, the two studies are probably best viewed as complementary to each other. Recent studies have demonstrated that the two exams may be equivalent in diagnosing dysphagia and implementing treatment strategies to facilitate safe and effective swallowing (Leder & Karas, 2000; Rees, 2006). Both exams have also been reported to be equally sensitive in identifying delayed initiation of swallow, penetration, aspiration, and post-swallow residue (Langmore, Shatz, & Olson, 1991; Leder, Sasaki, & Burrell, 1998). Aviv (2000) reported further that, whether dysphagic patients had their dietary and behavioral management directed by fluoroscopy or FEES with sensory testing, their outcomes with respect to the incidence of pneumonia or pneumonia-free time interval were essentially the same. In our view, there are a number of indications for FEES, some related to information provided by FEES but not videofluoroscopy, and others related to the exigencies of an endoscopic exam as opposed to a radiographic study.

Indications for FEES related to the unique type of information provided by the procedure include:

- Concerns about alterations in nasopharyngeal, oropharyngeal, or laryngeal anatomy that may not be apparent on videofluoroscopy. Certainly, the larynx and true vocal folds are better evaluated with endoscopy.
- Concerns about sensory integrity of pharyngeal and/or laryngeal structures.
- Concerns about the patient's ability to initiate and maintain airway protection over a given period of time.
- High risk of aspiration, where it is desirable to assess swallow function without food or liquid.

- Repeated swallows are of interest, as when there is a question of the patient fatiguing over time.
- It is desirable to assess symmetry of pharyngeal constriction, that is, differences from right to left. This can be done to some extent with fluoroscopy (in the anterior-posterior view), but endoscopy provides insights into the simultaneous contributions to constriction from both tongue and pharynx that are not possible with other techniques.
- It is desirable to provide "online" visual feedback to the patient or others.
- It is desirable to assess effects of various strategies, that is, head turning, breath holding, in a repeated fashion over time.

Indications related to the exigencies of the exam include the following:

- Patient cannot be transported to the site of a radiographic study.
- There are concerns about repeated exposure to radiation associated with videofluoroscopy, as when a patient's condition is changing rapidly over a brief period of time.
- Information is needed more quickly than scheduling a radiographic exam will permit.

Limitations of FEES

As noted, FEES cannot provide the examiner with all the same information that can be obtained from videofluoroscopy. For example, FEES does not allow evaluation of bolus management in the oral cavity. The patient's ability to form and hold a bolus in the mouth, transfer it from anterior to posterior oral cavity, and deliver it into the pharynx are better observed with fluoroscopy. Another limitation of FEES is that, during the moment of swallow, approximation of tongue and pharynx often precludes visualization of pertinent events. In addition, information regarding *degree* of pharyngeal constriction, opening of the upper esophageal sphincter, and hyoid/laryngeal elevation during the swallow is not available. This is important because the integrity of these gestures often explains the mechanics of dysphagia in an individual patient. Similarly, penetration or aspiration of the bolus, which occurs at, or in close proximity to, the time of swallow, may not be visualized, although it may be inferred after the swallow from inspection of laryngeal structures. Some clinicians would argue that FEES and fluoroscopy provide comparable information regarding subtle aspiration. In our experience, this depends on the quality of a FEES exam. We would suggest that, given comparable levels of exam quality and clinician skill, subtle aspiration is likely to be identified more often with fluoroscopy than with endoscopy. This may be particularly true when aspirated material is noted only below the vocal folds. In addition, most quantitative measures of timing and displacement, which can be obtained from radiographic studies, are not possible with FEES. Some clinicians have noted that endoscopy provides better information than fluoroscopy about the presence of secretions in the airway. In general, we would agree with this appraisal. However, if secretions are sufficiently copious, they may preclude endoscopic visualization of important structures. In such situations, fluoroscopy may be more useful.

FEES Versus Fluoroscopy in Assessment of Aspiration/ Penetration

Recently, investigators have considered the presence of penetration and/ or aspiration in normal subjects, using either FEES or fluoroscopy. Butler, Stuart, Markley, and Rees (2009) performed endoscopic evaluations on 20 normal elderly subjects (mean age 78.9 years), and observed a total of 520 swallows. Aspiration was identified in 6 of the subjects, on 3% of the swallows observed. Pentetration was observed in 15 of the subjects, on 15% of the swallows. Subsequently, we reviewed fluoroscopic studies performed on 149 normal subjects, approximately half under the age of 65 years and half over the age of 65 years (Allen, White, Leonard, & Belafsky, 2010). Across a total of 596 swallows, penetration was identified in 17 subjects and on 2.5% of swallows; aspiration was observed in only one subject, or .17% of swallows.

The explanation for such marked differences between studies is not completely clear, but two possibilities should be considered. First, the definition of penetration may differ depending on whether endoscopy or fluoroscopy is utilized. For example, bolus material observed on the laryngeal surface of the epiglottis is typically considered "penetration" on endoscopy. On fluoroscopy, however, bolus material may not be considered as "penetration" unless it more closely approximates the laryngeal vestibule, or violates the likely contact point between the arytenoids

and epiglottis during swallow (Figures 11–1, 11–2, and 11–3). Another problem, unique to fluoroscopy, is related to clinicians' efforts to minimize radiation

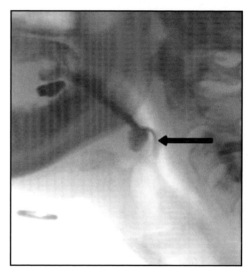

Figure 11–1. Bolus material on laryngeal surface of epiglottis would likely be defined as penetration on FEES; on our own fluoroscopy study, this would not be considered penetration.

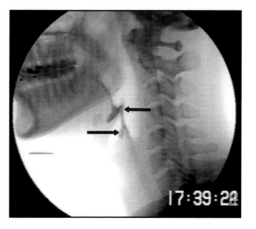

Figure 11–2. At upper arrow, bolus material would not be considered penetration on our fluoro study; material that penetrates laryngeal vestibule, shown at lower arrow, would be considered penetration.

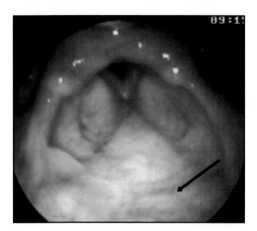

Figure 11–3. Material shown at arrow on endoscopic view would likely be considered penetration on endoscopy, and probably not on fluoroscopy.

exposure to patients. Typically, the fluoro unit is turned off immediately after completion of a swallow. If a patient aspirates *after* the swallow, when the airway is relaxed, the event may be missed. The problem can be minimized by first identifying patients who demonstrate residue after the swallow is completed. The fluoro unit can be turned off for a few seconds, and then turned on again, to determine if material has entered the airway. Our fluoro protocol calls for patients to be filmed, first, in lateral view, and turned for filming in the anterior-posterior view. In some instances, evidence of aspiration (again, of residue remaining after the swallow) can be observed when the patient is turned in this view.

Assessment Tasks

Specific tasks included in FEES will depend on a number of factors, including *how much the patient is able to tolerate without fatigue,* and *the direction the*

exam takes based on preliminary findings. In addition, some tasks may be included to address specific questions posed by the referring professional. Tasks designed to assess particular structures or functions are summarized below. In some instances, it may be both possible and desirable to perform all or most of them. But, as noted, the particular tasks included in the exam are very much dependent on the individual patient. What is reasonable in an outpatient who is recovering nicely from some incident or illness may be very different from what is possible in an inpatient who has been NPO (nothing by mouth) for days or weeks and is just being considered for limited oral eating. In all cases, the exam is begun when the patient is appropriately positioned, the scope has been inserted, and the structures of interest are in view. If the exam is being recorded and there is a need to provide feedback to the patient, the monitor should be placed so that both examiner and patient can easily refer to it. If the study is being performed by a sole examiner, it is, as noted previously, imperative to have all materials previously prepared and easily available.

Assessment of Valves and Chambers

One way to consider the structures of the upper airway is as a series of valves and chambers. Chambers, including the oral cavity, oropharynx, and hypopharynx, first expand to accommodate bolus material, and then compress. With compression, a gradient in favor of flow (from a region of higher pressure to a region of lower pressure) is established and bolus material is propelled and then cleared from the chamber. Failure of a chamber may thus impair both propulsion and clearing of bolus material. Valves, including the linguavelar, velopharyneal, laryngeal (including arytenoids and epiglottis, false vocal folds, and true vocal folds), and the pharyngoesopohageal segment (PES) regulate bolus flow from one chamber to the next. In doing so, they either appropriately permit or prevent bolus material from moving from chamber to chamber. Impairment in a valve may lead to early loss of the bolus, inappropriate entrance or reflux of bolus into a chamber and and/or ineffective bolus transmission. The first objective of FEES is to evaluate the integrity of these valves and chambers. Tasks for doing this are described next.

Tasks for Assessment of Velopharyngeal Valving

In a normal swallow, the velum first lowers, acting with the tongue to contain bolus material in the oral cavity. As the bolus is moved into the pharynx, the velum must then elevate to form another valve with the posterior and lateral pharyngeal walls. The rapid elevation of the velum may help to propel the bolus, and its valving action with the pharynx prevents bolus material from entering the nose. During speech, the area of the velopharyngeal orifice is typically less than 20 mm^2 for nonnasal sounds. At rest, this area is thought to be much larger; during speech, for example, areas greater than 100 mm^2 have been associated with the perception of extreme nasality (Warren & Mackler, 1968). During swallow, the area approximates zero. The tasks described here should allow the examiner to assess the valving function of the velum and corresponding lateral and posterior pharyngeal walls. (See "VPPORT" in Chapter 11 materials folder on DVD.)

- With the nasopharyngoscope between inferior and middle turbinates, the patient is asked to produce a sustained vowel sound, then a sustained /s/, and, if possible, a sentence that contains no nasal sounds ("Is Sassy sick?"). Elevation of the velum and constriction of the lateral and posterior pharyngeal walls are observed. Collectively, these structures contribute to closure of the velopharyngeal port during speech and swallow.

- Symmetry and contributions of each structure to closure are noted. Typically, one should see tighter closure for /s/ than for a vowel, and closure that is maintained for the duration of the sentence. Closure during a dry swallow can then be observed, and may be noted to be somewhat different from the closure for speech, for example, contact of structures may be lower. Following these tasks, the patient can be asked to swallow a small liquid bolus (1 to 3 cc). The velopharyngeal port is observed for any leakage of material into the nose. Alternatively, the examiner may elect to include this task in the evaluation of swallow function. (Figure 11–4)

Tasks for Assessment of Pharyngeal Chamber and Valve

The walls of the pharynx can constrict several millimeters in going from a relaxed to maximally constricted position.

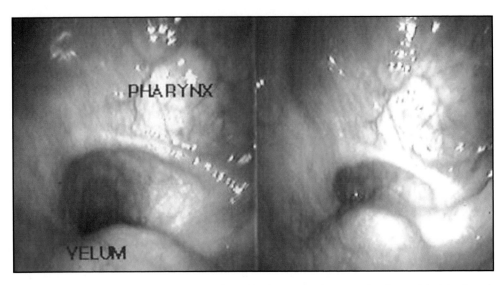

Figure 11–4. On left, velopharyngeal port is shown during production of /n/ (velum is at bottom, posterior pharyngeal wall at top, and lateral pharyngeal walls on right and left, respectively); on right, port is shown during closure for vowel /i/.

Normative data from our laboratory, in fact, suggest that mean pharyngeal area in a pseudorest position, measured in the lateral view from videofluoroscopic studies and thus representing only two of three dimensions of the pharynx (anterior-posterior and superior-inferior, but not lateral or left-right), approximates 8.5 cm^2 (measure corrected for age and gender) with a 1-cc bolus held in the oral cavity. At the point of maximum constriction and shortening during swallow, this value approximates zero. (These measures are discussed at length in Chapters 16 and 17.) During swallow, sequential changes in both size and shape of the pharynx help to propel the bolus from mouth to esophagus. The tasks described here should allow the examiner to observe the patient's potential for effecting appropriate pharyngeal dynamics. (The reader is encouraged to view the video clips "OROPHX" and "HYPOPHX" included in the Chapter 11 materials folder on the DVD while reviewing these tasks.)

- Scope is advanced along the floor of nose into the oropharynx, being sure to find a placement that will allow pharyngeal structures to be observed when the soft palate elevates. The patient is asked to produce /a/, pronounced "ah," and to then retract or move the tongue posteriorly in an attempt to produce pharyngeal frication, that is, fricative-like sound produced by forcing air across a constriction of posterior tongue to pharynx. Contact between tongue base and posterior pharynx is observed. Not all patients will be able to perform this task, but if they are able to attempt it, the information is very useful (Figures 11–5, 11–6, 11–7, and 11–8).

- Piriform sinuses, valleculae, pharyngeal walls, base of tongue, and

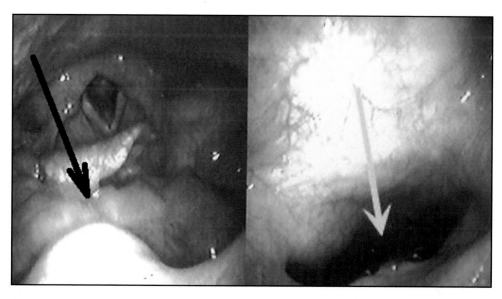

Figure 11–5. Oropharynx expanded (*left*) and then compressed (*right*) as subject moves tongue (*at arrows*) posteriorly. Scope is just above oropharynx, at about the velum.

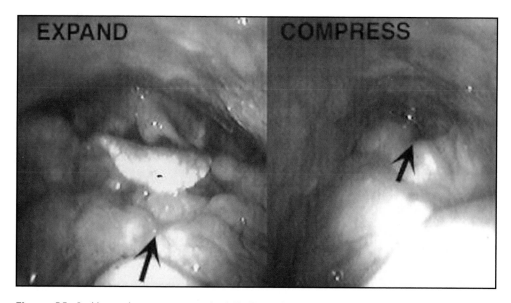

Figure 11–6. Hypopharynx expanded (*left*) and compressed (*right*); scope tip is below velum.

postcricoid area are examined for evidence of pooled secretions (Figure 11–9). At sites of pooling, examiner may want to lightly touch the tissue with the scope tip and ask the patient to respond when the stimulus is felt. In the normal case, there should be no or

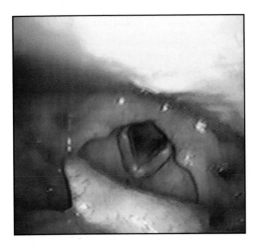

Figure 11-7. Scope tip is just above epiglottis. Pharynx is expanded.

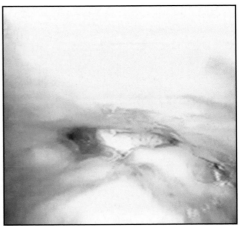

Figure 11-8. Scope tip above epiglottis; pharynx compressed (not a swallow). Upper portion of epiglottis can be seen between tongue base and posterior pharyngeal wall.

minimal secretions at these sites, perhaps only a few bubbles, and even light touch with the scope tip should elicit a response. The presence of pooling may indicate poor sensation, or poor ability to clear tissues. If pooled secretions clear well with swallow, sensation may be implicated. Secretions that do not clear with swallow, on the other hand, may suggest incomplete or ineffective movements of structures. In some patients, sensory and motor functions may both be impaired.

■ Ask patient to elevate vocal pitch to as high a level as possible. Observe pharyngeal constriction. Note presence or absence, and whether there is a difference from one side to the other. Typically, the pharynx does constrict during this task. The maneuver is sometimes described as a surrogate measure of pharyngeal strength, but this has yet to be documented. However, intact pharyngeal squeeze has been associated with a reduced

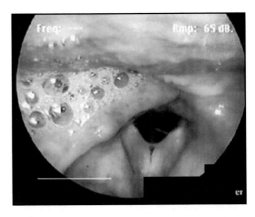

Figure 11-9. Thin secretions in right piriform sinus; thick secretions appear as folds in left piriform sinus and postcricoid area.

risk of aspiration on pureed foods, independent of laryngopharyngeal sensation (Perlman, Cohen, and Setzen, et al., 2004).

■ Ask patient to hold the nose and bear down. Observe piriform sinuses for maximal opening. Have patient relax and observe return of sinuses to rest.

■ Ask patient to turn head from one side to the other. Observe closure of piriform sinuses (Figure 11–10). Note, in particular, asymmetries from right to left that may suggest weakness.

Tasks for Assessment of Laryngeal Chamber and Valves

Typically, the larynx acts to protect the airway and assist in opening of the PES during swallow. The tasks described here allow the examiner to assess the ability of the larynx to close, thereby protecting the airway, and to elevate, further protecting the airway and facilitating opening of the PES. The tasks also consider the ability of the larynx to respond to bolus materials that may come in contact with its structures.

■ With the scope lowered to approximately the epiglottis, ask the patient to sustain a vowel sound for several seconds (a high, front vowel sound, such as "ee," typically causes the larynx to elevate, and facilitates visualization of laryngeal structures). If good visualization of the larynx is dif-

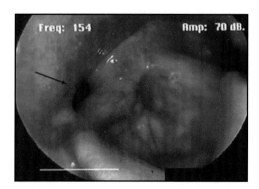

Figure 11–10. Piriform sinus on right is compressed with head turned to right.

ficult because of elevation of the soft palate, a nasal sound, such as a sustained "mmm," may be used for this task. Observe the mobility of the true vocal folds, the completeness of closure of the true vocal folds along their anterior to posterior dimension, and the length of time they remain in an adducted position (patients with impaired swallow may need to protect the airway for several seconds). Note the quality of the voice produced. Incomplete closure, inability to maintain closure, and weak, breathy voice quality may be indicative of vocal fold dysfunction and compromised ability to protect the airway.

■ With the scope held in as constant position as possible, ask the patient to produce a vowel at a low vocal pitch, and to then shift to as high a pitch as possible. Note changes in length of vocal folds, any elevation of laryngeal structures, and patient's ability to raise pitch (Figure 11–11). Typically, raising pitch (fundamental frequency) is associated with the larynx elevating, and often, with pharyngeal constriction. An inability to alter pitch in this way may indicate some dysfunction of the superior laryngeal nerve, or cricothyroid muscle, or of the suprahyoid muscles of the larynx.

■ Observe patient's ability to produce a series of brief /i/ sounds ("i" is pronounced as the vowel in "P*e*te"), each of which is followed by inspiration (preferably, through the nose). Instructing the patient to sniff after vocalization may facilitate the task. Watch for

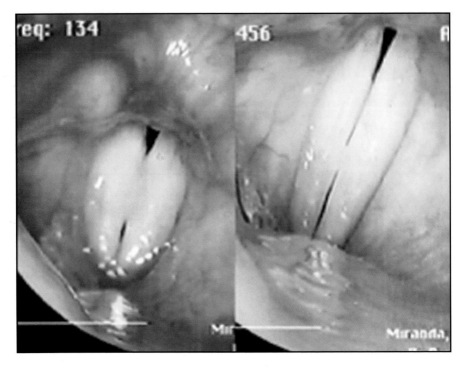

Figure 11-11. With scope held in place at patient's nostril, patient is asked to alternate between low (*on left*) and high-pitched (on right) /i/s. True folds elongate and also appear to elevate on high-pitched production (note enlarged size of superior arytenoid cartilages, as well as of true folds).

obvious or subtle asymmetries in abduction and adduction of the true vocal folds that could indicate a paralysis or paresis of one fold.

■ Ask the patient to hold his or her breath (Figure 11–12). Observe degree of adduction of true folds, as well as any constriction/medialization of the false folds, and/or approximation of the arytenoids to the epiglottis. Typically, the false folds are closed during breath holding. With tight breath holding, the larynx may appear sphincteric, with the false folds constricted and arytenoids approximating the epiglottis. This task is a good way to evaluate all the valves of the larynx. In Figure 11–13, a

patient has gagged and the larynx has rocked forward, opening the PES. This rocking action of the larynx is also associated with opening of the PES valve during swallow, which is not typically observed during FEES.

■ Observe effectiveness of true fold adduction for throat clearing and cough.

Tasks for Assessment of Swallow Function

Requirements for normal swallow include the transfer of a bolus quickly and safely from the oral cavity through the pharynx to the upper esophagus. The tasks described here allow the examiner

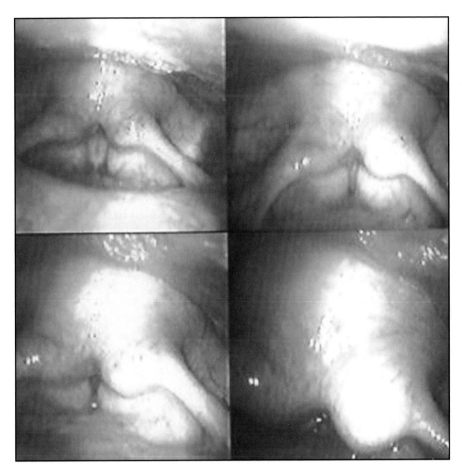

Figure 11–12. During tight breath holding, true vocal folds close, then false folds constrict, followed by approximation of arytenoids to epiglottis.

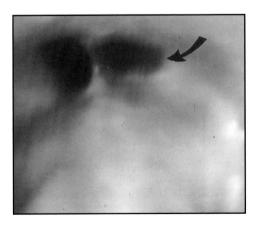

Figure 11–13. During gag, the cricoid can be seen to rock forward, and the PES opens (*at arrow*).

to assess several events before and after swallow that are critical to this process.

With the scope positioned back in the oropharynx, bolus materials are introduced, starting with a small amount of liquid that has been colored green with food coloring (i.e., edible vegetable dyes). In our clinic, the standard exam is begun with a 1 to 3-cc liquid bolus, or a small amount of ice chips. Ice chips may be particularly helpful in patients who have not been eating orally for a period of time (Rees, 2006). With the scope positioned appropriately for observing relevant structures, the patient is asked to perform the following:

- Hold the bolus in the mouth until the examiner counts to three, then swallow. Any early loss of the bolus into the valleculae or piriform sinuses, or any penetration or aspiration of bolus material prior to the swallow, is noted.
- Following the swallow, sites previously examined (i.e., nose, valleculae, piriform sinuses, tongue base, pharyngeal walls, postcricoid area, and true and false vocal folds) are examined for evidence of residue. Sites and sidedness of residue material, and estimate (if possible) of how much of bolus introduced appears as residue, are noted.
- If residue is observed, evidence of repeat swallow is noted. If none is observed, the patient is asked to repeat the swallow. Any clearing that takes place during the repetition is noted.
- If residue is present on the vocal folds, cough or throat-clearing responses are noted. If no response is noted, the patient is asked to cough and then repeat the swallow. Effectiveness in clearing residue is assessed.
- If the swallow approximates normal, the examiner is unlikely to actually observe the instant of swallow because constriction of tongue and pharynx obscures visualization. In patients with weak tongue–pharynx constriction, however, it may be possible to obtain more information.

Following swallow of the small bolus, the patient repeats the tasks with a 3 to 5-cc liquid bolus, and then a larger self-selected bolus in a cup. For the latter task, the patient selects how much of the bolus material he or she wants to attempt. These tasks are repeated for the larger liquid boluses if it appears safe to do so, and with pudding if difficulties are encountered on any of the liquid swallows. If the liquid swallows are managed without incident, the pudding bolus is replaced with a paste bolus (e.g., peanut butter).

These assessment tasks represent similar tasks, in the same order, as those used in videofluoroscopic studies at our institution. Bolus materials used for FEES typically do not contain radiopaque material, but they do represent similar consistencies and a similar order of presentation. The reason for this is twofold. If you anticipate following a patient over time, the ability to repeat at least some of the same tasks from exam to exam permits more uniform assessment of progress or deterioration over time. Furthermore, if both fluoroscopy and endoscopy studies are performed on a patient, completion of a portion of the same or very similar tasks on both provides some basis of comparison across evaluation techniques.

When these protocol swallows are complete, specific foods that have been identified as causing particular difficulty for a patient can be tried. Or, if the objective is to determine if a patient's diet needs to be altered, either advanced or restricted, the exam can be tailored to answer these questions. In following patients serially, it is important to maintain a balance between identifying changes in integrity of structures and functions, and changes in swallowing capabilities. Attempting to adhere to a protocol, that is, some uniformity in tasks and task order across exams, can in our opinion usually be accomplished even with patients whose tolerance for the exam is quite limited.

Implications of Findings

By the completion of the FEES evaluation, the examiner should have good insights into the integrity of oropharyngeal and laryngeal structures and functions for food management and swallowing. For example, the patient's ability to effect linguavelar, velopharyngeal, linguapharyngeal and laryngeal *valving actions* necessary for safe and effective swallowing should be well understood. Impressions gained will lead to therapeutic strategies directed at improving, bypassing, or compensating for any deficits identified. Similarly, indications of *diminshed sensation* identified during the examination will require consideration of strategies that may enhance sensory stimulation, as by manipulating bolus characteristics or redirecting bolus materials to a more intact side or site. In like manner, the patient's *ability to compensate* for the early loss of bolus material, or residue remaining after an attempted swallow, will have been sampled across bolus materials, and in terms of both sites and amounts of loss or residue noted. The resulting observations will enter into decisions regarding whether oral feeding is safe, or under what conditions it can be made safer.

As noted, a particular appeal of FEES is the opportunity it provides for assessing the likely benefit of behavioral strategies via *therapeutic probes* (including the effects of positional changes, voluntary maneuvers, bolus manipulation,

etc.) The length of the examination is constrained by the patient's comfort and attention levels, but not greatly by concerns about hazards associated with the examination technique, itself. Trial probes performed with both examiner and patient observing the consequences on the video monitor are particularly useful. The ability to make *observations over time* is another feature of FEES that adds to its value. Evidence of fatigue in valving functions, consequences of collective swallows, or residue buildup, over precise periods of time, are examples of the kinds of time-delay observations that can have implications for treatment planning and can be explored more thoroughly with endoscopic evaluation than with other assessment techniques.

FLEXIBLE ENDOSCOPY AS A THERAPEUTIC TOOL

Endoscopy is an extremely valuable assessment tool, and an equally useful tool in the management of dysphagic patients. Very often in our setting, patients who have undergone fluoroscopy studies, and for whom particular strategies have been identified as potentially useful, are brought in for at least one therapy session to explore in depth the strategies previously identified. During these sessions, the emphasis is on assessing the effects of strategies, and on providing clinician, patient and other caregivers with feedback regarding these techniques. The conduct of these sessions is different from an assessment with FEES, particularly if they occur in close proximity to the fluoroscopy evaluation and there is no evidence of significant change in the patient's capabilities.

Noted below are therapeutic swallowing strategies, that is, strategies designed to facilitate safe swallowing. Visual feedback provided to the patient during their performance may be useful in teaching their effectiveness and in improving the patient's control of volitional gestures involved. (The reader is directed to the "FEESPT1" clip in the Chapter 11 materials folder on the DVD for an example. The patient in this clip has undergone base of tongue/pharynx resection for head and neck cancer.)

- Tongue–pharynx constriction: Ask the patient to produce "ah" or "uh," and to then move the tongue posteriorly until pharyngeal frication can be produced.
- Pharyngeal constriction by producing high-pitched vocalization.
- Laryngeal elevation by raising pitch, or rapid alternation of high and low pitches.
- Breath holding, with true vocal folds, and with sphincteric closure involving true and false vocal folds, and arytenoid to epiglottis approximation.
- Effects of postural changes, such as head turning or sidelying. Note changes in voice and breath holding, but also any closing off of piriform sinuses.

Equally important in attempting strategies that have been identified as potentially helpful to safe or effective swallow is the determination of any *aversive* consequences of these strategies. For example, the reader is directed to video clip "FEESPT2" in the Chapter 11 materials folder on the DVD. In this clip, a patient for whom airway protection has been determined to be impaired is counseled to hold his breath during swallow. Because his transit times have been determined (via dynamic fluoroscopic swallow study) to be prolonged, he is encouraged to hold his breath tightly for several seconds, thereby protecting his airway throughout the swallow. With the patient complying with this instruction, that is, "Hold your breath, tighter . . . tighter . . . " for a few seconds, a massive reflux event occurs that imperils his airway. This was not observed on fluoroscopy and, had we not scheduled the endoscopic follow-up to assess the effectiveness and safety of our recommendations, the strategy would have been recommended to the patient with no recognition of the potential aversive consequences it posed to his safe swallowing. We view this type of postevaluation appraisal of any behavioral strategies recommended as a necessary and valuable part of our management plan for a patient.

ISSUES AND CONCERNS

Major issues associated with endoscopic examination include the examiner(s), the setting in which the exam is performed, the use of a topical anesthetic, and other risks posed by the procedure. The examiner, whether physician or speech pathologist, should be skilled in the use of flexible endoscopy, and, of course, knowledgeable about both head and neck anatomy, and the particular physiology of swallowing. The setting or settings in which the exam is performed should have both staff and equipment resources to respond appropriately to a medical emergency. Some states, including California, require that speech-language pathologists complete a certification program beyond licensure in order to perform endoscopy procedures (details are specified in California Senate Bills 1379 and 1285). Specific requirements (in California) include the speech pathologist's mentoring by an otolaryngologist during the completion of 25 flexible endoscopic procedures. The physician must then document the speech-language pathologist's competency to perform the exam. Beyond this requirement, settings in which the procedure can be performed must meet certain requirements regarding the availability of medical professionals and resources for the management of a medical emergency.

Potential risks associated with the procedure include vasovagal responses, nose bleed, and a reaction to the topical anesthetic (if used). Much can be done to minimize the likelihood of any of these risks, for example, by taking pains to put the patient at ease before proceeding with the exam, careful insertion of the scope, limitation of the anesthetic agent to the nasal mucosa (and away from the larynx), or performing the exam without an anesthetic. Precautions for cleaning and maintaining equipment must be observed strictly, as well. Even with careful adherence to these guidelines, however, the potential risks associated with the procedure require that it be undertaken, in our opinion, in a setting with resources available for handling any emergencies that might arise. In our setting, all patients who are undergoing bedside, clinical, radiographic, or endoscopic evaluations for dysphagia are followed by a team of professionals, all of whom share in the evaluation of diagnostic studies and treatment planning for each patient. Similarly, specific guidelines for use of topical anesthetic agents, responses to medical emergencies, and cleaning and maintenance of equipment have been developed by our institution. Beyond this, our team has invested considerable time and energy in continuing education activities, both formal and didactic, to ensure that specialists who are performing endoscopic examinations are well-qualified to do so. Depending on individual specialists, patient populations, and settings, different approaches to endoscopic swallow studies may be applicable and appropriate. However, in our opinion, any approach must maximize the patient's safety and ensure the most accurate information possible.

STUDY QUESTIONS

1. What is the difference between FEES and FEEST?
2. What are the concerns about using a topical anesthetic agent in assessing dysphagic patients with FEES? What other risks are associated with FEES?
3. What aspects of swallowing typically *cannot* be observed during FEES that can be observed with fluoroscopy?
4. Name five indications for using FEES rather than the MBS/DSS.
5. Name the physiologic "valves" and "chambers" involved in swallowing. What tasks might you use to assess the integrity of each with endoscopy?
6. How might you use endoscopy to implement information about a patient's swallow learned from a fluoroscopic study?

7. What is the advantage of using a standard protocol when assessing dysphagia with FEES?
8. What might explain differences in judgments of aspiration and penetration on FEES and fluoroscopy, respectively?

REFERENCES

Allen, J. E., White, C. J., Leonard, R. J., & Belafsky, P. C. (2010). Prevalence of penetration and aspiration on videofluoroscopy in normal individuals without dysphagia. *Otolaryngology-Head and Neck Surgery, 142*, 208–213.

Aviv, J. (2000). Prospective, randomized outcome study of endoscopy versus modified barium swallow in patients with dysphagia. *Laryngoscope, 110*, 563–574.

Aviv, J. E., Martin, J. H., Keen, M. S., Debell, M., & Blitzer, A. (1993). Air pulse quantification of supraglottic and pharyngeal sensation: A new technique. *Annals of Otology Rhinology and Laryngology, 102*, 777–780.

Bastian, R. W. (1993). The videoendoscopic swallowing study: An alternative and partner to the videofluoroscopic swallowing study. *Dysphagia, 8*, 359–367.

Butler, S. G., Stuart, A., Case, L. D., Rees, C., Vitolins, M., & Kritchevsky, S. B. (2009). Effects of liquid type, delivery method, and bolus volume on penetration-aspiration scores in healthy older adults during flexible endoscopic evaluation of swallowing. *Annals of Otology, Rhinology, and Laryngology, 120*, 288–295.

Butler, S. G., Stuart, A., Markley, L., & Rees, C. (2011). Penetration and aspiration in healthy older adults as assessed during endoscopic evaluation of swallowing. *Annals of Otology, Rhinology, and Laryngology, 118*, 190–198.

Hyodo, M., Nishikubo, K., & Hirose, K. (2010). New scoring proposed for endoscopic swallowing evaluation and clinical significance. *Nihon Jibiinkoka Gakkai Kaiho, 113*, 670–678.

Johnson, P. E., Belafsky, P. C., & Postma, G. N. (2003). Topical nasal anesthesia for transnasal fiberoptic laryngoscopy: A prospective, double-blind, crossover study. *Otolaryngology-Head and Neck Surgery, 128*, 452–454.

Kidder, T. M., Langmore, S. E., & Martin, B. J. (1994). Indications and techniques of endoscopy in evaluation of cervical dysphagia: Comparison with radiographic techniques. *Dysphagia, 9*, 256–261.

Langmore, S. (2003). Evaluation of oropharyngeal dysphagia: which diagnostic tool is superior? *Current Opinion in Otolaryngology-Head and Neck Surgery, 11*, 485–489.

Langmore, S. E., & McCulloch, T. M. (1997). Examination of the pharynx and larynx and endoscopic examination of pharyngeal swallowing. In A. Perlman & K. Schulze-Delrieu (Eds.), *Deglutition and its disorders* (pp. 201–226). San Diego, CA: Singular.

Langmore, S. E., Schatz, K., & Olson, N. (1988). Fiberoptic endoscopic evaluation of swallowing safety: A new procedure. *Dysphagia, 2*, 216–219.

Langmore, S. E., Schatz, K., & Olson, N. (1991). Endoscopic and videofluoroscopic evaluations of swallowing and aspiration. *Annals of Otology and Rhinology, 100*, 678–681

Leder, S. B., & Karas, D. E. (2000). Fiberoptic endoscopic evaluation of swallowing in the pediatric population. *Laryngoscope, 110*, 1132–1136.

Leder, S. B., Sasaki, C. T., & Burrell, M. I. (1998). Fiberoptic endoscopic examination to identify silent aspiration. *Dysphagia, 13*, 19–21.

Perlman, P. W., Cohen, M. A., Setzen, M., Belafsky, P. C., Guss, J., & Mattucci, K. F., & Ditkoff, M. (2004). The risk of aspiration of pureed food as determined by flexible endoscopic evaluation of swallowing with sensory testing. *Otolaryngology-Head and Neck Surgery, 130,* 80–83.

Rees, C. (2006). Flexible endoscopic evaluation of swallowing with sensory testing. *Current Opinion in Otolaryngology-Head and Neck Surgery, 14,* 425–430.

Setzen, M., Cohen, M. A., Perlman, P. W., Belafsky, P. C., Guss, J., Mattucci, K. F., & Ditkoff, M. (2003). The association between laryngopharyngeal sensory deficits, pharyngeal motor function, and the prevalence of aspiration with thin liquids. *Otolaryngology-Head and Neck Surgery, 128,* 99–102.

Suiter, D., & Moorehead, M. K. (2007). Effects of flexible fiberoptic endoscopy on pharyngeal swallow physiology. *Otolaryngology-Head and Neck Surgery, 137,* 956–958.

Warren, D., & Mackler, S. B. (1968). Duration of oral port constriction in normal and cleft palate speech. *Journal of Speech and Hearing Research, 11,* 391–401.

12

Radiographic Evaluation of the Pharynx and Esophagus

Jacqui Allen

INDTRODUCTION

Radiographic examination of the pharynx is typically referred to as a dynamic swallowing study, and is accomplished by videofluoroscopy, or videoradiography. Other radiographic methods that can be used for examination of the pharynx include cineradiography and rapid sequence digital radiography, ultrasound (USS), computed tomography (CT) or magnetic resonance imaging (MRI). Recently, dynamic MRI techniques (cine-MRI, turbo-FLASH MRI), which are free of ionizing radiation, have been described to assess swallow (Amin, Lazarus, Pai, Mulholland, Shepard, Branski, & Wang, 2012; Hartl, Kolb, Bretagne, Marandas, & Sigal, 2006; Kitano, Asada, Hayashi, Inoue, & Kitajima, 2002; Kreeft, Rasch, Muller, Pameijer, Hallo, & Balm, 2012). However, technical limitations, that is, poor temporal resolution, supine position-

ing, and expense have to date limited their wide application. Radiographic examination of the esophagus is termed a barium meal or swallow, or esophagram. This study is often combined with examination of the stomach and duodenum. The pharynx and esophagus may be examined together in one sitting or may be examined separately. To obtain optimal information from the examination and minimize radiation exposure, it is important to have an understanding of the indications and technique for each of these examinations.

Description of Equipment

Examination of the pharynx and esophagus is generally performed in a fluoroscopy suite that is equipped with a system for rapid sequence filming. The rapid sequence recording is necessary because the process of swallowing occurs quickly (pharyngeal phase is typically less than 1s), and in order to analyze the swallowing process, this capability must be available. Previously, cineradiography was utilized but with the advent of digital processing this has largely become obsolete. Cineradiography has been replaced by videofluoroscopy, which is a recording of the fluoroscopic image by a videorecorder and magnetic tape, or frequently now onto digital media. Although spatial resolution is less than with cineradiography, it is generally adequate for most studies. It has the advantages of less radiation exposure, easier manipulation of the images, and the ability to record sound. More recently, rapid sequence digital radiography which is capable of rapid sequence filming of up to six frames per second has become available. Advantages of this system include excellent spatial resolution, easy manipulation of the images, including brightness and contrast changes, and relatively low radiation exposures. The chief disadvantages are too few frames per second for some studies, and its lack of availability in many departments. Newly developed cine-MRI and turbo-FLASH MRI sequences can acquire up to 24 frames per second. This may offer the opportunity to examine deglutition with less (or no) ionizing radiation. However, a large magnet (3T) MRI machine is required, which (as yet) is not commonplace in most radiology departments.

Radiation Exposure and Safety

Exposure to radiation occurs with examination of both the pharynx and esophagus. For this reason, patients should be carefully evaluated before these studies are done to determine with certainty that the examination is indicated. This is of particular concern with younger patients and female patients. Younger patients are up to 10 times more susceptible to injury from radiation exposure than older patients. Radiation dose is cumulative and the National Council for Radiation Protection (NCRP) and International Atomic Energy Association (IAEA) support the linear non-threshold theory. This states that there is no "safe" dose of radiation and that all medical radiation should conform to the ALARA principle—As Low As Reasonable Achievable (http://www.imagegently.org; http://www.acr.org). It is now estimated that between 1 to 2% of cancers are induced by medical radiation (Smith-Bindman, Lipson, Marcus, Kim, Mahesh, Gould, Berrington de González, & Miglioretti, 2009; Berrington de Gonzalez, Mahesh, & Kim et al, 2009) and that the lifetime relative risk of cancer from screening radiological procedures may range from 4 to 7 per 1,000 for men and 6 to 13 per 1,000 for women (Berrington de González, 2011). All clinicians ordering tests involving ionizing radiation must be cognizant of the risks and benefits of the procedure.

The referring physician, radiologist, and speech pathologist should all be involved in the decision to perform a study. In addition, individuals conducting the examination should have knowledge of radiation exposure and use appropriate protection from radiation, for both the patient and the individuals conducting the examination. Radiation exposure to the patient can be measured in several ways, including skin exposure, gonadal dose, and total body exposure, and expressed in different units including gray, rads, or seiverts. The seivert is preferred as it is a unit that has been normalized for the tissue effects of radiation. Different tissues have different levels of susceptibility to radiation and this is normalized by the seivert measurement allowing comparison of doses independent of the site receiving the radiation. An alternative method is to use the dose area product (DAP) which is a measure of effective radiation dose. When combined with a standardized multiplier determined by the tissue characteristics of the exposed tissue, the DAP can yield information regarding the true tissue exposure.

Of particular concern in examination of the pharynx and upper esophagus is radiation exposure to the thyroid. Radiation exposure of the lens of the eye is also an important issue when the head and neck are exposed to radiation. A comparison of radiation exposure for the techniques used for radiographic swallowing studies is seen in Table 12–1. Factors affecting radiation dose include: kilovolt peak (kVp), which is the peak voltage across the x-ray tube; milliampere seconds (mAs), which is the tube current multiplied by exposure time; image field size; source to skin distance; source to detector distance; and use of a grid. Most modern fluoroscopic machines incorporate safety features to minimize radiation such as beam coning, last frame hold, automatic kVp adjustment, grid removal, and adjustable frame rates. Operators should employ appropriate shielding, reduce screening time to the minimum needed to achieve the required information, and avoid backscatter by removing objects within the beam path. The patient should always be positioned closest to the detector and staff should stand a minimum of 5 feet from the beam emitter whenever possible.

During a normal year we are exposed to approximately 3 mSv of background radiation. One chest x-ray imparts an additional 0.01 mSv of radiation, while travelling on an international trans-Atlantic flight would expose passengers to 0.04 mSv of additional radiation. Most fluoroscopic swallowing studies are estimated to deliver doses in the range of 0.04 to 1 mSv depending on total fluoroscopy time (Table 12–2). Chau and Kung recently measured VFSS dose using the DAP in patients undergoing studies for neurological abnormalities or after radiation to the head and neck. They demonstrated a mean DAP of 2.42 ± 2.04 Gy cm² for an effective dose of 0.31 (± 0.26) mSv for all studies, well within the quoted range (Chau & Kung, 2009). Mean fluoroscopy time was 4.23 minutes (± 2.56 minutes). When they compared the dose and screening time for stroke patients versus patients treated with radiation for nasopharyngeal cancer the mean dose and screening time was significantly greater in the stroke patients: 2.61 versus 1.80 Gy cm², and 4.26 versus 3.65 minutes.

Table 12–1. Radiation Dose Rate During Videofluoroscopy Swallowing Study (mGy/min)*

Projection	Skin	Thyroid
Posterior-anterior	9.5	.27
Lateral	7.7	.99

*Exposure factors include: Automatic brightness control with 65 kVp, 1.1 mA, 8:1 grid, source to skin distance—46 cm, source to detector distance—86 cm, 9″ field of view.

Table 12–2. Radiation Dose Comparison

Test Situation	Radiation Dose (mSv)
Chest x-ray	0.01
Annual background radiation	3
Trans-Atlantic aircraft flight	0.04
Videofluoroscopic swallowing study	0.04–1
CT scan (head)	2
CT scan (abdominal)	5

Indications

History and clinical examination provide invaluable information in assessing the dysphagic patient; however, they are unable to detect silent aspiration: one of the leading causes of disability and death in patients with neurological conditions, head and neck cancer, head and neck trauma, or following surgery (Garon, Sierzant, & Ormiston, 2009; Ramsey, Smithard, & Kalra, 2003, 2005). An instrumental examination is required to fully assess the pharyngeal and esophageal phases of swallowing. This may be accomplished endoscopically or radiographically. The optimal radiographic procedure is the DSS. DSS provides critical information regarding the transit and pathway of the bolus through the oropharynx, hypopharynx, pharyngoesophageal segment, and esophagus. This examination is indicated in patients presenting with persistent dysphagia, odynophagia, aspiration, pulmonary pathology, chronic cough, regurgitation, or weight loss, after surgery or radiotherapy to the head and neck, and, in some cases, for those with symptoms of reflux or esophageal pathology (chest pain or pressure).

The study should only be requested after assessment by either a physician or speech language pathologist (or preferably both). Because radiation exposure is involved careful consideration must be given to performing the optimal study in the shortest possible time. Although a protocol is essential, the clinician performing the procedure must be familiar with the patient's symptoms, signs and indications for the examination. In this way the DSS can be tailored to answer the clinical question and minimize screening time. Specific maneuvers or strategies can be tested during the study to enable safe treatment recommendations. Contraindications to esophageal examination with standard barium swallow and esophagram include inability of the patient to swallow, obstruction of the pharynx or esophagus, and a strong likelihood of aspiration. These problems are minimized with the dynamic swallow study.

Examination Technique

Because of its general availability and ability to demonstrate motion, videofluoroscopy is the method most often used for swallowing studies and other examinations of the pharynx. The examination is performed in the standing or sitting position using a standard fluoroscopy table in the upright position. For patients who are unable to support themselves, chairs have been developed that provide support for the patient's head and neck. The examination is usually performed first in the lateral position. The patient takes a bolus of barium (about 60% weight/volume) into the mouth and is instructed to swallow while a recording is made from the oral cavity to the cervical esophagus. Structures that are visualized include the base of the tongue, valleculae, epiglottis, piriform sinuses, pharyngoesophageal segment, and cervical esophagus (Figure 12–1) (Dodds, 1989; Dodds, Stewart, & Logemann, 1990). In the normal person, the passage of a bolus of barium from the mouth to the cervical esophagus takes approximately one second. A similar recording of a swal-

low is then done in the frontal (anteroposterior, AP) projection (Figures 12–2 and 12–3). The valleculae and piriform sinuses are usually better seen in this projection, whereas the epiglottis and cricopharyngeus muscle are less well visualized. Some pathologies, such as Zenker's diverticulum, may be better viewed from this position, as well (Figure 12–4). Asymmetries reflecting unilateral weakness, for example, of the pharynx, are also likely to be better appreciated in the frontal view. In both projections recordings are made while

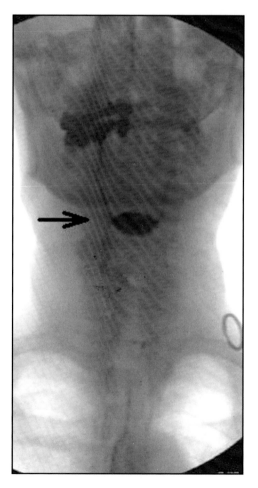

Figure 12-1. Lateral view of the pharynx. The base of the tongue and uvula are indicated by arrows. The cricopharynx muscle is completely relaxed and therefore not seen.

Figure 12-2. Anterior posterior view of the pharynx. Residue is noted in the valleculae.

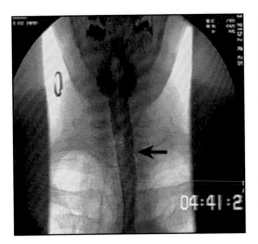

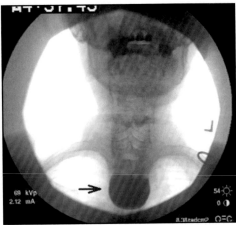

Figure 12–3. Slight narrowing in anterior posterior view reflects location of cricopharyngeus m.

Figure 12–4. Zenker's diverticulum (*at arrow*) is filled with barium in anterior posterior view.

the patient swallows several different quantities and consistencies of barium, and in some cases, swallowing is evaluated with a bolus of food mixed with barium.

Findings of particular interest that may be observed during DSS in the oropharynx include inadvertent passage of barium into the airway, termed penetration (when material remains above the vocal folds) or aspiration (when material passes through the vocal folds). DSS is an extremely sensitive tool in identifying airway violation, in particular when aspiration occurs without a response from the patient. This is termed silent aspiration and is common in patients with neurological deficits or disorders and sensory impairments (such as after radiotherapy or surgery to the head and neck). Silent aspiration can have significant clinical consequences including pneumonia, lung abscess and death (Garon et al., 2009; Ramsey, Smithard, & Kalra, 2003, 2005). Because there is no obvious response from the patient, silent aspira-

tion cannot be detected during clinical examination. A change in voice quality after a swallow may indicate presence of bolus material on the vocal folds, but as noted, silent aspiration may happen with no clues. Instrumental evaluation is the only reliable method of detection.

Other findings that should be observed include hyolaryngeal elevation, epiglottic retroversion, vallecula and piriform sinus residue and posterior cricoid (PC) region findings. The posterior cricoid region may show a variety of indentations in the barium stream (Allen, White, Leonard, & Belafsky, 2011). Outlining of the posterior cartilaginous lamina of the cricoid gives a slightly flattened indentation on the anterior wall of the PC region. This is a normal anatomical finding. A thin shelf-like indentation may be seen on the anterior wall of the PC region just below the cricoid lamina. This typically is an esophageal web. These are often small (1–2 mm) and nonobstructive, but can become larger, circumferential and then narrow the esophageal inlet. Finally a small rounded impression may be seen on the anterior wall of the PC region, termed the posterior cricoid plication. This is mobile with the larynx, nonobstructive, and caused by mucosa overlying prominent muscle strips and veins beneath the pharyngoesophageal mucosa (Allen et al., 2011). This is also a normal anatomic variant and is asymptomatic.

Once the pharyngeal phase has been assessed in the AP plane the patient is asked to swallow a large bolus (20 cc) of barium and this is followed right through to the stomach. We term this the esophageal screen (Allen et al., 2012). Because it is possible for an abnormality in the esophagus to cause pharyngeal symptoms, in most cases this organ should be evaluated along with the pharynx (Smith, Ott, Gelfand, & Chen, 1998).

As part of the esophageal screen the patient is administered a 13-mm barium tablet to swallow and this is again followed from oral cavity to the stomach. Hold-up of the tablet at any point is noted. During the esophageal screen particular note is made of the transit time to the stomach (normal = <10s), completeness of bolus transfer, that is, whether residue remains in the esophagus, intraesophageal reflux, intraesophageal stasis, constrictions of the barium stream or presence of hiatal hernia. Extra screening time required to perform this view is only 10 to 15s. The esophageal screen has a sensitivity and specificity of greater than 70% for common esophageal pathologies and may allow the clinician to direct further investigations more appropriately (Allen et al., 2012). For example if a constriction is noted the patient may be sent for endoscopy to delineate the nature of

the mechanical obstruction, or if there is significant intraesophageal stasis or reflux, manometry may be warranted. The esophageal screen does not replace formal esophagram but may give valuable information regarding the cause of patient symptoms and direct further appropriate investigations, for example, transnasal esophagoscopy, manometry, pH probe, without the increased radiation exposure associated with formal esophagram. Examples of findings on the esophageal screen are presented in Figures 12–5 and 12–6.

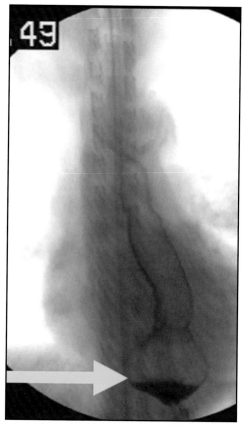

Figure 12–5. Hiatal hernia is noted on A/P esophageal screen. Hernia is indicative of a portion of the stomach that pushes upward through a small opening called the hiatus into the esophagus.

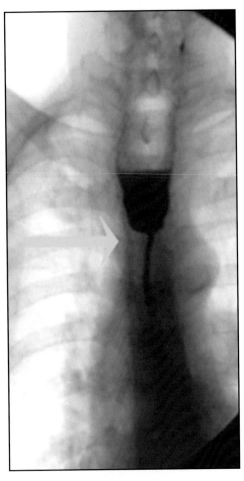

Figure 12–6. Large bolus swallow on A/P screen reveals esophageal stricture.

Formal esophageal evaluation (esophagram/barium swallow) is generally examined by fluoroscopy and spot films, which can be obtained either by standard films or digital recording of individual frames. This examination is also done by observing a bolus of barium as it passes through the esophagus from the level of the cricopharyngeus to the stomach. The examination is performed in the frontal, lateral, and oblique projections, and observations are made both in the upright and recumbent positions.

The esophagus is a tubular structure that measures approximately 23 to 25 cm in length and 1 to 2 cm in diameter. The upper limit of the esophagus is at the upper esophageal sphincter at the level of the cricopharyngeus muscle and the lower border is the cardiac orifice where the esophagus joins the stomach. The aorta causes an indentation on the left side of the mid-portion (Figure 12–7), and just below this level, there is often an indentation caused by the left mainstem bronchus. The anatomy of the distal esophagus is somewhat complex but important to understand when evaluating clinical problems. In the distal esophagus there is an area of increased pressure known as the lower esophageal sphincter (LES). The increased pressure in this area can be measured by intraluminal manometry and an area of intermittent narrowing is often seen during barium studies. Approximately 2 cm above the LES a second ring is often visualized, which is typically at the junction of the esophageal mucosa and the gastric mucosa (squamocolumnar junction, SCJ). This mucosal indentation is referred to as a Schatzki's ring. If this ring is above the diaphragm, the SCJ and gastroesophageal junction are elevated and an esophageal hiatus hernia is present. The anatomy of this region is seen in Figure 12–8.

In addition to evaluation of the esophageal anatomy, peristalsis is observed in the prone position. The types of peristalsis that are seen include the primary wave (initiated by swallowing), secondary peristalsis (initiated by retained barium in the esophagus), and tertiary contractions (nonpropulsive contractions of the distal third of the esophagus) (Laufer, 1994; Megibow, 1994).

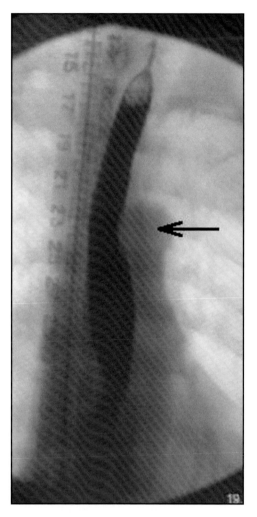

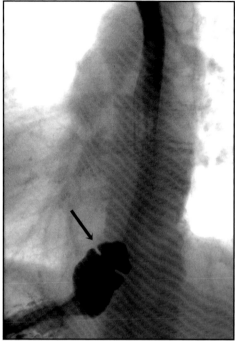

Figure 12–8. Anatomy of the distal esophagus demonstrated by barium swallow. Schatzki's ring is well demonstrated (*at arrow*).

Figure 12–7. Barium in esophagus; arrow indicates indentation of aortic arch on left.

An important part of this examination is the evaluation for possible reflux of barium from the stomach into the esophagus. Reflux of stomach contents into the esophagus is a very common condition that usually causes pain in the epigastric or substernal regions, but occasionally produces dysphagia or odynophagia. In addition, reflux into the hypopharynx may result in aspiration, hoarseness, and cough. The examination is done in the supine position after the patient has consumed about 300 to 400 mL of barium solution. While the examiner observes the gastroesophageal junction fluoroscopically, the patient is asked to cough, do a Valsalva maneuver, and raise both legs above the x-ray table. All of these techniques increase intra-abdominal pressure and thus may produce reflux. Some radiologists advocate using the "water siphon test," which consists of observation for reflux with the patient in the Trendelenburg position while drinking water. Although this test is more likely to induce reflux, the argument against its use is that it is highly nonphysiologic and no one would be likely to eat or drink in this position.

This maneuver results in more false positive results.

Common abnormalities that may be seen during the examination of the esophagus include hiatal hernia, with or without reflux; evidence of esophagitis; and motility disorders of the distal esophagus. Less common abnormalities include benign and malignant tumors, strictures, and achalasia. When abnormalities are seen on the esophagram, the findings must be correlated with the findings of the dynamic swallowing study and the patient's clinical symptoms to determine the clinical significance. These patients are often referred for further evaluation (including endoscopy) and treatment.

STUDY QUESTIONS

1. How is radiation exposure to a patient measured?
2. What factors affect radiation dose?
3. What are some contraindications for a barium esophagram?
4. What structures, and pathologies, may be better viewed from a frontal (A/P) projection than a lateral projection?
5. What are the findings one might see on barium screening of the esophagus?
6. What are the typical dimensions of the esophagus?
7. Can esophageal dysmotility be appreciated on an esophagram?
8. Can the aorta be appreciated on an esohpagram?
9. If a Schatzki's ring is identified, where is its location?
10. What is the difference between primary and secondary peristalsis in the esophagus?
11. What techniques are used during esophagram to test for reflux?
12. How much radiation exposure occurs with a typical DSS?

REFERENCES

Allen, J., White, C., Belafsky, P. C., & Leonard, R. J. (2012). Comparison of esophageal screen findings on videofluoroscopy with full esophagram. *Head and Neck, 34*, 264–269. (Epub April 2011)

Allen, J., White, C. J., Leonard, R. J., & Belafsky, P. C. (2011). Posterior cricoid region fluoroscopic findings: The posterior cricoid plication. *Dysphagia, 26*, 272–276.

Amin, M. R., Lazarus, C. L., Pai, V. M., Mulholland, T. P., Shepherd, T., Branski, R. C., & Wang, E. Y. (2012). 3-tesla turbo-FLASH magnetic resonance imaging of deglutition. *Laryngoscope, 122*, 860–864.

Berrington de González, A. (2011). Estimates of potential risk of radiation-related cancer from screening in the UK. *Journal of Medical Screening, 18*, 163–164.

Berrington de González, A., Mahesh, M., Kim, K. P., Bhargavan, M., Lewis, R., Mettler, F., & Land, C. (2009). Projected cancer risks from computed tomographic scans performed in the United States in 2007. *Archives of Internal Medicine, 169*, 2071–2077.

Chau, K. H. T., & Kung, C. M. A. (2009). Patient dose during videofluoroscopy swallowing studies in a Hong Kong public hospital. *Dysphagia, 24*, 387–390.

Dodds, W. J. (1989). The physiology of swallowing. *Dysphagia, 3,* 171–178.

Dodds, W. J., Stewart, E. T., & Logemann, J. A. (1990). Physiology and radiology of the normal oral and pharyngeal phases of swallowing. *American Journal of Roentgenology, 154*, 953–963.

Ekberg, O., & Nylander, G. (1983). Pharyngeal dysfunction after treatment for pharyngeal cancer with radiotherapy. *Gastrointestinal Radiology, 8*, 97–104.

Garon, B. R., Sierzant, T., & Ormiston, C. (2009). Silent aspiration: Results of 2000 videofluoroscopic evaluations. *Journal of Neurosciences and Nursing, 41*, 178–187.

Hartl, D. M., Kolb, F., Bretagne, E., Marandas, P., & Sigal, R. (2006). Cine magnetic resonance imaging with single-shot fast spin echo for evaluation of dysphagia and aspiration. *Dysphagia, 21*, 156–162.

Jones, B., Kramer, S. S., & Donner, M. W. (1985). Dynamic imaging of the pharynx. *Gastrointestinal Radiology, 10*, 213–224.

Kitano, H., Asada, Y., Hayashi, K., Hiroshi, I., & Kitajima, K. (2002).The evaluation of dysphagia following radical oral and pharyngeal carcinomas by cine-magnetic resonance imaging (cine-MRI). *Dysphagia, 17*, 187–191.

Kreeft, A. M., Rasch, C. R., Muller, S. H., Pameijer, F. A., Hallo, E., & Balm, A. J. (2012). Cine MRI of swallowing in patients with advanced oral or oropharyngeal carcinoma: A feasibility study. *European Archives of Otorhinolaryngology, 2269*, 1703–1711.

Laufer, E. I. (1994). Barium studies: Principles of double contrast diagnosis. In R. M. Gore, M. S. Levine, & E. I. Laufer, (Eds.), *Textbook of gastrointestinal radiology* (Chap. 4). Philadelphia, PA: W. B. Saunders.

Levine, M. S., &. Rubesin, S. E. (1990). Radiologic investigation of dysphagia. *American Journal of Roentgenology, 154*, 1157–1163.

Megibow, A. J. (1994). Computed tomography of the gastrointestinal tract: Techniques and principles of interpretation. In R. M. Gore, M. S. Levine, & E. I. Laufer, (Eds.), *Textbook of gastrointestinal radiology* (Chap. 8). Philadelphia, PA: W. B. Saunders.

Ramsey, D., Smithard, D., & Kalra, L. (2005). Silent aspiration: What do we know? *Dysphagia, 20*, 218–225.

Ramsey, D. J. C., Smithard, D. G., & Kalra, L. (2003). Early assessments of dysphagia and aspiration risk in acute stroke patients. *Stroke, 34*, 1252–1257.

Smith, D. F., Ott, D. J., Gelfand, D. W., & Chen, M. Y. M. (1998). Lower esophageal mucosal ring: correlation of referred symptoms with radiologic findings using a marshmallow bolus. *American Journal of Roentgenology, 171*, 1361–1365.

Smith-Bindman, R., Lipson, J., Marcus, R., Kim, K. P., Mahesh, M., Gould, R., . . . Miglioretti, D. L. (2009). Radiation dose associated with common computed tomography examinations and the associated lifetime attributable risk of cancer. *Archives of Internal Medicine, 169*, 2078–2086.

13

Other Technologies in Dysphagia Assessment

Peter C. Belafsky
Catherine J. Rees Lintzenich

Technological developments over the past 10 years have greatly enhanced our ability to diagnose and subsequently care for individuals with swallowing disorders. In order to provide comprehensive treatment for individuals with dysphagia, a broad understanding of these emerging diagnostic modalities is necessary.

AMBULATORY REFLUX TESTING

Reflux disease is a major contributor to pharyngeal and esophageal phase swallowing disorders. Extraesophageal or laryngopharyngeal reflux (LPR) has been implicated in symptoms such as intermittent dysphonia, chronic cough, excessive throat mucus and throat clearing, otitis media, chronic sinusitis and postnasal drip (Koufman, 2002). LPR has been causally linked to cricopharyngeal dysfunction and Zenker's

diverticulum (Sasaki, Ross, & Hundal, 2003). The ability to accurately diagnose reflux disease is essential to the care of persons with dysphagia. Many consider ambulatory pH testing to be the gold standard for the diagnosis of reflux. The diagnosis of gastroesophageal reflux disease (GERD) and LPR on pH testing differs.

In order to diagnose GERD on pH testing the pH sensor must be placed 5 cm above the upper border of the lower esophageal sphincter (LES). The location of the LES may be determined by endoscopy or manometry. The distal sensor may be hardwired to a Transnasal catheter or may be wireless. Hard-wired reflux testing can be uncomfortable and unsightly, and it has been shown to cause dysphagia and decrease reflux-provoking behavior. Wireless pH testing is more comfortable and has the advantage of routinely collecting 48 hours of data (Belafsky, Allen, et al., 2004). A wireless pH telemetry capsule is placed 5 cm above the LES or 6 cm above the endoscopic determination of the esophagogastric junction (Figures 13–1A and 13–1B). The wireless capsule transmits to a data receiver worn on the belt or kept in a purse. The capsule falls off spontaneously in 7 to 10 days and is then passed harmlessly through the GI tract.

In order to diagnose extraesophageal reflux or LPR, a pH sensor must be placed outside of the esophagus 1 to 2 cm above the upper esophageal sphincter (UES) in the hypopharynx (Merati, Lim, Ulualp, & Toohill, 2005). The wireless pH sensor cannot be safely placed in the hypopharynx. Therefore, in order to accurately diagnose LPR on reflux testing, a hard-wired pH catheter must be used. Most pH labs that use dual probe pH testing place a distal sensor 5 cm above the LES and a proximal sensor 10 or 15 cm cephalad. This places the proximal sensor somewhere in the mid or upper esophagus. In order to diagnose extraesophageal reflux, however, a sensor must be outside the esophagus in the hypopharynx. The

reason most pH labs do not place the upper sensor above the UES is that it is technically more difficult to do so. It requires a large inventory of catheters with different interprobe differences to accommodate individuals of different sizes. In addition, it also requires the manometry technician to perform manometry on the UES to accurately place the extraesophageal sensor. This adds more time to an already lengthy procedure. Figure 13–2 displays the appropriate placement of the dual-probe pH catheter.

We all experience reflux. Up to 46 reflux episodes per day can be considered normal. This "normal" amount of reflux is referred to as physiologic reflux. The normal pH of the esophagus approaches 7. A reflux episode on pH testing is registered when the pH drops below 4. Normative reflux data have been established for GERD based on a pH sensor 5 cm above the LES. Normative data for LPR based on hypopharyngeal pH values suggest that some "acid" in the hypopharynx is normal. Although controversial, most clinicians consider a

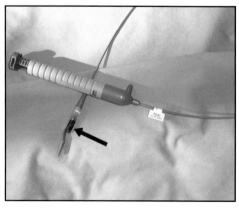

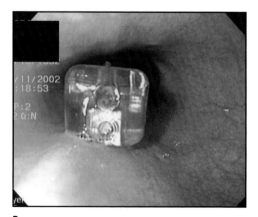

A   **B**

Figure 13–1. A. Wireless pH telemetry capsule (*at arrow*) with introducer. **B.** Endoscopic view of capsule in the esophagus.

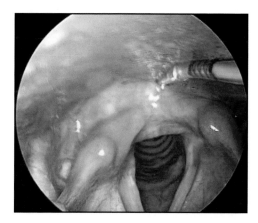

Figure 13–2. Endoscopic view of the proximal sensor (1 to 2 cm above the upper esophageal sphincter) in dual-probe pH testing.

pH test for LPR to be abnormal when there is more than one reflux episode in the hypopharynx.

New technologies have recently emerged for reflux testing, and further research is needed to define their role in LPR. A nasopharyngeal pH catheter that measures pH in the gaseous form (Respiratory Technology Corporation, San Diego, CA) may provide improved sensitivity for reflux events in the laryngopharynx. Furthermore, there is increasing evidence to suggest that the most injurious component of gastric refluxate is the activated gastric enzyme pepsin (Johnston, Knight, Dettmar, Lively, & Koufman, 2004; Roh & Yoon, 2006). In the near future, it may be possible to detect pepsin levels in saliva to diagnose LPR.

MULTICHANNEL INTRALUMINAL IMPEDANCE

Not all symptoms of reflux are caused by damage from acid and pepsin.

Regurgitated pH neutral gastric contents (nonacid reflux) can still cause symptoms in the upper aerodigestive tract. Nonacid reflux has been implicated in chronic cough and aspiration, dysphagia, throat clearing and globus. Standard pH testing cannot measure nonacid reflux. Combined multichannel intraluminal impedance and pH (MII-pH) testing is a novel method of reflux testing that can quantify acid and nonacid reflux. Impedance measures resistance to current flow. Intraesophageal content with high ionic concentrations (food/refluxate) have a low resistance (high conductivity). When food from the pharynx or refluxate from the stomach enters the esophagus, impedance drops. Thus, MII provides a measure of antegrade or retrograde bolus transit within the esophagus. MII can be coupled with manometry or ambulatory pH testing. MII-pH has been particularly helpful in evaluating persons with persistent reflux symptoms on acid-suppressive therapy. Of individuals on reflux medication with persistent symptoms, 20% will have symptoms from persistent acid reflux, 40% will have symptoms from nonacid reflux, and 40% will have symptoms not related to reflux (Tutuian & Castell, 2005). Figure 13–3 displays an MII tracing of a nonacid reflux event.

TRANSNASAL ESOPHAGOSCOPY

Distal chip videoscopes are now available that can provide high-resolution images of the esophagus through ultra-thin transnasal endoscopes. Typical esophagoscopy is performed through the mouth with a rigid or flexible scope in a sedated individual. Transnasal

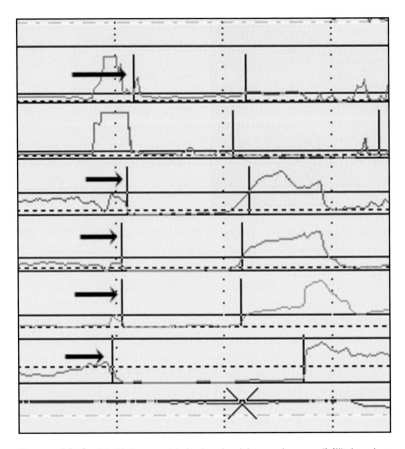

Figure 13-3. Multichannel Intraluminal Impedance (MII) tracing of a non-acid reflux event. In this trace, time is represented along the horizontal axis, and information from each of 6 sensors is represented along the vertical axis. Vertical lines (*at arrows*) in the traces represent changes in impedance recorded by the respective sensors as material passes over them. It can be seen that the first set of lines (at impedance drops), on the left, proceed in time (*left to right*) from the lowest to the highest, indicating material moving in a direction consistent with retrograde flow. In contrast, impedance changes that proceed in time from top to bottom are consistent with swallow.

esophagoscopy (TNE) may now be performed reliably and comfortably through the nose without sedation. We introduced TNE in 2000. Since that time we have reported our experience of over 700 cases (Postma, Cohen, Belafsky, et al., 2005). The most frequent indications for TNE were esophageal screening in persons with reflux, globus, and dysphagia. Only 17 procedures had to be aborted because of a tight nasal vault. The most serious complication has been self-limited epistaxis (<2%). In our practice, TNE has replaced radiographic imaging of the esophagus in patients with reflux, globus, and dysphagia. It has greatly enhanced our ability to diagnose esophageal pathology in persons with dysphagia. The most common findings encountered on TNE in persons with dysphagia are peptic esophagitis, hiatal hernia, Schatzki's ring, candida esophagitis, Barrett's metaplasia, and carcinoma. Patients are not very accurate at localizing the site of their swallowing problem. Approximately one-third of individuals who localize the site of their dysphagia above the clavicle will have an esophageal etiology to their symptom. Therefore evaluation of the esophagus is a critical component of a comprehensive dysphagia evaluation.

GUIDED OBSERVATION OF SWALLOWING IN THE ESOPHAGUS

The fiberoptic endoscopic evaluation of swallowing (FEES) is a tool to endoscopically evaluate the oropharyngeal phase of deglutition. Because TNE is performed in an unsedated, upright individual, we now have the ability to endoscopically evaluate the esophageal phase of swallowing. The Guided Observation of Swallowing in the Esophagus (GOOSE) is the esophageal counterpart to the FEES (see videoclip of GOOSE in media clips folder for Chapter 5 on the DVD accompanying the text). In the clip, patient is given applesauce and its passage through the esophagus is observed. In the last portion of the clip, the scope is inserted through the lower esophageal sphincter and retroverted to watch a pill exit the esophagus into the stomach). The ultrathin endoscope is passed through the nose and placed at the level of the soft palate approximately 3 cm above the tip of the epiglottis. FEES is performed as per a previously established protocol (see Chapter 11). If an obvious source of the patient's swallowing problem is encountered during the FEES, the GOOSE may be deferred. If the FEES is normal and no oral or pharyngeal disorder responsible for the patient's dysphagia is encountered, or a comorbid esophageal disorder is suspected, the endoscope is passed through the upper esophageal sphincter into the cervical esophagus. Normal esophageal transit time is less than 13 seconds. Any residue from the previously performed FEES in the esophagus suggests delayed esophageal transit. With the scope in the esophagus the patient is first given a 15-cc bolus of thin liquid impregnated with blue or green food coloring. Esophageal peristalsis is visualized as the liquid passes. The lumen of the esophagus should obliterate around the endoscope as the liquid is transported through. The esophagoscope is promptly advanced to follow the food bolus as it moves through the entire length of the esophagus. The bolus is visualized until it passes into the stomach. If the liquid traverses the esophagus without difficulty the person is fed a puree (applesauce) and then a solid (marshmallow, cracker, or bagel) consistency. If the patient has a problem with pills or any particular food, they are administered as well. At the end of the examination a retroflexed view of the gastric cardia is obtained from within the stomach. The patient is given a 15-cc bolus of thin liquid and the timing from the initiation of the swallow to the entry of the bolus into the stomach is noted. A transit time >15 seconds suggests an esophageal transit problem.

PHARYNGEAL AND ESOPHAGEAL MANOMETRY

In an individual with profound dysphagia, it is often difficult to distinguish between pharyngeal weakness, poor pharyngeal/cricopharyngeal coordination, and incomplete upper esophageal sphincter (UES) relaxation. Simultaneous pharyngeal and UES manometry provides valuable information about pharyngeal strength, UES resting pressure and relaxation, and pharyngeal-UES coordination.

Solid-state pharyngeal-UES manometry is performed with a 4.5-mm-diameter catheter that has two circumferential solid-state pressure sensors spaced 3 cm apart and a third directional sensor placed 2 cm above the proximal circumferential sensor (Sandhill Scientific Inc., Highlands Ranch, CO). This places one sensor at the level of the UES, one in the hypopharynx, and one in the pharynx (Figures 13–4A and 13–4B). The catheter is inserted transnasally into the esophagus just below the UES. Baseline intraesophageal and pharyngeal pressures are then established. The UES pressure is determined by a 0.5-cm station pull-through technique. A smaller 2.1-mm diameter catheter is also available for pharyngeal manometry (Gaeltak, Hackensack, NJ) (Hiss & Huckabee, 2005).

Esophageal manometry is typically performed with a 4.5-mm-diameter catheter that has two circumferential solid-state pressure sensors at 5 and 10 cm from the tip and three unidirectional pressure sensors at 15, 20, and 25 cm. This places 4 sensors in the esophagus and one in the LES. High resolution manometry (HRM) has recently been introduced (Sierra Scientific Instruments, Los Angeles, CA). In comparison to only 5 solid-state sensors with traditional manometry, HRM incorporates 36 circumferential sensors at 1 cm spacing to provide a unique high fidelity measurement of pharyngeal, sphincteric, and esophageal body physiology and pathophysiology. The role of HRM in the diagnosis and management of swallowing disorders is currently being defined (Ghosh, Pandolfino, et al., 2006).

STUDY QUESTIONS

1. What is the advantage of impedance testing as compared to traditional manometry?
2. Does wireless pH testing measure proximal reflux, distal reflux, or both?
3. What is considered a "normal" esophageal transit time in the supine position?
4. In true dual-probe pH testing, sensors are located where?
5. What percentage of patients who localize their site of dysphagia to the area above the clavicle will actually have an esophageal etiology to their symptoms?

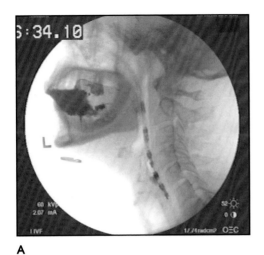

A

Figure 13–4. A. Fluoroscopic image indicating the correct positioning of the sensors for pharyngeal/upper esophageal sphincter manometry. **B.** Normal manometric tracing in the pharynx and upper esophageal sphincter.

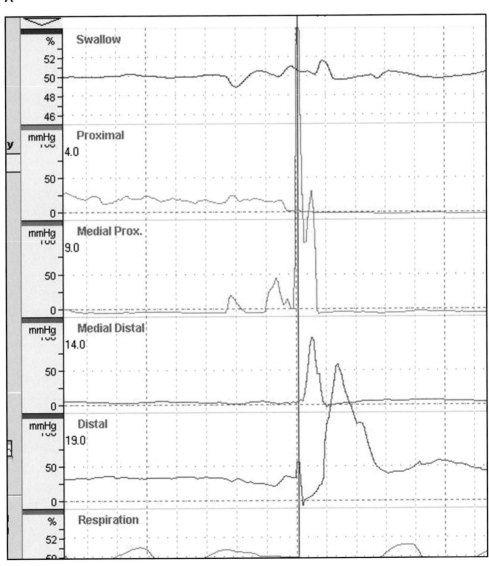

B

REFERENCES

Belafsky, P. C., Allen, K., Castro-Del Rosario, L., & Roseman, D. (2004). Wireless pH testing as an adjunct to unsedated transnasal esophagoscopy: The safety and efficacy of transnasal telemetry capsule placement. *Otolaryngology-Head and Neck Surgery, 131*, 26–28.

Ghosh, S. K., Pandolfino, J. E., Zhang, Q., Jarosz, A., Shah, N., & Kahrilas, P. J. (2006). Quantifying esophageal peristalsis with high-resolution manometry: A study of 75 asymptomatic volunteers. *American Journal of Physiology: Gastrointestinal and Liver Physiology, 290*, G988–G997.

Hiss, S. G., & Huckabee, M. L. (2005). Timing of pharyngeal and upper esophageal sphincter pressures as a function of normal and effortful swallowing in young healthy adults. *Dysphagia, 20*, 149–156.

Johnston, N., Knight, J., Dettmar, P. W., Lively, M. O., & Koufman, J. (2004). Pepsin and carbonic anhydrase isoenzyme III as diagnostic markers for laryngopharyngeal reflux disease. *Laryngoscope, 114*, 2129–2134.

Koufman, J. A. (2002). Laryngopharyngeal reflux 2002: A new paradigm of airway disease. *Ear Nose and Throat Journal, 81* (Suppl. 2), 2–6.

Merati, A. L., Lim, H. J., Ulualp, S. O., & Toohill, R. J. (2005). Meta-analysis of upper probe measurements in normal subjects and patients with laryngopharyngeal reflux. *Annals of Otology, Rhinology and Laryngology, 114*, 177–182.

Postma, G. N., Cohen, J. T., Belafsky, P. C., Halum, S. L., Gupta, S. K., & Bach, K. K. (2005). Transnasal esophagoscopy: Revisited (over 700 consecutive cases). *Laryngoscope, 115*, 321–323.

Roh, J. L., & Yoon, Y. H. (2006). Effect of acid and pepsin on glottic wound healing: A simulated reflux model. *Archives of Otolaryngology-Head and Neck Surgery, 132*, 995–1000.

Sasaki, C. T., Ross, D. A., & Hundal, J. (2003). Association between Zenker diverticulum and gastroesophageal reflux disease: Development of a working hypothesis. *American Journal of Medicine, 115* (Suppl. 3A), 169S–171S.

Tutuian, R., & Castell, D. O. (2005). Reflux monitoring: role of combined multichannel intraluminal impedance and pH. *Gastrointestinal Endoscopy Clinics of North America, 2*, 361–371.

14

Dynamic Swallow Study
A Swallow Evaluation with Videofluoroscopy

Susan McKenzie
Rebecca Leonard

Known in our center as the Dynamic Swallow Study and in others as the Modified Barium Swallow, this well known procedure was initially described by Logemann, Boshes, Blonsky, and Fisher (1977). When we began doing these studies, we chose the name Dynamic Swallow Study (DSS) to reduce confusion with other barium swallow studies and to indicate our focus on oral, pharyngeal and laryngeal movements during the swallow, as well as on anatomy. Recording and imaging technologies have advanced significantly, with improvements both in image quality and ease of analysis.

INDICATIONS

Patients are referred for DSS whose complaints, signs/symptoms, and/or histories suggest oral, pharyngeal, laryngeal, or pharyngoesophageal segment dysfunction. Ideally, all will have undergone evaluation, at least by their primary physician, and perhaps treatment for underlying diseases, most frequently directed by a gastroenterologist, neurologist, or otolaryngologist. In our practice, which includes both out- and inpatients, the dysphagia may be acute or chronic, obvious or subtle, severe or mild. The DSS is undertaken to identify risks to respiratory/pulmonary and nutrition/hydration health, and to target behavioral, surgical or medical intervention more precisely and effectively. Because standard protocols and objective measures are used, repeated DSS can be used to assess changes in dysphagia due to surgical, medical or behavioral treatment, or deterioration due to progression of disease/condition. DSS is not indicated in situations where performance status might fluctuate rapidly due to expected improvement or deterioration in health condition or when moving the patient is dangerous.

FOCUS

Fluoroscopy studies in dysphagic patients are intended to identify swallowing disorders that threaten pulmonary/respiratory and nutrition/hydration health. The perfoming clinician seeks not only to identify aspiration (which can be done during other barium swallows) but to clarify the reasons for aspiration in order to direct treatment (Logemann, 1983).

DSS differs from other fluoroscopic swallow studies in that it is not considered a "feeding evaluation," but a protocol of standard tasks testing a range of swallow capabilities that can be compared to performance by normal swallowers. Although under some circumstances real food and drink (mixed with contrast) is included in the study, in all cases the DSS begins with a standard protocol of swallow tasks, with standard instructions. Emphasis is on identifying a patient's risks, and also potential, for oral eating.

LIMITATIONS

Limitations of the use of fluoroscopy in dysphagia assessment and management have to do with its invasive nature (limiting length of observation and frequency of repetition), its lack of correspondence to real-life feeding (limiting generalization of observations), and its technical limitations, for example, two-dimensional, restricted to observation of mechanical events, and poor visibility of secretions.

Use of fluoroscopy in dysphagia assessment and management must be limited due to its invasive nature. In our facility, fluoroscopy time is limited to <3 minutes. Prior review of patient history, and a thorough clinical evaluation, will optimize time spent in the fluoro suite. Review of the recorded DSS after the study is completed also helps to retrieve maximum information from a limited period of observation. Frequency of repetition of the DSS is similarly limited due to the risks of radiation exposure.

Fluoroscopy provides an excellent examination of swallow mechanics, but other aspects of swallow, such as pressures generated by the mechanical events observed, are not directly assessed, although some may be accurately inferred (Leonard, Rees, & Belafsky, 2007). Other limitations include the clinician's inability to assess sensation of tissues during the study (possible with endoscopic evaluation), and inability of some patients to undergo the study. And, as noted, pooled or adherent secretions are not readily visible on fluoroscopy.

Finally, the conditions of a fluoroscopic swallow study, including the setting, the use of bolus material, and time and positioning constraints, can have an effect on swallow performance, rendering the study only faintly similar to real-life eating or drinking. Additionally, young children and others who require and are used to being held or otherwise supported physically during feeding are usually denied this because of radiation exposure concerns. These dissimilarities reduce the power of generalizations to eating/drinking in other settings.

BALANCING ASPIRATION RISK WITH FULL ASSESSMENT

The dysphagia evaluation, including the comprehensive DSS, is an attempt:

- to determine risks to the subglottic respiratory system during eating/drinking;
- to clarify and characterize behaviors that lead to such risks, and
- to modify them, if possible
- in determining the above, to elaborate an individual patient's potential for oral eating.

As stated throughout this text, because fluoroscopy is an invasive tool, the obligation to extract information fully is greater. Yet, the need for complete assessment must be balanced with the risks to respiratory health associated with aspiration. Each step of the dysphagia exam is a way of collecting information that defines aspiration risk for an individual patient. During parts of the clinical evaluation and throughout the DSS, the clinician must decide, following swallow of each bolus, whether to proceed with the exam, or to discontinue the DSS due to excessive risk.

Ability to make risk assessments during the DSS is based in part on prior knowledge regarding:

- patient history, especially respiratory, fragility/tolerance;
- performance on clinical evaluation of oral, pharyngeal, laryngeal tasks;
- effects of diseases and/or their interventions on swallow; and
- cognitive/behavioral conditions that interfere with instruction or self-control.

In addition to the above, the ability to make risk assessments during DSS is based on patient awareness of any failure, as well as the vigor and success of compensatory or protective responses to this failure.

Clearly, as the above conditions and behaviors will be different for each patient, the DSS is not a pass/fail (or doesn't/does aspirate) exam. If the swallow is not fully assessed because historical or clinical information is unknown beforehand, if all the above factors are not taken into account, if feeding decisions are based only on presence or absence of aspiration during fluoroscopy, then risks to respiratory and nutrition/hydration health can be over- or understated with obvious consequences to the patient.

THE DYNAMIC SWALLOW STUDY

Standard DSS Protocol

A protocol in this case refers to a standardized approach to the fluoroscopy study. That is, the same set of tasks is presented, in the same way, to every patient seen. In order to accommodate every patient, it must begin with tasks that all (or certainly most) patients are likely to be capable of (Logemann, 1983), and then advance in terms of volumes and consistencies/textures of bolus materials presented until the protocol is completed or must be abandoned due to the clinician's judgment of excessive risk. At that point, systematic diagnostic probes, including mixing particular foods with the contrast, can be explored.

A successful protocol is one that will elucidate the mechanical nature of the patient's dysphagia, subtle or severe. In our setting, two protocols for DSS are utilized. One is comprehensive; the other is limited. The comprehensive DSS is appropriate for all patients with suspected or known risk factors for oral-pharyngeal dysphagia. A more limited, but still standardized, set of tasks is used for patients who are referred primarily for esophagrams, but for whom there is still some concern about oral-pharyngeal dysphagia. By completion of either protocol, the clinician should have an understanding of the patient's risks for safe and effective oral eating. As noted, the standardized portion of the DSS can then, as indicated, be followed by tasks tailored to an individual patient's specific impairments. Typically, strategies attempted on these tasks would be designed to either facilitate bolus flow or improve airway protection.

There are many advantages of a standardized approach to the DSS. First, performance of a uniform protocol on every study allows a patient's performance to be compared:

- over time or treatment,
- to other patients or patient populations, and
- to normative data, if available.

Other benefits of a protocol relate to the clinicians involved, and include the following:

- Adherence to the imposed structure of a protocol facilitates learning a new procedure.
- The use of a protocol facilitates the teaching of a procedure to another clinician. In fact, it seems unlikely that teaching could occur without imparting some semblance of

structure or order to the individual trying to learn a new procedure. A mentor/instructor's ability to review and assess the trainee/student's facility with the procedure, decision-making, technical competence, and so forth. is critically dependent on this structure, and on comparing the student's performance against this standard.

- Adherence to a protocol ensures that critical features of the assessment/therapy are not overlooked in the heat/noise/stress of the test/treatment situation.
- If one clinician is unavailable, and another performs the procedure, adherence to a shared protocol facilitates communication regarding the procedure, its results, and so forth, and ensures some consistency in the service provided.
- If a patient may require 2 (or more) different procedures, such as a DSS and a FEES (or DSS and manometry), the use of similar bolus size/amounts (for example) for a portion of both tests allows for some comparison between them.

Participants

Currently, in our setting (an ENT clinic) the Dysphagia/Speech Pathologist conducts the DSS assisted by a Radiology Technologist who is supervised by a medical doctor with a fluoroscopy license. Because the invasive nature of the exam imposes additional responsibilities beyond dysphagia assessment, a physician familiar with head/neck anatomy should review the images for pathology of the anatomy. As noted, in our own setting, physician orders may include DSS (comprehensive or limited) and esophagram. If findings on a limited DSS reveal significant oral-pharyngeal dysphagia, the limited exam can be expanded to comprehensive DSS. If triage, clinical evaluation or events during the DSS indicate, the evaluation may be extended to include a full esophagram. Because of known relationships between oral-pharyngeal and esophageal dysfunction (Triadafilopoulos, Hallstone, Nelson-Abbott, & Bedinger, 1992), most DSS studies will include at least a screening observation of the esophagus (see Chapter 8). The esophageal portion of the fluoroscopic exam is read and reported separately by the physician. If additional documentation of aspiration is desired, a chest film taken by the technologist is read by the physician.

Image Views and Fluoroscopy Time

The DSS routinely includes observation in both lateral and anterior-posterior (A/P) views. The use of other views is dictated by the questions that arise during study. Optimally, in the lateral view, the fluoroscopy field includes the lips anteriorly, the palate superiorly (including enough of the nasopharynx to account to palatal knuckling) the cervical spine from the atlas to the cervical esophagus posteriorly and inferiorly. The A/P view provides the best means of assessing asymmetry from left to right, and is critical when patients with possible unilateral weakness or obstructive processes are evaluated. In the A/P view, the field includes the nasopharynx superiorly to the cervical esophagus inferiorly, and the walls of the pharynx laterally. Fortunately, current fluoroscopy technology permits imaging of all these various densities without "burnout" of the larynx. For the A/P esophageal screen, a view from above the upper esophageal sphincter to the lower esophageal sphincter is required.

Our protocol includes a 3-minute limitation on total fluoroscopy time. The technologist or radiologist warns the clinician when the time limit approaches.

Positioning

Care in establishing and maintaining the standard position should be part of any swallow assessment protocol. For the DSS, the patient is seated upright with head/neck and upper body as symmetrically within the fluoroscopy planes as possible and with neither flexion nor extension of the neck. If the patient is unable to maintain position, external support is provided. If the patient is unable to achieve good lateral position, this must be taken into account during analysis and interpretation of the results. In addition to reducing the strength of the observations, failure to control patient head/neck and upper body position changes biomechanics of the swallow. Even slight head or upper body leaning or rotation or neck extension affects the biomechanics of the swallow (Castell, Castell, Schultz, & Georgeson, 1993; Ohmae, Ogura, Kitahara, Karaho, & Inouye, 1993), complicating interpretation and diagnostic probing if the effects of position on biomechanics are to be systematically explored.

Calibration

A metal ring of known diameter placed on the midline under the chin is used in calibration for spatial measures obtained after the study. If the relationship between the patient and the fluoroscopy arm is changed during the study, the image must be recalibrated.

Contrast: Bolus Sizes and Consistencies on Comprehensive DSS

Since 1983 (for most tasks), we have followed this standard protocol for adults:

In the lateral view:

1–1-cc bolus of liquid contrast

1–3-cc liquid contrast

1–20-cc liquid contrast

1–3-cc paste contrast

1–1/4 Lorna Doone cookie coated with paste contrast

1–60-cc liquid contrast by straw-drinking (added in 1998)

In the A/P view:

1–1-cc liquid contrast

1–3-cc paste contrast (possibly)

1–20-cc liquid contrast

1–13-mm barium capsule

The DSS limited (performed with esophagram) involves two liquid bolus swallows filmed in lateral view: a 1-cc and a 20-cc bolus. Again, this study is limited in our setting to patients referred primarily for esophagram, but for whom the referring physician wants to "rule out" the possibility of oral-pharyngeal dysphagia. If evidence of oral-pharyngeal dysphagia is identified, from interview or the limited DSS, the study can be expanded.

The standard protocol for infants is as follows:

Normative information regarding swallow performance of normal infants on fluoroscopy is scant. The protocol we use is similar to the adult protocol in that it follows a sequence of maximum caution to maximum challenge. The focus is on pharyngeal, particularly hypopharyngeal, performance.

Position: swaddled, head stabilized, reclining only adequate for head stability.

Bolus: see below

First task: trace contrast on nipple/pacifier

Second task: undiluted liquid contrast from a bottle; sustained suck-swallow sequence

Third task: 1/2 sterile water–1/2 contrast; sustained suck-swallow sequence.

For both age groups, if oral transit is inadequate delivery is modified to achieve

- stable preswallow position in adults;
- bolus control in both infants and adults while
- either provoking or instructing posterior oral bolus control behaviors as much as possible. In adults, if this is not possible, instructing preswallow laryngeal closure is important.

Instruction (Adults and Children)

The bolus is offered by spoon, cup, or straw by the clinician. The patient is instructed to hold the bolus on the tongue (or the straw at the lips) and wait. When a stable baseline/hold position is established, the patient is instructed to "swallow all at once." If a stable hold position is not achieved the patient can be reinstructed or support strategies to achieve a stable position can be introduced.

As long as swallow performance is adequate on a given bolus, the exam proceeds to the next step in the protocol. Instructions are repeated each time a bolus is offered. Otherwise, feedback, except for general encouragement (e.g., "you're doing great," "do your best") should be avoided because it can change behavior. Similarly, the monitor should be positioned out of the patient's field of view unless instruction regarding feedback is intended. If the swallow is not successful due to biomechanical failure but does not threaten airway safety for the next bolus step, then the protocol should proceed without changes in instruction.

- Instructions for liquid, pudding and paste boluses from spoon or cup: "Put this in your mouth, hold it in your mouth (or the front of your mouth) and, when I tell you to, swallow it all at once."
- Instructions for solid boluses: "Chew this and swallow when you are ready."
- Instructions for straw-drinking: "Put the straw in your mouth and, when I tell you, drink this as fast as you can."

Oral, pharyngeal, or laryngeal failure that results in aspiration during the DSS justifies systematic alteration of the protocol. Compensations to avoid aspiration can be instructed so that the swallow can be evaluated as completely as possible. As all compensations change swallow biomechanics, they must be taken into account during interpretation of objective and subjective results.

DIAGNOSTIC AND THERAPEUTIC PROBES

Replicate the Symptoms

All DSSs begin with the standard protocol, which is followed as far as the patient can tolerate. Whether or not the standard protocol appears to reveal biomechanical failure, an attempt may be made to replicate the complaint. For example, if dysphagia symptoms indicate dysphagia is bolus specific, swallow of the problem bolus (including capsules or tablets) can be observed. Similarly, if dysphagia symptoms vary with position, this can be systematically observed during fluoroscopy.

Tasks Not Requiring Additional Contrast

If introduction of additional boluses appears too risky, swallow and nonswallow behaviors that do not require contrast can be observed. For example, speech tasks targeting behaviors important to swallow can be observed, that is, "k" repetition to assess posterior linguapalatal valving, sustained sibilants, and repeated plosive+vowel syllables (ka, pa) to assess velopharyngeal valving. Nonspeech tasks might include effectiveness of hawk-spit to clear the pharynx, or cough to see if material in the larynx or trachea can be cleared. In the A/P view, tasks requiring blowing against resistance can reveal asymmetry in lateral wall tone, if unilateral weakness is suspected.

COMPENSATION/FACILITATION BY CHAMBERS AND VALVES

General Principles

If abnormalities in timing, clearing and/or valving have been detected during the standardized protocol, compensatory strategies targeting the specific impairment are systematically explored. The ability of the clinician to apply compensations/facilitations during the DSS is dependent on ongoing interpretation of swallow biomechanics, and identification of effective and defective components (see Chapter 15). Compensation and facilitation strategies are aimed at maximizing intact components and minimizing or avoiding failures. Strategies include:

- changing the size and relationships of pharyngeal spaces and structures;
- changing the effects of gravity on bolus flow; or
- increasing effort to increase range, timing or vigor of swallow gestures.

The effectiveness of the strategy should always be compared to the performance on the task where failure is noted. For example, if head turning is used to reduce residue, the success of the compensation can only be compared if the head is returned to the original position, and the swallow repeated. Additionally, the effectiveness of the strategy can only be assessed if the goal of the

strategy is clear. For example, the goal of head rotation may be to clear hypopharyngeal residue, avoid it in the first place, or both.

The compensatory tasks or strategies available to a given patient depend on cognition; upper aerodigestive tract sensory integrity; head/neck oral, pharyngeal and laryngeal anatomy and range of motion, control and strength; respiratory health/resilience; and upper body postural stability and control. Again, as progression through both the standard protocol and exploration of strategies involves constant risk assessment, this information must be compiled *prior to the DSS*.

Compensations of Oral Chambers and Valves

As many observations of the mouth can be made without fluoroscopy, the DSS is most valuable in assessing the competence of the posterior oral cavity (OC). Nevertheless, inadequate oral bolus management has implications for airway safety; all observations are thus valuable in combination with clinical findings. In the OC, a bolus is prepared, created and maintained as it is transferred toward the pharynx. These competencies are dependent on lingual shaping and agility of a muscular floor within a hard-walled chamber of bone and, usually, teeth. Successful oral transit also requires sensation for judgment (bolus readiness in consistency and size) and mucosal wetness.

When ability to control and propel the bolus in the oral cavity is poor, compensatory tasks or "tools" available to he therapist include *bolus consistency, bolus placement*, and *gravity*.

Site of placement of the bolus on the tongue and/or head/neck flexion and/or extension may be used to manipulate bolus position and flow. If necessary, the OC can be bypassed by using a syringe with a short catheter to deliver the bolus to the posterior tongue (an example of this strategy is included in the materials folder for Chapter 18 on the DVD accompanying this text). If oral transit must be bypassed in this manner, competent bolus control is less likely and the patient should be instructed for preswallow breath-holding to prevent the uncontrolled bolus from entering the airway before glottic closure for swallow. Very lateral bolus placement and side-lying may also reduce the likelihood of aspiration during this maneuver. It should be remembered that the decision to undertake manipulation of OC events that facilitate oral transit is dependent on the competence of events in the pharynx. That is, oral transit impairments cannot be fully assessed if pharyngeal transit and laryngeal airway protection are intractably incompetent.

Observation of Nonswallow Tasks

When the amount of contrast must be very limited because of airway threat, speech and other oral nonswallow tasks may provide insight. Speech tasks require different but perhaps no more demanding range of motion and agility than oral deglutitive tasks, especially mastication of hard solids. Observations of speech tasks can be helpful in clarifying subtle limitation in the lingual and palatal range for movement. Our standard protocol includes repetition of vowel extremes (/i/ as in "heat," /a/ as in "hot," and /u/ as in "hoot")

as well as consonants whose production requires lingual tip (/t/, /d/) or posterior palatal contact and palatal closure (/k/, /g/). If historical or clinical findings leave questions regarding posterior lingual or palatal competence, additional tasks can be added to the DSS without adding much more time to the study. Techniques to measure palatal anatomy and competence using multiview fluoroscopy have long been available and aid in differentiating between anatomic and movement failures when valving for swallow is incompetent.

The Linguapalatal Valve

The anatomy and physiology of the oral and pharyngeal chambers are linked by the linguapalatal valve (or retro-oral portal [Bosma, 1956]), which is created by posterior tongue elevation against the bony palate or against the tensed and lowered soft palate. This valve acts alternately to contain the bolus within the oral cavity and then release it into the pharynx.

The linguapalatal valve differs from other pharyngeal valves in the complexity of its relationship with oral preparatory and oral transit components of deglutition, and because it is central in the relationship between the initiations of swallow gestures and initiation of pharyngeal transit. During swallow of liquids, especially boluses >1 cc, failure to coordinate onset of bolus transit with swallow gestures is likely to result in nasal reflux, aspiration, or regurgitation. In swallows of other consistencies and perhaps very small liquid boluses, particularly those associated with mastication, the linguapalatal valve may open repeatedly to allow small amounts of the bolus into the pharynx some time before swallow gestures are initiated. Because of this normal variability, interpretation of linguapalatal valving failure can only be made if instructions are clearly understood and the patient is able and attempting to comply. Failure of linguapalatal valving may result in absent pharyngeal transit or in discoordination of onset of pharyngeal transit with initiation of the sequence of swallow gestures.

If linguapalatal valving failure results in bolus entry into the pharynx prior to initiation of swallow gestures, strategies that can delay or prolong bolus flow or employ pharyngeal anatomy and gravity to deflect the bolus from the airway are useful. Such strategies include *head/neck flexion and/or rotation, upper body reclining on one side or the other (the degree depending on the impact desired), increasing bolus viscosity (the degree depending on the need)*, and *limiting bolus size to the capacity of the valleculae and piriform sinus*. Alternatively or additionally, *voluntary preswallow laryngeal closure* can protect the airway until pharyngeal transit is complete. Strategies believed to facilitate timely initiation of pharyngeal gestures by enhancing sensory information are widely used and involve manipulation of the characteristics of the bolus (size, temperature, texture, taste) or presenting other stimulation (e.g., cold touch to the faucial pillars) just before offering the bolus (see Chapter 18 for discussion of the effects of various stimuli on swallow).

When failure of linguapalatal valving results in initiation of pharyngeal transit after initiation of swallow gestures, the bolus will fall into the pharynx partway through the sequence of swallow gestures, or after they have been completed. Depending on the impairment, strategies may be aimed at slowing or deflecting the bolus, or at facilitating bolus flow. Strategies to slow or deflect the bolus include limiting the amount of the bolus falling into the piriform sinuses (side-leaning and head rotation) until repeated swallow gestures can complete pharyngeal transit. Strategies to facilitate bolus flow include head/neck extension with voluntary preswallow airway closure followed by flexion and head (not upper body) tilting or rotation.

Compensations of Pharyngeal Chambers and Valves

The pharynx switches from respiratory to deglutitive physiology by altering the shape of its chamber and the configuration of its valves. Most of the time, the pharynx is an airway: the linguapalatal valve may be open or closed, the velopharyngeal valve is open, the laryngeal valve is open and pharyngoesophageal valve is closed. Failure of any of these valves and/or failure to maintain pharyngeal patency for respiration can at least disturb respiration and negatively impact deglutition.

During normal swallow, the switch from respiratory to deglutitive valving begins immediately, often before, the bolus is delivered to the oropharynx (see Chapter 1). During pharyngeal transit the pharyngeal airspace first expands and then is obliterated (completely in young normal swallowers). In the oropharynx, expansion to accommodate the bolus is achieved by forward movement of the tongue base and flexibility of the lateral walls and obliteration by medial movement of these structures. In the hypopharynx, expansion is accomplished by forward movement of the hyolaryngeal complex and lateral wall, including the flexible pharyngoesophageal segment. At the same time, elevation/foreshortening of these structures helps to engulf the bolus and draw it into the esophagus (Kennedy & Kent, 1985).

Pharyngeal Valves

The Velopharyngeal Valve. Failure of velopharyngeal valve timing or extent of *closure* results in leakage of the bolus (or of air) into the nasopharynx and diminished ability to generate adequate oropharyngeal pressures to propel the bolus through the oropharynx for swallow (or to divert air through the mouth for speech). Observation of velopharyngeal function during speech (plosives and fricatives) may yield insights into velopharyngeal function for swallow. Strategies to compensate for or improve velopharyngeal valve closure include *head/neck rotation* and *manipulation of bolus size and/or viscosity*. When compensatory strategies fail, other therapies, either prosthetic or behavioral, can be guided by findings of the dynamic swallow study.

Failure of timing or extent of velopharyngeal valve *opening* results in competition between respiration and deglutition, particularly during mastication. This can slow meals and decrease the comfort and ease of eating or drinking. Strategies to compensate for diminished velopharyngeal airway are those that increase the time allowed for respiration between swallows. Techniques that accomplish this objective include *limiting the size and viscosity of the bolus,* *the rate of bolus presentation,* and *the total number of boluses given.*

The Laryngeal Valves. Dysphagia due to structural or sensory-motor laryngeal valve dysfunction can be one of the least amenable to behavioral compensations during the DSS. This is, after all, the last line of defense against aspiration. If the patient's history or clinical evaluation suggests laryngeal dysfunction contributes to dysphagia or breathing problems, the dysphagia evaluation must include otolaryngology exam.

Failure of timing or extent of supraglottic and glottic laryngeal valve *closure* results in leakage into the trachea and in decreased ability to generate adequate hypopharyngeal pressure to propel the bolus through the pharyngoesophageal segment (PES) and into the esophagus. Strategies available to compensate for ineffective laryngeal closure will depend on the etiology, that is, sensation, movement, structure. These strategies aim to deflect bolus flow around the larynx and/or optimize laryngeal elevation and closure. These potentially include *head/neck flexion and/or rotation, upper body side-reclining,* and *increased effort and prolongation of laryngeal closure* and/or *elevation.*

Failure of timing or extent of supraglottic and glottic laryngeal valve *opening* may or may not be obvious during quiet breathing and swallowing small boluses. In other cases, stridor may be present even in these situations. However, even subtle laryngeal airway obstruction, like other conditions that result in air hunger, can result in intolerance for the obligatory respiratory pause during swallow, thus interfering with adequate nutrition and the subtle relationships between deglutition and respiration (Hiss, Strauss, Treole, Stuart, & Boutilier, 2003).

The Pharyngoesophageal Valve (pharyngoesophageal segment or PES). Failure of extent or timing of PES opening (expansion) due to changes in the PES valve structure itself may be due to neuromuscular impairment or decreased tissue compliance (fibrosis.) Inadequate opening limits the amount of food or liquid entering the esophagus per swallow.

Strategies to compensate for decreased PES patency aim at prolonging maximum opening or increasing the number of swallows per bolus, and protecting the laryngeal airway from residue after/between swallows. Strategies include *repeated swallows per bolus on a single respiration, increased and prolonged maximum hyoid-laryngeal elevation and closure, head/neck rotation, flexion or extension,* or *upper body reclining.*

When the PES never closes completely, the pharynx and larynx are vulnerable to reflux of just-swallowed material in the esophagus or to gastroesophageal reflux (GER). Compensatory strategies are aimed at maximizing the effects of gravity on the bolus to keep it in the esophagus. These include *slowing the rate of bolus presentation,* and *adhering to behavioral precautions,* that is, postprandial maintenance of upright posture and caution in the ingestion of substances that may reduce lower esophageal sphincter (LES) pressures or otherwise increase the likelihood of GER. Unlike the laryngeal valve, the PES valve appears less amenable to behavioral compensation. The finding of PES valve dysfunction requires teaming with ear, nose, and throat (ENT) and gastrointestinal medicine (GI) physicians.

Pharyngeal Chamber

Failure of pharyngeal chamber obliteration results in contrast residue that falls into the available distal pocket (valleculae or piriform sinuses) after/between swallows. Selection of strategies depends on identification of site of incompetence. Strategies to compensate for incomplete pharyngeal clearing can be aimed at diversion of the bolus away from the failure site, increased effort (extent or duration) of pharyngeal constriction or of PES opening, and prevention of aspiration when clearing takes longer to achieve. These strategies may include *head/neck rotation or flexion, prolonged and increased laryngeal elevation, repeated swallows, postswallow voluntary laryngeal clearing,* and *upper body reclining.*

Failure of pharyngeal expansion due to pharyngeal wall stiffness reduces the size of the bolus that can be accommodated. If wall stiffness affects the size or presence of essential pharyngeal spaces (the "gutters" lateral to the epiglottis and the piriform sinuses) the bolus is diverted into, rather than around the larynx. Compensation for these structural changes includes *effort strategies aimed at early, prolonged, and vigorous laryngeal closure.* Observation of the pharynx during vocal pitch change and other speech and nonspeech aerodynamic tasks may offer insight into pharyngeal tone and movement range.

TEAMWORK

The upper aerodigestive tract is remarkable for the number of professionals whose patients can be profoundly affected by dysphagia, and who have their own particular and nuanced insights into diagnosis and management of dysphagia (the dysphagia therapist, the radiologist, the laryngologist, the physiatrist and neurologist, the gastroenterologist, and the pulmonologist). We believe that the fluoroscopic swallow study should contribute to diagnosis and management of dysphagia beyond the bailiwick of the behavioral therapist.

STUDY QUESTIONS

1. What aspects of the DSS make it "standardized"?
2. Can you name three benefits of using a protocol when conducting a DSS?
3. Ideally, what structures would you like to visualize in lateral view fluoroscopy?
4. What strategies might you try with a patient who has difficulty getting bolus material out of the oral cavity? What concerns would you have about using these?
5. Can speech tasks be helpful in understanding swallowing deficits?
6. What strategies might you use to facilitate initiation of pharyngeal gestures?
7. Why would poor velopharyngeal opening interfere with swallowing?
8. What strategies may be helpful in deflecting bolus flow around the larynx? In optimizing laryngeal elevation and closure?
9. What techniques might facilitate decreased PES opening?
10. What might you try in a patient with poor pharyngeal clearing?

REFERENCES

Bosma, J. F. (1956). Myology of the pharynx of cat, dog, and monkey with interpretation of the mechanism of swallowing. *Annals of Otology, Rhinology and Laryngology, 65,* 981–992.

Castell, J. A., Castell, D. O., Schultz, A. R., & Georgeson, S. (1993). Effect of head position on the dynamics of the upper esophageal sphincter and pharynx. *Dysphagia, 8,* 1–6.

Hiss, S. G., Strauss, M., Treole, K., Stuart, A., & Boutilier, S. (2003). Swallowing apnea as a function of airway closure. *Dysphagia, 18,* 293–300.

Kennedy, J., & Kent, R. D. (1985). Anatomy and physiology of deglutition and related functions. *Seminars in Speech and Language, 6,* 257–272.

Leonard, R., Belafsky, P. C., & Rees, C. J. (2006). Relationship between fluoroscopic and manometric measures of pharyngeal constriction: The pharyngeal constriction ratio. *Annals of Otology, Rhinology and Laryngology, 115,* 897–901.

Logemann, J. (1983). *Evaluation and treatment of swallowing disorders,* San Diego, CA: College-Hill Press.

Logemann, J. A., Boshes, B., Blonsky, E. R., & Fisher, H. B. (1977). Speech and swallowing evaluation in the differential diagnosis of neurologic disease. *Neurologia, Neurocirugia, and Psiquiatria, 18*(2–3 Suppl.), 71–78.

Ohmae, Y., Ogura, M., Kitahara, S., Karaho, T., & Inouye, T. (1993). Effects of head rotation on pharyngeal function during normal swallow. *Annals of Otology, Rhinology and Laryngology, 107,* 344–348.

Triadafilopoulos, G., Hallstone, A., Nelson-Abbott, H., & Bedinger, K. (1992). Oropharyngeal and esophageal interrelationships in patients with nonobstructive dysphagia. *Digestive Diseases and Sciences, 37,* 51–57.

15

DSS Analysis and Interpretation

A Systematic Approach for the Clinician

Susan McKenzie

The normal oral-pharyngeal-laryngeal swallow, observed fluoroscopically or otherwise, is one smoothly coordinated, highly skilled event (Martin-Harris, Michel, & Castell, 2005). Nevertheless, assessment of the dysphagic patient involves analysis to determine (1) whether one or more of the many oral, pharyngeal or laryngeal events required to accomplish a swallow are abnormal; and (2) the implications of that abnormality for a patient with a unique pattern of medical, surgical, neurological and social histories. The more narrowly and accurately abnormalities can be described and interpreted, the more likely treatment will be successful.

The number of swallow events and their requisite speed, normal variability, and adaptability are obstacles to specifying and interpreting abnormalities on fluoroscopic swallow studies. For this reason, we have adopted a standard approach to directing, analyzing and interpreting fluoroscopic swallow studies (for us, the Dynamic Swallow Study) described earlier. This approach aims to control many of the conditions that affect swallow performance, facilitating analysis and interpretation.

Analysis of the swallow observed fluoroscopically aims at systematic objective and subjective description of critical aspects of swallow. Observations are organized by chamber (oral, oropharyngeal, and hypopharyngeal) and kinetic categories including timing, movement of critical structures, and valve competence. Events that are measured can be compared to the performance of normal swallowers on the same task, making determinations of normal versus abnormal possible even for less experienced clinicians. Events for which DSS does not provide normative data may be rated on a 5-point scale as a supplement to subjective description. If objective comparisons between swallows by the same patient are desired, normative data are not needed for measurements to be informative.

Interpretation of fluoroscopic observations, whether an abnormality is detected or not, involves correlation of the observed performance to a complex array of contexts. The first correlation might be with other swallows observed (clinically or fluoroscopically) or with the patient's complaint; for example, does the patient complaint predict performance on fluoroscopy? Or, does performance change with the swallow task? When detailed analysis such as DSS can be made, correlation of individual events within the same or different swallows has implications for swallow safety (e.g., pharyngoesophageal [PES] opening time with laryngeal closure). Correlation of different swallowing tasks within the same fluoroscopy session can reveal conditions that provoke decompensation. Correlation with broader contexts, including the nutritional, medical, surgical, and neurological histories and the social/cultural history reveals consistencies or inconsistencies with implications for prognosis and medical/surgical management. For a given patient, additional contexts might be relevant. Thus, interpretation of fluoroscopic swallow studies determines consistency or "fit": is the observed behavior predictable based on what is known about the patient? For

example, if fluoroscopy demonstrates nasopharyngeal incompetence, what evidence in the complaint, the clinical observation, behavioral history, surgical history, and so on would predict that finding? If the observation is not explained by what it known about the patient, further investigation (fluoroscopic, clinical, or historical probing) may be warranted.

Clearly, accurate interpretation of fluoroscopy findings is dependent not only on accurate analysis but also on appreciation of the wide variety of conditions and variables that might affect swallow performance of a given patient. Although thorough discussion of these is beyond the scope of this chapter, some important variables are listed below.

Interpretation of swallow events must take into account factors that might facilitate or complicate swallow performance. Several examples follow.

BIOMECHANICAL INTERRELATIONSHIPS

Although only kinematic (movement) observations can be made from fluoroscopy, other biomechanical elements (e.g., kinetics [force] and friction) can be inferred. Such inferences can be strengthened by studies that assess these elements directly, such as manometry. (Leonard, Belafsky, & Rees, 2006)

Distinguishing primary or causal from secondary swallow events depends on knowledge of kinematic interrelationships. For example, absence of epiglottic retroversion can be related to failure of timing or range of movements that constrict the oropharynx, or movements that foreshorten the hypopharynx, or both. On the other hand, a primary event such as incomplete PES opening can be associated with multiple secondary observations within an individual swallow, such as incomplete pharyngeal clearing and velopharyngeal valve failure.

Position

Position of the torso, the head and neck, and the oral, pharyngeal, and laryngeal structures within the head and neck influence swallow performance by altering the effects of gravity on the bolus, the relationships of structures, and shapes of the oral, pharyngeal, and laryngeal chambers.

Position of the torso changes the swallow task in the head/neck. For example, oral transit in a patient with kyphosis can be more or less against gravity and bolus flow through the pharynx is biased toward the larynx.

Position of the head/neck affects the shape of the pharyngeal chamber and structural relationships. Well-recognized examples include rotation of the head to increase or decrease the size of the piriform sinus spaces or neck flexion aimed at changing the shape of the vallecular space. Another example is head/neck extension (as in the kyphotic patient trying to look forward) where the relationship between hyoid movement direction and the PES is altered.

Dysphagic patients may decompensate when head/neck position changes. For example, a patient with tenuous velopharyngeal valving may experience reflux into the velopharynx when leaning over to drink from a fountain or extending the neck to take the last drops from a cup.

Posture Stability and Flexibility

Fine movements such as those associated with swallow depend on a stable support structure. In patients with neurological conditions, the effectiveness of external postural support is widely appreciated. In the case of swallow, postural stability of the pharyngeal (including nasopharyngeal) and laryngeal airways is essential. Difficulty in achieving an adequate pharyngeal and laryngeal airway might preclude swallow without respiratory alternatives such as tracheostomy.

Often, applied postural compensatory strategies such as side-reclining, neck flexion, and head/neck rotation are dependent on the flexibility of the upper body, the head/neck, and component structures. The importance of flexibility for adaptive strategies is seen in patients fitted with stabilizing appliances whose mild dysphagia is exaggerated by reduced flexibility.

Respiratory Sufficiency

It hardly needs to be said that immediate respiratory needs trump swallow, but this condition is sometimes overlooked when assessment is confined to the fluoroscopic suite.

Stamina and Endurance

Similarly, when assessment is focused on the events of swallow themselves (as happens during fluoroscopy) the effects of poor stamina and endurance associated with some neurological conditions or with prolonged illness can be overlooked.

Lubrication

The health of oral, pharyngeal, laryngeal, and esophageal mucosa and the presence and condition of saliva is not assessed directly by fluoroscopy, but can have dramatic effects on swallow timing and clearing performance (see Chapter 2).

Bolus Characteristics

In addition to size and thickness, multiple variations of bolus taste, texture, viscosity, and temperature facilitate or complicate timing, valving, and clearing performances during swallow. The potential for variation should be considered when interpreting swallowing performance. Normative data on performance during a standard set of swallow tasks is valuable because fluoroscopy time constraints prevent exploration of the infinite combinations of food, drink, and saliva that a dysphagic patient may face. (See Chapter 18 for a discussion of the therapeutic use of these types of variables in dysphagia management.)

COMPETING BEHAVIORS AND STATES

Multiple behaviors and state share with, or affect responses of, the oral, pharyngeal, and laryngeal structures during swallow: Gagging, sneezing, hiccupping, laughing, crying, speech, startle, fear—essentially any distraction—can affect swallow performance. Clinician direction during the fluoroscopy studies should take this into account.

Environmental Variables

Some environmental circumstances, even the presence of pictures (Maeda, Ono, Otsuka, Ishiwata, & Kuroda, 2004), promote interest in eating or drinking but others do not. The fluoroscopy suite likely represents the latter category for most people. The influence of environment is one of the many reasons why we do not consider the fluoroscopic swallow study a feeding assessment.

Adaptability

In view of the number and complexity of variables affecting swallow, adaptability must be a signature characteristic of the normal swallow. Indeed, when a swallower's ability to adapt is overwhelmed or unavailable, dysphagia results. Evidence of spontaneous adaptability is one of the most important pieces of information available on fluoroscopic swallow studies. Clues to patient awareness of real or potential swallow failures can be inferred from behaviors that could be called precautionary, protective, or adaptive. Cough in response to aspiration or supraglottic penetration is the most recognized protective response, but there are spontaneous preventative behaviors less appreciated (e.g., early lingual retraction and early laryngeal closure among them). Spontaneous compensations have been observed for many years (Bosma, 1957a, 1957b) and more recently encouraged. Observations of older non-dysphagic patients who demonstrate change in swallow performance with age support the idea that adaptability of swallow movements is essential

(Kendall & Leonard, 2002; Leonard, Kendall, & McKenzie, 2004a, 2004b).

Conversely, recognition of a patient's maladaptive or excessive responses during fluoroscopy, leads to more appropriate intervention. With evidence of good adaptability in a dysphagic patient, both swallow assessment and therapeusis can be more aggressive.

CHAMBERS DIVIDED BY VALVES—A PERSPECTIVE FOR ANALYSIS

Analysis of the oral, pharyngeal, and laryngeal spaces as a series of mutable chambers (tubes or cavities) and valves is an accepted tool for the analysis of speech or voice (Fant, 1970, 1980; Flanagan, 1972). Kennedy and Kent (1985) proposed a similar model of tubes and valves for description of swallow. They divided the oral and pharyngeal chambers based on spatial orientation (horizontal and vertical), the differences in their function, and on the presence of a functional valve between them, the posterior linguapalatal or retro-oral valve (Bosma, 1957a, 1957b). We have found this model to be valuable in approaching analysis and interpretation.

During analysis of fluoroscopic studies, we have also found it insightful to further subdivide the pharynx into the oropharynx (mesopharynx) and the hypopharynx (laryngopharynx). In our experience conducting and analyzing fluoroscopic swallow studies, this division has become apparent to us in the following ways:

- Airway threat escalates significantly as the bolus passes from one chamber to another. Contrast retained in the oral cavity is least likely to be aspirated and most easily expelled. Contrast retained in the oropharynx is more threatening, but can be expelled by hawk-spit or suctioned fairly easily. Contrast retained in the hypopharynx cannot be voluntarily expelled unless it is at the entry to or in the larynx (and cough is effective) and it is very difficult to suction. Awareness of the progression of risk is helpful when directing the swallow study.

- The oropharynx and hypopharynx differ in their actions for swallow. Bolus flow through the oropharynx is normally midline propelled by the retracting tongue and the medializing constrictors. In the hypopharynx, bolus flow is deflected around the larynx, primarily laterally, by the epiglottis as the pharynx foreshortens to engulf and draw the bolus distally.

- Finally, in our experience, patients appear to use the midpharyngeal deflecting structures, the valleculae/epiglottis as a functional valve, the opening and closing of which can be controlled, if need be. Certainly, patients lacking the means to control, even stop, the bolus at that point are severely impaired.

In any case, as noted, we have found the perspective of the oral, pharyngeal, and laryngeal spaces as a series of chambers and valves a useful model in our analysis and interpretation of the fluoroscopic swallow study. What follows is a discussion of our approach to analysis and interpretation using this model.

DSS Analysis: Bolus Transit Time Versus Swallow Gesture Times

The goal of swallow gestures (movements of the chamber and valve structures) is to move the bolus quickly and completely from the mouth, through the pharynx, and into the esophagus, without leaks into the trachea or nasopharynx (or backflow into the mouth from the pharynx or into the pharynx from the esophagus). DSS analysis considers swallow gestures separately from their effects. In this case, timing of swallow gestures is considered separately from timing of bolus transit through the pharynx. (See detailed discussion in Chapters 16 and 17.)

Comparing timing of swallow gestures with timing of bolus positions reveals breakdowns in sequence that are associated with increased aspiration risk, for example, arrival of the bolus in the PES more than 0.10 sec before completion of supraglottic closure (Kendall, Leonard, & McKenzie, 2004a, 2004b; Leonard, unpublished data). Gesture timing versus bolus transit timing highlights competent, as well as failed, performance. An excellent example of this is a swallow in which the bolus moves no further than the oropharynx (i.e., remains in the valleculae), while hypopharyngeal swallow gestures (including hyoid and laryngeal displacement and PES opening and closing) continue on in a timely manner. Although it is true in this case that the swallow has failed to be effective

(in transferring the bolus to the esophagus), it must be said that a swallow sequence was completed. The distinction between gestures and their effects helps to specify incompetent gestures while appreciating competencies: information that is valuable in planning treatment and developing prognoses.

DSS Analysis: Displacement

DSS analysis offers tools to determine whether range of motion (apart from time) of some critical swallow gestures is normal for age and gender. Distinction between range of movement and timing of movement clarifies whether failure of a component is due to poor movement, or to lack of coordination of movements with each other or with position of the bolus as it moves through the pharynx. Movements chosen to be measured (e.g., hyoid and laryngeal displacement, opening of the pharyngoesophageal segment [PES]), pharyngeal space obliteration, are difficult to judge subjectively, but readily lend themselves to objective measurement. Measures of hyoid and laryngeal displacement target individual structures. PES opening and pharyngeal clearing measures are comprised of movement of multiple structures with a single goal (i.e., expansion of the PES and obliteration of the pharyngeal chamber space).

DSS Analysis: Discussion by Chamber and Valve

As noted earlier, DSS analysis begins by describing each chamber in terms of timing, clearing, and valving. If one of these functions has failed, components of that chamber that would normally contribute to successful timing, valving, or clearing are inspected. For example, if oropharyngeal clearing is incomplete, lingual or pharyngeal wall medialization, velopharyngeal, and/or epiglottic valving may have failed. Each component is judged objectively or subjectively, with the goal of determining relative contribution to the clearing failure. Not infrequently, in our experience, designation of incompetence or competence cannot be made with confidence without objective measurement of both timing and displacement. (Detailed descriptions of measures developed by our team, and how to make them, are presented in Chapters 16 and 17.)

The following is a discussion of our approach to systematic analysis of chambers and valves in the mouth to esophagus sequence associated with swallow.

Oral Cavity: Oral Chamber, Linguapalatal Valve

As noted in Chapter 14, fluoroscopic observations are most valuable for assessment of the posterior oral chamber, especially linguapalatal valving, since that is least available to clinical observation. Other observations (e.g., bolus creation, containment [including labial] and control), the nature of searching or groping lingual behaviors and so forth are helpful in correlation with clinical oral motor and speech evaluations and the particular history (medical, surgical, neurological, etc.) of the individual patient.

Oral Preparation and Transit Time

Analysis: DSS analysis does not provide norms for timing of oral preparation or transit. Subjective observations are recorded for comparison to input from other evaluations.

Interpretation: Oral transit time is especially subject to wide normal variation in response to a wide range of variables (see discussion of variables affecting swallow). Performance on fluoroscopy has meaning only when correlated with clinical evaluations and relevant histories as noted above.

Oral Clearing

Analysis: Similarly, DSS analysis does not provide norms for measurement of oral clearing. Subjective descriptions should include rating of severity, location, and variation in performance with changes in bolus characteristics. Clearing of the oral chamber is probably less normally variable than transit time.

During some DSS tasks (i.e., swallow of 1 and 3 boluses of liquid), the bolus should be almost completely transferred to the pharynx on one swallow, as instructed. A slight to mild amount of residue, especially for larger or thicker boluses would not be considered abnormal but should prompt spontaneous, immediate repeated swallow.

When oral clearing is incomplete, the site of residue is more likely to be related to the site of impairment than it is in the pharynx where analysis can be clouded by the effects of gravity. Components to inspect when oral clearing is incomplete include the chamber walls (labial and buccal movement and sensation, palatal anatomy, and sensation), condition of the mucosal covering and, of course, the tongue (size relative to its chamber, symmetry, range of motion, agility, or shaping, strength, and coordination).

Interpretation: Determination of the meaning and implications of fluoroscopic observations of oral clearing is dependent on correlation with detailed patient complaint, clinical oral motor and speech evaluations, and the various histories (feeding/dietary, dental, developmental, neurological, surgical, medical, etc.) of the individual patient. Poor clearing can be due to xerostomia postradiation therapy, to structure deficits associated with oral cancer surgery, and to movement deficits either due to restriction because of scarring or sensation and movement deficits associated with neurologic diagnoses.

Posterior Linguapalatal Valving

Analysis: Posterior linguapalatal or "retro-oral portal" (Bosma, 1957a, p. 901) valving is central to DSS analysis because, in this scheme, timing of all subsequent events is compared to the beginning of bolus entry into the oropharynx. Timing of linguapalatal valving is the only oral chamber event that is measured.

Normally, if the patient is instructed properly, once the linguapalatal valve is opened, all remaining events will proceed apace. Confidence that the instruction is understood and that the patient is doing his or her best to comply are essential, since there are normal variations in bolus transfer to the pharynx during eating and drinking. For example, it is not abnormal to let some part of the bolus fall into the oro- or hypopharynx prior to initiation of swallow gestures when eating, especially during chewing, unless one has been instructed to prevent it. Inability to attend to or understand the instruction complicates interpretation of linguapalatal valving.

Assessment of linguapalatal valving competence requires that, at least at the beginning of the fluoroscopic study, the position of the head/neck should be neutral (not flexed or extended). Even small changes in head/neck position can alter the valving task. A dysphagic patient may spontaneously flex his neck prior to swallow. Because this would compensate for incompetent valving it should not be allowed during the DSS until it has been demonstrated to be necessary for swallow safety.

Standardized control of valving initiation and head/neck position facilitates determination of linguapalatal valve competence or incompetence in its major functions:

1. Closure achievement and maintenance
2. Opening range adequate for the task (bolus size)
3. Coordination of opening with onset of pharyngeal swallow gestures.

Interpretation: If linguapalatal valving fails in the above functions even though the patient is able to follow the instruction, components of the valve to be inspected include palatal anatomy and sensation, lingual anatomy (especially relative to posterior oral space), movement range, strength, and control, and sensation. Suspected impairment of any component should correlate with detailed patient complaint, clinical oral motor and speech evaluation, and the multiple relevant histories of the particular patient (see previous discussions). Complaints associated with impaired linguapalatal valving can be nonspecific (potentially due to several kinds of failure), for example, coughing on liquids and mixed consistencies. Findings on oral sensory motor and, especially, speech evaluations can be very specific (e.g., poor posterior tongue elevation strength or distortion, absence of, or compensatory articulation of back stops [k/g]).

If fluoroscopic and clinical findings are consistent with each other, they should in turn be consistent with history, depending on the impairment identified. For example, poor linguapalatal valving would be consistent with neurologic diagnoses that affect movement and/or sensation, or with surgical therapies that might affect the size or movement of the posterior tongue or palatal anatomy. If no consistencies in the constellation of histories of a given individual patient can be found, referral to a physician should be considered.

Oropharynx: Oropharyngeal Chamber, Nasopharyngeal Valve, Epiglottis

Timing

Transit Time: Oropharyngeal transit begins when the linguapalatal valve begins to open, that is, when the soft palate and tongue separate, giving up control of the bolus to the oropharynx. Oropharyngeal transit ends when the head of the bolus passes the base of the valleculae.

Analysis: Pharyngeal gestures that contribute to timing of bolus transit include linguapalatal valving behaviors (see previous discussion), lingual retraction capability, posterior and lateral wall anatomy and medialization capability, and the influence of these on the epiglottis and on the lateral gutters between the sides of the epiglottis and the lateral pharyngeal walls.

When oropharyngeal transit time is prolonged, the following components should be inspected:

- Competence of linguapalatal valving: failure, either of bolus control or of coordination of onset with onset of other gestures
- Anatomic abnormalities of the pharyngeal tongue, lateral and posterior pharyngeal walls, and epiglottis affecting chamber shape and impeding bolus flow
- Mucosal dryness may slow movement of the bolus, especially when combined with other abnormalities
- Changes in head/neck and body position that alter the effects of gravity

Prolonged oropharyngeal transit associated with complete bolus control and evidence of precautionary closure can also be a voluntary caution strategy in some patients.

Interpretation: The presence and relative contribution of abnormalities identified in the components above, as well as plans for intervention and/or counseling, are developed by correlation with what is known about the patient from clinical evaluations and historical reviews. Because of the potential for behavioral interference (such as fearfulness), prolonged oropharyngeal transit that is not explained by impairments identified as above, and/or consistent with clinical or historical findings might be judged as precautionary.

Oropharyngeal Clearing. Because of the effect of gravity on whatever residue might remain, incomplete oropharyngeal clearing of liquids is often characterized by residue in the valleculae after or between swallows. The actual site of failure is best identified and measured at the time of maximum chamber space obliteration.

Analysis: Because incomplete clearing can fall within the normal range for age, determination of clearing abnormality requires measurement (see Chapter 17). When clearing is abnormally incomplete, the range of movement and coordination of movement of chamber structures should be inspected, including:

- Retraction of the pharyngeal tongue. Incomplete lingual retraction can be bilateral or unilateral, and consistent with neurological conditions, surgical and trauma histories that change lingual or mandibular anatomy and development of scarring, and radiation therapies for head/neck cancer.
- Lateral and posterior pharyngeal wall medialization. Lingual retraction alone is unlikely to be sufficient if the pharyngeal chamber walls do not medialize or lack tone. Normally, a descending wave of medialization is identifiable in the posterior and lateral walls. A prominent (perhaps compensatory) posterior wall wave may be associated with inadequate lingual retraction.
- Size of the oropharyngeal chamber or space in baseline position. Chamber space, when a component of dysphagia, is generally larger than normal, but occasionally is abnormally small. Measurement of lateral area at baseline is necessary to determine whether size is abnormal. Changes in chamber size can be seen in neurological conditions where pharyngeal constrictor and/or suspensory muscles are weakened, and in head/neck cancer patients where structures have been removed or irradiated. Abnormally small chamber size, when present, is generally post head/neck or spinal surgeries, frequently when observed acutely.
- Complete obliteration of the oropharyngeal space is the goal, but is insufficient if lingual and pharyngeal wall gestures are not appropriately sequenced. When oropharyngeal obliteration is complete but not sequenced, some or all of the bolus may be forced back into the mouth or into the nasopharynx. Inability to sequence constriction for swallow is seen most often in patients whose anatomy is distorted by surgical intervention or trauma. It can be distinguished from voluntary pharyngeal constriction during nonswallow tasks (i.e., hawking) if it occurs during attempts to swallow and is coupled in a timely fashion to gestures essential to swallow, namely, hyoid and laryngeal displacement and PES opening.

- Mucosal dryness can result in diffuse pharyngeal wall residue. Xerostomia is not uncommon in patients post radiation therapy for head/neck cancer. Many medications can cause some dryness and some medical diagnoses are associated with changes in the mucosa.
- Competent velopharyngeal or epiglottic valving (see next section)

Interpretation: It should be obvious from the examples above that the meaning and implications of pharyngeal events observed fluoroscopically really cannot be determined without correlation with history. In addition, as noted earlier, swallow events affect each other and the primary event may not be obvious on fluoroscopy. Knowledge of relationships between events, as well as knowledge of patient histories that might bear on pharyngeal structure and function are necessary before fluoroscopic observations can be interpreted. For example, when incomplete clearing is due to incomplete posterior tongue-posterior pharyngeal wall contact, determining whether lingual retraction or pharyngeal wall medialization (or both) are impaired can be difficult. Clarification that will guide prognosis and intervention is often dependent on correlation with what is known about the patient. In this case, patient complaint and speech and dietary histories may be nonspecific but neurological and head/neck surgical histories may reveal consistencies. Similarly, prior knowledge of relevant diagnoses and details of interventions may guide more careful inspection and diagnostic probing of specific gestures during fluoroscopy.

Oropharyngeal Valving. The linguapalatal, velopharyngeal, and epiglottic valves divert the bolus to and out of the oropharynx, enable development of descending pharyngeal pressures driving the bolus, and prevent "leaks" into adjacent chambers (oral cavity, nasopharynx, and hypopharynx.)

Analysis: The role of these valves is to switch, completely and at just the right times, from respiratory to deglutative positions and back again. Valve opening extent must be adequate for the task and closure must be firm enough to resist pressure on the bolus during swallow. This is even true of the epiglottis which is only arguably a pharyngeal valve: The pharyngeal walls at the level of the epiglottis must provide adequate opening around it for respiration and bolus transfer, but can close against it to prevent bolus entry into the hypopharynx.

The linguapalatal valve (discussed in the oral chamber section):

- opens in a manner adequate for bolus size to begin oropharyngeal transit
- prevents backflow of the bolus into the mouth
- prevents oral contrast residue (after or between swallows) from falling into the pharynx uncontrolled (without initiation of a second swallow) where it would increase potential for aspiration

The velopharyngeal valve closes during swallow and opens during respiration.

- During the swallow, when the bolus in the oropharynx is under pressure, this valve prevents backflow or reflux of contrast into the nasopharynx. If contrast is extruded into the nasopharynx, some or all of it is likely to fall back into the oro- or hypopharynx after or between swallows, increasing aspiration risk. Backflow during the period of maximum velopharyngeal closure is due to bi- or unilateral weakness or anatomic insufficiency of the palate or excessive lateral or A/P dimension of the velopharyngeal space. Cephalometric norms for these structures have long been available.

- After or between swallows, but also important for eating and drinking, the velopharyngeal valve opens adequately to support nasal respiration. When opening is inadequate, nutrition/hydration and respiration compete for the oral chamber, and both activities require more time and work.
- When backflow of contrast is seen as the velopharynx begins to reopen post swallow, it is more likely due to a more distal event, such as obstruction, than to valve dysfunction.

The epiglottis, whether it retroverts or not, is an important obstruction to bolus flow, that is, it diverts the bolus to the lateral pharyngeal gutters, away from the larynx. When the epiglottis fails to retrovert, more or less obstruction results. Absence of epiglottic retroversion for swallow of a very small bolus may not be abnormal. When failure to retrovert combines with changes in the lateral and/or posterior walls that reduce the space around the epi-

glottis, however, obstruction of bolus flow can be excessive, resulting in dysphagia. The epiglottis may retrovert incompletely or not at all due to:

- inadequate or ill-timed (relative to bolus position) lingual retraction
- inadequate extent of posterior and lateral pharyngeal wall medialization or lack of descending sequencing of medialization
- inadequate hyoid and laryngeal displacement (Fink & Demarest, 1978)
- inadequate space between the epiglottis and posterior pharyngeal wall due to anatomic changes in the pharyngeal wall or the spine (or to cervical appliances). Because head/neck position affects chamber size and shape, neck extension may decrease this distance as well.
- inadequate flexibility of the epiglottis.

Interpretation: Clearly, judgment about which of the many potential causes for inadequate valving is dependent on a detailed description of the abnormality and identification of historical consistencies that explain the particular fluoroscopic observation. Speech and feeding or dietary histories, as noted previously, should be consistent with linguapalatal and velopharyngeal findings. Developmental and/or neurological diagnoses and histories of head/neck (including spinal) abnormalities, surgical intervention, or trauma should reveal consistencies with fluoroscopic observations that will, again, guide decisions regarding prognosis and intervention. If consistencies are not identified, further investigation, including more thorough speech and swallow evaluation and referral to a physician should be considered.

Hypopharynx: Hyopharyngeal Chamber, Laryngeal Valves, and Pharyngoesophageal Valve

The presence of the bolus in the hypopharynx is associated with increased aspiration risk.

Hypopharynx: Timing

Transit Duration

Analysis: Transit time must be measured to identify abnormality. Hypopharyngeal transit time begins when the bolus head (or some part of it) exits the valleculae and ends with the clearing of its tail from the PES into the esophagus. As in the oropharynx, hypopharyngeal time can be prolonged by failure of gestures that propel the bolus and anatomic or movement abnormalities that impede bolus flow.

Interpretation: Prolonged hypopharyngeal transit may be due to:

■ failure to coordinate position of the bolus with onset of hypopharyngeal elevating and medializing (engulfing) gestures. When bolus entry to the hypopharynx is uncontrolled, the bolus may enter the hypopharynx prior to initiation of hypopharyngeal swallow gestures. Such a lag between gestures and bolus position is likely if the epiglottis is all or partially absent but is also the result of poor bolus containment in the oropharynx.

■ incomplete obliteration of the hypopharyngeal space due to inadequate medialization of the posterior and lateral walls and/or inadequate foreshortening, or to excessive hypopharyngeal space. Poor obliteration of the hypopharyngeal space is associated with reduced ability to propel the bolus so that bolus flow is dependent on gravity, increasing time for transfer. Unilaterally or bilaterally, poor or absent pharyngeal wall movement might be consistent with neurological diagnoses, and immobility of the wall is consistent with a history of treatment for head/neck cancer.

■ obstruction due to changes in anatomy of the wall, the larynx, the pharyngoesophageal (PES) valve or the spine (including large osteophytes and cervical appliances). More time is required for transit if space at any level is inadequate for bolus size, and the bolus must flow around an obstruction (e.g., impingement on the space by a cervical appliance or associated thickened posterior wall). Obstruction at the PES, discussed later in this section, may prolong hypopharyngeal transit by slowing bolus transfer to the esophagus. The condition of Zenker's diverticulum is an extreme example. In this case, hypopharyngeal transit is prolonged due to 2 factors: PES obstruction and poor space obliteration because of the diverticulum proximal to the PES.

Interpretation: Interpretation of timing abnormalities in the hypopharynx is dependent on recognizing the consequences of abnormalities in the oral and oropharyngeal chambers for swallow demands on the hypopharynx. For example, poor control of oral residue requires that the hypopharynx and larynx adopt defensive postures and be habitually wary of bolus material even after or between swallows. During fluoroscopic observation of swallow, timing relationships between events can be insightful and predictive. For example, closure of the laryngeal valve normally occurs within 0.10 sec of bolus entry into the PES (Kendall, Leonard, & McKenzie, 2004). In stroke patients, failure to achieve this degree of coordination between laryngeal closure and bolus position in the PES has been demonstrated to increase the likelihood of aspiration during fluoroscopy (Leonard, unpublished data).

Hypopharynx: Clearing. Because of its proximity to the airway hypopharyngeal clearing failures, like timing failures, can be associated with greater risk than in the oral and oropharyngeal chambers. As noted, voluntary and passive (suctioning) expulsion of residue is easier when residue is in the latter. Hypopharyngeal residue can be difficult to remove if it can't be swallowed. Fortunately, the lateral gutters (around the epiglottis) and the piriform sinuses divert and store residue if they are intact. When these spaces are missing because of changes in the pharyngeal walls or due to impingement, their value for laryngeal protection is obvious. When the piriform sinus spaces are filled due to changes in the hypopharyngeal wall, the bolus may be funneled directly into the larynx.

Analysis: Because some residue is normal, especially in elderly patients, determination of abnormally incomplete clearing is dependent on measurement. Because of gravity effects, site of incomplete clearing may be best identified at the point of maximum pharyngeal constriction. A/P observation is especially helpful in specifying asymmetry. Additionally, overlap between the piriform sinuses and the larynx in the lateral view, occasionally a source of confusion, can be more clearly understood by comparison to the A/P view. Hypopharyngeal clearing abnormalities can be due to:

- inadequate bilateral or unilateral pharyngeal wall tone or descending sequential medialzation. Pulsion diverticulae may contribute to residue, but their contribution to dysphagia may or may not be significant.
- inadequate pharyngeal foreshortening associated with incomplete anterior-superior hyoid and laryngeal displacement. Reliable determination of abnormality requires measurement. If hyoid and laryngeal displacement is not correctly judged, incomplete clearing may be incorrectly attributed to obstruction at the PES.
- insufficient mucosal lubrication
- obstruction at any level, due to thickening of structures (laryngeal cartilages, pharyngeal walls, impingement by spinal abnormalities or appliances on the spine). Obstruction can be acute or

chronic, depending on the etiology. Secondary effects such as proximal dilation and backflow into the oro- or nasopharynx or mouth will suggest the degree of obstruction. Although safety may preclude it, obstruction can only be completely assessed by swallow of a large bolus.

- laryngeal and pharyngoesophageal valve failures (see next section)

Interpretation: Suspected abnormalities leading to incomplete hypopharyngeal clearing must be correlated with neurological, surgical (including head/neck and spine), and trauma histories. Because of the health risks and implications of abnormalities in the hypopharynx, referral to an ENT physician is indicated.

Hypopharynx: Valving. The epiglottic, laryngeal, and pharyngoesophageal valves divert the bolus away from the airway and draw it into the esophagus. Failure of adequate opening of the pharynx at the epiglottis and PES will slow bolus flow and may prevent complete bolus clearing. Inadequate PES closure increases potential for backflow of material in the esophagus (either a just-swallowed bolus or material refluxed from the stomach). Inadequate supraglottic closure is associated with supraglottic residue. Of course, inadequate glottic valving increases the likelihood of aspiration.

As discussed previously, the epiglottis with its surrounding pharyngeal walls diverts, controls, and at times prevents transfer of the bolus into the hypopharynx. Please see that discussion.

Laryngeal Valve: Supraglottic and glottic laryngeal valving provides primary defense for the trachea and lungs. Compared to other valves involved in swallow, this valve differs markedly in complexity and behavioral capabilities. Competence of the laryngeal valve for swallow requires, in addition to range, agility, and coordination of movement, intact sensation and ability to respond to stimulation protectively, even to anticipate a threatening situation. Laryngeal closure adequate to withstand bolus pressures during swallow depends on sensory as well as motor competence. Laryngeal reopening and maintenance of a sufficient laryngeal airway is required for oral nutrition/hydration.

Analysis: Supraglottic penetration (contrast material that stays above the glottis) is judged to be abnormal when it is frequent and/or is not extruded during the swallow.

Aspiration during fluoroscopy is defined as contrast material that passes into and through the glottis. By far the most helpful construct for describing aspiration timing is that developed by Logemann (1983, p. 65). In our experience, however, rather than referencing aspiration timing relative to "the swallow" or triggering of the swallow reflex, we have found it more useful to specify aspiration timing relative to achievement of laryngeal closure, once the bolus has entered the pharynx (regardless of other swallow gestures). Logemann's description, with this modification, is as follows:

- Aspiration before laryngeal closure for swallow, after the bolus has entered the pharynx.

- Aspiration during maximum laryngeal closure for swallow, as the bolus passes the laryngeal aditus
- Aspiration after or between swallows, following reopening for respiration

Interpretation: Aspiration *prior* to laryngeal closure for swallow is considered a failure of timing due to inadequate bolus control, inability to coordinate initiation of swallow gestures or altered structural (such as epiglottic) protection. The longer the bolus takes to transit the pharynx, the more likely it will be aspirated. In patients post CVA, prolonged pharyngeal transit has been shown to increase the risk of developing aspiration pneumonia, even if aspiration is not detected during the fluoroscopy (Johnson, McKenzie, & Sievers, 1993). Risk of aspiration during the DSS also increases when closure is not coordinated with bolus arrival in the PES (Leonard, unpublished data). Aspiration prior to laryngeal closure for swallow is almost always associated with abnormalities of other swallow events: among them, inadequate control of the bolus, inability to coordinate onset of pharyngeal gestures with onset of pharyngeal transit due to movement or sensory deficits, structural deficits that direct bolus flow toward instead of away from the larynx. Cognitive deficits (poor attention, distractibility, difficulty suppressing other behaviors) and unstable head/neck posture make aspiration prior to laryngeal closure more likely as well.

Aspiration *during* laryngeal closure for swallow is due to incompetent laryngeal valving and may only become apparent when the maximally closed valve is exposed to pressure from the bolus as it passes the aditus. Thus, if it is judged unsafe to swallow a large liquid contrast bolus during fluoroscopy, this valve cannot be completely tested. Aspiration during laryngeal closure is, of course, more likely when both supraglottic and glottic closure is incompetent. The observation of aspiration during the swallow should be consistent with the findings of voice evaluation, patient complaint, and feeding, especially drinking history. Management of patients with laryngeal dysfunction is directed by the ENT physician. If incompetent laryngeal valving is suspected, referral should be made immediately.

Aspiration *after* the swallow is always of oropharyngeal or hypopharyngeal residue so is a consequence of inadequate pharyngeal clearing (discussed in previous sections).

Hypopharynx: PES Valve: The pharyngoesophageal segment (PES) valve opens to draw the bolus into the esophagus, expands depending on bolus size and closes, preventing backflow of bolus material into the pharynx from the esophagus. Between swallows the PES remains closed to prevent any gastroesophageal reflux from reaching the airway. During DSS, questions most often arise regarding timing and extent of PES opening. Occasionally, PES closure is inadequate.

Analysis: Determination of PES opening abnormality is not always clear. Prominence of the PES on fluoroscopy (cricopharyngeal bar) does not necessarily mean opening is restricted. Atrophy of the pharyngeal wall just above the PES complicates interpretation by making the PES appear more prominent. If swallow safety does not permit swallow of a large liquid bolus, the PES cannot be completely tested. In addition, the standard deviation for normal opening extent is large. Thus, measurement of the PES in both A/P and lateral views increases confidence in identifying restriction. Consequences of obstruction (proximal dilation and backflow) may help to confirm poor PES opening in the absence of other obstruction. Abnormal timing of PES opening cannot be determined without measurement and comparison to other timing measures. For example, PES opening that appears delayed relative to bolus arrival in the hypopharynx may be normally timed relative to other swallow gestures. In this case, then, arrival of the bolus may be early (due, perhaps to poor control) rather than PES opening being late.

Determination of PES closure abnormality is fairly clear: contrast should be entirely cleared from the walls of the PES once the swallow is complete.

Interpretation: Abnormal PES opening extent may not be due to failure to relax or structural abnormalities of the PES but to inadequate movement of structures that pull the relaxed PES open (hyoid and laryngeal displacements) and structures that propel the bolus through the PES (tongue and pharyngeal walls). (Please see previous discussions of these components.) If these components are normal, structural, or neuromuscular aspects of PES function are implicated. If the PES is indeed obstructive, consistencies should be found in detailed patient complaint and dietary history. PES obstruction in patients without histories of surgical intervention, radiation therapy, and so forth is often attributed to chronic GER.

The finding of abnormal PES closure should correlate with neurological, surgical, or radiation therapy history.

REPRISE

Accurate analysis of swallow during fluoroscopic studies like DSS is dependent on detailed knowledge of the biomechanical relationships between normal swallow events, and the ability to distinguish normal from abnormal behaviors despite the variability associated with different swallow tasks and multiple additional influences on swallow performance. Accurate assessment is also best guided by prior knowledge of performance on speech, feeding, and voice evaluations; detailed patient complaint; and a complex array of histories (neurological, developmental, dietary, medical, and surgical among them) that are particular to an individual patient. This means having a working knowledge of what the potential impacts of various diagnoses and conditions might be on swallow and on the direction of the fluoroscopic study.

Interpretation, or derivation of meaning and implications from analysis, is the process of correlating fluoroscopic observations with what is known about the individual patient from historical review, interview, and clinical performances and ferreting out consistencies and inconsistencies, both of which will guide recommendations and interventions. If consistencies are not identified, analysis may suggest additional investigation. Accurate interpretation of fluoroscopic swallow studies like DSS cannot be achieved in isolation, but leans heavily on awareness of the roles and interests of a variety of medical specialties and interaction with those professionals.

Most important for the patient, accurate analysis and interpretation of fluoroscopic swallow studies improves efficacy of dysphagia management by improving specificity of intervention.

REFERENCES

Bosma, J. (1957a). Studies of the pharynx. I. Poliomyelitic disabilities of the upper pharynx. *Pediatrics, 19,* 881–907.

Bosma, J. (1957b). Deglutition: Pharyngeal stage. *Physiological Reviews, 37,* 276–299.

Fant, G. (1970). *Acoustic theory of speech production.* The Hague, Netherlands: Mouton.

Fant, G. (1980). The relations between area functions and the acoustic signal. *Phonetica, 37,* 55–86.

Fink B. R., & Demarest, R. J. (1978). *Laryngeal biomechanics.* Boston, MA: Harvard University Press.

Flanagan, J. (1972). *Speech analysis, synthesis, and perception.* Berlin, Germany: Springer-Verlag.

Johnson, E. R., McKenzie, S. W., & Sievers, A. (1994). Aspiration pneumonia in stroke. *Archives of Physical Medicine and Rehabilitation, 74,* 665.

Kendall, K. A., & Leonard, R. J. (2002). Videofluoroscopic upper esophageal sphincter function in elderly dysphagic patients. *Laryngoscope, 112,* 332–337.

Kendall, K. A., Leonard, R. J., & McKenzie, S. (2004). Airway protection: Evaluation with videofluoroscopy. *Dysphagia, 19,* 65–70.

Kennedy, J. G., & Kent, R. D. (1985). Anatomy and physiology of deglutition and related functions. *Seminars in Speech and Language, 6,* 257–272.

Leonard, R., Belafsky, P. C., & Rees, C. J. (2006) Relationship between fluoroscopic and manometric measures of pharyngeal constriction: The pharyngeal constriction ratio. *Annals of Otology, Rhinology and Laryngology, 115,* 897–901.

Leonard, R., Kendall, K., & McKenzie, S. (2004a). Structural displacements affecting pharyngeal constriction in nondysphagic elderly and nonelderly adults. *Dysphagia, 19,* 133–141.

Leonard, R., Kendall, K., & McKenzie, S. (2004b). UES opening and cricopharyngeal bar in nondysphagic elderly and nonelderly adults. *Dysphagia, 19,* 182–191.

Logemann, J. (1983). *The evaluation and treatment of swallowing disorders.* San Diego, CA: College-Hill Press.

Maeda, K., Ono, T., Otsuka, R., Ishiwata, Y., Kuroda, T., & Ohyama, K. (2006). Modulation of voluntary swallowing by visual inputs in humans. *Dysphagia, 19,* 1–6.

Martin-Harris, B., Michel, Y., & Castell, D. O. (2005). Physiologic model of oropharyngeal swallowing revisited. *Otolaryngology-Head and Neck Surgery, 133,* 234–240.

McConnel, F. M. (1988). Analysis of pressure generation and bolus transit during pharyngeal swallowing. *Laryngoscope, 98,* 71–78.

16

Dynamic Swallow Study

Objective Measures and Normative Data in Adults

Rebecca Leonard
Katherine A. Kendall
Susan McKenzie

INTRODUCTION

This chapter is divided into two main sections. First, a brief history of our team's use of objective measures obtained from dynamic swallow studies (DSS) is presented. Though we have subsequently used these measures for research purposes, our initial interest in them arose primarily from a shared dissatisfaction with the credibility of our fluoroscopy (DSS) interpretation and recommendations for treatment, based as they were on subjective observations. Even though our team included very experienced medical, surgical, and radiology professionals, as well as speech pathologists and nurses, no one at that time had broad experience in observing and interpreting these types of evaluations. As soon as objective measures appeared in the literature, we incorporated them in our patient studies. As more information was published on swallow and as our experience grew, we adjusted and developed new measures to reflect new developments in the literature, our understanding of swallow and the particular problems presented by the head and neck cancer population. Our experience in this pursuit may be of interest to other clinicians, and is included here for this reason.

In the second portion of the chapter, the specific measures we collect, and the rationale for each, are discussed. Normative values and reliability data for each measure are also provided, as are differences according to age, gender, and bolus size or consistency. Our own experience with the clinical utility of particular measures is discussed.

BACKGROUND AND RATIONALE

The Path to Objective Measures

Our interest in making objective measures started at about the same time our team began meeting weekly to discuss patients. In reviewing their dynamic swallow studies, it became apparent that we sometimes disagreed about what we were seeing, even when we watched a recording repeatedly, and in slow motion. In general, and consistent with many subsequent literature reports (Ekberg et al., 1988; Gibson & Phyland,1995; Karnell & Rogus, 2005; Kuhlemeier, Yates, & Palmer, 1998; McCullough et al., 2001; Perlman, Booth, & Grayhack, 1994; Scott, Perry, & Bench, 1998), we were usually in agreement for binary observations, for example, whether or not there was aspiration, penetration, velopharyngeal reflux, or significant postswallow residue. Swallows that appeared greatly prolonged typically produced consensus, as well. Times that were possibly prolonged, on the other hand, were problematic. For other observations —how normally did the hyoid move, the pharynx constrict, or the pharyngoesophageal segment (PES) open—our judgments frequently differed. Beyond our problems with subjective reliability,

and in fact even when we did agree, there was a strong feeling within our team that, without objective information, our impressions and recommendations lacked credibility.

In the interest of harmony, improved objectivity, and enhanced credibility, we searched available resources for information that would lead to improved assessments. We had been performing fluoroscopy studies in our craniofacial anomaly patients, and referred frequently to the cephalometric literature for help in evaluating velopharyngeal function in a quantitative manner. When the fluoroscopic evaluation of swallow was introduced by Logemann and her colleagues (Blonsky, Logemann, Boshes, & Fisher, 1975; Logemann, 1983; Logemann, Boshes, Blonsky, & Fisher, 1977), we recognized that it also lent itself to quantitative analysis. We adopted Logemann's recommended protocol with its emphasis on standardization, and have been employing it with little change ever since. With the exception of some work on timing, however, which began to emerge in the 1980s, quantitative guidelines pertinent to swallowing were slow to emerge. Although limited, the data available were quite useful; very quickly, we added timing information to our studies.

Initially, we used conventions described by Logemann (1983) for measuring transit times, but the parameters she was using were not always present or identifiable in our studies. For example, the faucial pillars were not easily visualized, and neither the angle of the mandible nor the faucial pillars were always present in patients who had undergone head and neck resections. In time, we modified our scheme to facilitate measurement, in particular, in our head and neck population. Our first effort to collect normative timing data was in a group of 16 adults who were undergoing upper gastrointestinal (GI) studies for distal esophageal GI complaints (unpublished data, 1988; Johnson, McKenzie, Rosenquist, Liberman, & Sievers, 1993). The resulting data were consistent with those reported by other investigators (Cook et al., 1989; Curtis, Cruess, Dachman, & Maso, 1984; McConnel, 1988a, 1988b), and our standard deviations were small, which encouraged us to move forward.

Soon after adding timing information to our studies, we explored possibilities for displacement measures. Our explorations led us to strategies for getting video images into a computer (or "digitizing" them). Fortunately, the technology for doing this easily, relatively inexpensively, and effectively improved just as our interest piqued. Once the digitization problems were solved, we worked on techniques for measuring hyoid displacement and PES opening. When several members of our own team, as well as outsiders recruited for the task, made measurements that demonstrated good inter- and intrajudge reliability, we again felt we were moving in the right direction. As always, we incorporated measurements into routine patient assessments and our measurement techniques reflect this perspective. When our data appeared comparable to values reported by other investigators using different techniques (Dantas et al., 1990; Dejaeger, Pelemans, Ponette, & Joosten, 1997; Dodds, Man, Cook, Kahrilas, Stewart, & Kern,1988; Ekberg, 1986; Jacob, Kahrilas, Logemann, Shah, & Ha, 1989;

Kahrilas, Dodds, Dent, Logemann, & Shaker, 1988; Perlman, VanDaele & Otterbacher, 1995), our confidence improved further.

Normative Data

Ultimately, we collected additional normative data, using the same equipment and measurement strategies we used for patients. In time, we performed fluoroscopy studies on large groups of younger and more elderly normal subjects, respectively (Kendall, 2002; Kendall & Leonard, 2002; Kendall, Leonard, & McKenzie, 2001, 2003, 2004a, 2004b; Kendall, McKenzie, Leonard, Gonçalves, & Walker, 2000; Kendall, Leonard, & McKenzie, 2004a, 2004b; Leonard, Kendall, McKenzie, Gonçalves, & Walker, 2000). As a team, we were now able to use our particular measurement scheme to compare patient data to nondysphagic subjects according to age and gender. Observations from these studies also provided us with a much better idea about normal variability, and of the range of behaviors, both times and displacements, that characterize normal swallow. Normative data for the measures we obtain, for adults younger than 65 years of age, and for a more elderly population of adults over 65 years, are presented in Table 16–1.

Data Display

Having now worked out strategies for both timing and displacement measures, and having collected these measures for normal subjects, we needed to

Table 16–1. Normative Values for Timing, Duration and Displacement Measures for Subjects Under and Over Age 65 Years

NORMAL DISPLACEMENT mean with 2 SD

< AGE 65 yrs

MEASURE (cm)	1 CC		3 CC		20 CC	
Hmax (M)	2.00	1.42	2.12	1.38	2.4	1.36
Hmax (F)	1.39	1.0	1.62	1.12	1.81	1.46
HL (M)	1.33	.92	1.30	1.08	1.25	.83
HL (F)	1.10	1.48	1.08	1.17	1.07	1.10
PESmax	.39	.38	.30	.30	.90	.55
Pamax (M)	.13	.22	.22	.36	.28	38
Pamax (F)	.10	.18	.12	.23	.17	.33
Pam/Pah (M)	.02	.04	.04	.05	.06	.12
Pam/Pah (F)	.02	.03	.02	.04	.03	.06
Hmax+HL (M)	3.33	1.86			3.72	1.82
Hmax+HL (F)	2.49	1.7			2.88	.86

PA HOLD (M) 7.9 (4.2) (F) 6.5 (3.4)

> AGE 65 yrs

MEASURE (cm)	1 CC		3 CC		20 CC	
Hmax (M)	1.98	1.41	2.08	1.62	2.48	2.04
Hmax (F)	1.63	1.06	1.79	1.54	2.07	.45
HL (M)	1.50	.68	1.71	1.43	1.58	1.35
HL (F)	1.27	.87	1.24	1.2	1.23	1.30
PESmax	.37	.34	.50	.37	.80	.40
Pamax (M)	.24	.49	.35	.46	.90	1.06
Pamax (F)	.25	.46	.52	1.04	1.38	3.33
Pam/Pah (M)	.02	.04	.03	.04	.13	.28
Pam/Pah (F)	.02	.06	.07	.15	.14	.28
Hmax+HL (M)					4.06	.98
Hmax+HL (F)					3.30	.55

PA HOLD (M) 11.4 (6.0) (F) 8.09 (4.0)

Morphometry of the Cartilaginous Larynx (mm)

	(M)	(F)
Cric	24.6±1.9	21.6±1.5
Aryt	16.6±1.9	12.6±2.1
Total =	41.2 mm ±15.1 mm	34.2 mm ±13.6 mm

Sprinzl GM, et al. Head & Neck, December (1999).

Increased aspiration pneumonia risk post CVA

2–3 sec = 33%
3–5 sec = 48%
>5 sec = 90%

Hyoid to mandible @ baseline (cm)

	<65	>65	>65+bar
(M)	2.67 (.8)	2.68 (.62)	2.63 (.84)
(F)	1.86 (.53)	2.02 (.68)	2.08 (.53)

Hyoid to larynx @ baseline (cm)

	<65	>65
(M)	3.79 (.54)	4.20 (.74)
(F)	2.95 (.59)	3.36 (.55)

NORMAL DURATION *mean with 2 SD*

MEASURE (cm)	< AGE 65 yrs			MEASURE (cm)	> AGE 65 yrs		
	1 CC	3 CC	20 CC		1 CC	3 CC	20 CC
H max	.22 .20	.21 .21	.20 .24	H max	.13 .12	.12 .14	.12 .20
PES max	.34 .16	.41 .14	.50 .21	PES max	.47 .20	.62 .50	.64 .21
AE closed	.53 .28	.60 .30	.72 .50	AE closed	.66 .28	.84 .62	.85 .93
OP transit	.50 .33	.41 .34	.23 .26	OP transit	.50 .64	.49 .46	.42 .36
HP transit	.41 .46	.43 .34	.64 .24	HP transit	.65 .37	.76 .62	.77 .26
AEcl-Aest.	.27 .18	.27 .29	.25 .31	Aecl-Aest	.48 .65	.50 .66	.54 .69
Em	1.07 .59	1.01 .24	1.0 .36	Em	1.30 .88	1.30 .95	1.30 .57

Maximum phx expansion, a-p (cm)

	<65	>65
(M)	3.60 (.44)	3.99 (.59)
(F)	3.07 (.43)	3.41 (.50)

Invariant Sequence Pairs

AEs before Pop

AEc no more than .1 sec after Pop, BP1

HL after Pop

PAmax after PESmax

Pop before/same time as BP1

Pcl after/same time as BP2

UES Max Openings, a-p (cm)

	<65	>65	>65+bar
(M)	1.69 (.18)	1.54 (.32)	.65 (.17)
(F)	1.35 (.25)	1.40 (.32)	1.21 (.21)

display the information in a clinically useful way. After several attempts, we arrived at the method currently used and illustrated in Figure 16–1. In the objective measures plot, *bolus transit* times are tracked separately from *swallow gesture* times. Bolus movement through the pharynx for a 20-cc swallow is represented along the lower portion of the plot by hatched lines and small circles. The *"B"* values on this axis (*B1, BV1*, etc.) represent bolus arrival or departure from certain anatomical sites.

The timing of various swallow gestures is also indicated along the horizontal axis. These points represent structural movements critical to swallow, for example, onset of hyoid elevation (H1), point of maximum pharyngoesophageal opening (PESmax), and closure of the supraglottic airway (AEclose). For both *bolus transit* and *swallow gestures*, an individual patient's values, in red, are plotted against our normative mean values (± 1 SD), in blue. This presentation allows us to consider both the coordination between bolus transit and the timing of various swallow gestures, and also how our individual patient compares to normal.

Displacement and duration data, respectively, appear in boxes inserted at the bottom of the plot (see Figure 16–1). As before, an individual patient's values, in red, are plotted on vertical lines representing the normative mean (± 1 SD) for each measure, in blue. Patients' data are graphed separately for ages under and above 65 years, respectively, and for gender, when appropriate. Again, the plot permits ready comparison of the patient's performance to a group of comparable normal subjects.

Our team discussions now included presentation of the objective measures we had obtained from the DSS, and the advantages of this were several. We had anticipated that improved objectivity would reduce our disagreements and enhance our credibility, and this proved true. The ability to compare our patients to normal subjects was, of course, a significant development as well. Other benefits became apparent over time.

Data Storage

Once we had a large amount of patient data (a few hundred patients per year), we wanted to be able to store the information, preferably in a database. This option allows the user to retrieve results quickly, and even link them to a report generator, a definite timesaver in clinical situations (Figures 16–2A, 16–2B, and 16–2C). But perhaps the real power of a database is that, once patient information is added to it, the program can be "queried" to organize and summarize the data in a particular manner. If it is of interest to review transit times in all patients with cerebrovascular accident (CVA), or all patients with reduced PES opening size, or even all the patients seen in a certain time interval who are of a certain age or gender, the information can be produced in minutes (Figure 16–3). If we are discussing a particular patient, and want to know how other patients with similar pathologies or impairments compare to this individual, we simply query the database (see Figure 16–3). Generalizations about given populations, or insights into the unique characteristics of certain types of patients, are possible.

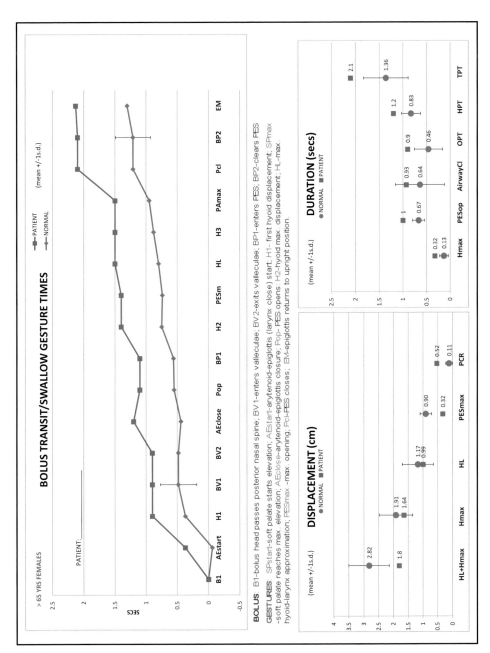

Figure 16-1. Plot (in Excel) displays objective data from fluoroscopic study.

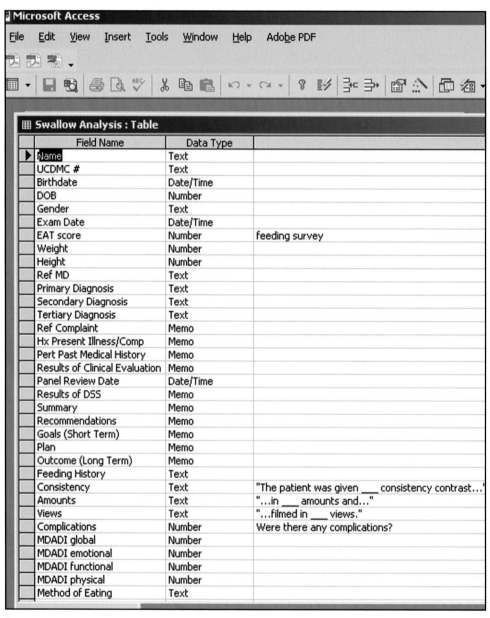

A

Figure 16–2. A. Database fields for which information will be obtained. *(continues)*

Swallow Analysis | Pre99 | Open Obj Measures | Panel | 0-4 Definitions

Name: ▮▮▮▮▮▮▮▮ **UMC #:** 012 28 58 **DOB:** 7 /26/1942 **Gender:** m

Exam Date: 4 /5 /2006 **Age:** 63 yr 9 mo **Ref MD:** Roberto RolandoMD, Peter BelafskyMD

DOB 1 **EAT:** 44

Panel Review Date: 4/11/2006 ☐ **Record is incomplete**

Primary Diagnosis: GI **Esophagram:**

Secondary Diagnosis: Spine **Height (in):** 60

Tertiary Diagnosis: **Weight (lbs):** 106

Complaint on Referral: 63 y.o. cheerful woman with severe rheumatoid arthritis and solid food dysphagia.

History of Present Complaint: Chief complaint is food sticking in her mid chest. She says she eats with a "quart of water" beside her. She takes a bite and a sip. She, or someone helping her, cuts up food into small pieces. She eats 3 meals/day and it takes her about 45 min-1 hour to eat which she believes is a long time. She reports

Pertinent Medical History: ENT visit 3/0/06 revealed normal vocal fold function, pharyngeal strength appeared normal, paroxysmal laryngospasm. She is scheduled for spine surgery in 5 days for some revision fusion C7-T1 as she has developed a more kyphotic position and had increase in pain and parasthesias recently. Hypoglycemia,

Clinical Eval Results: Patient wears a soft neck collar as prescribed over the past year due to neck pain. Normal oral mechanism examination. Articulation precise, voice quality is clear, normal resonance.

The patient was given liquid, paste and solid **consistency contrast in** 1-20cc

amounts and filmed in lateral and AP **views. The evaluation was completed with:**

◉ **no complications** ○ **the following complications:**

DSS Results: As included with an esophagram, the DSS protocol is altered and only liquid contrast is offered.

Oral transit is WNL. Mild oral residue prompts immediate spontaneous repeat swallow.

Total pharyngeal transit time (Pcl-B1) for 1cc is mildly prolonged for age @ 3.04 sec. Swallow of 20cc liquid bolus is slightly prolonged age @ 1.50 sec. due, entirely, to prolonged hypopharyngeal transit and slow PES clearing. Maximum hyoid elevation duration is, also, prolonged, perhaps as a compensatory strategy.

Pharyngeal clearing is complete. Epiglottic retroversion is absent but compensated for by a mildly prominent posterior pharyngeal wall wave. Moderate kyphosis and anterior & posterior cervical spine hardware are present. PES open extent is low NL for age @ .45 cm due to marked PES bar. In the AP

Oral Function Reset Oral Ranges

Oral bolus control is characterized by ▦ oral continence ▦ lack of oral continence **and**

to ability to form/hold a bolus. Oral transit is characterized by residue: to

Record: 1679 of 1720

B

Figure 16-2. *(continued)* **B.** Form created in Access database is used to enter pertinent patient information, including objective measures. *(continues)*

BERKELEY : DAVIS : IRVINE : LOS ANGELES : RIVERSIDE : SAN DIEGO : SAN FRANCISCO : SANTA BARBARA : SANTA CRUZ

DYNAMIC VIDEOFLUOROSCOPIC SWALLOW STUDY
Speech Pathology Report

Name: **Referral:**
UCDMC #:   **Birth Date:**
Exam Date: **Panel Review Date:**

ASSESSMENT: **EAT:** 44   **WT(lbs):** 106   **HT(in):** 60

Complaint on Referral:

    63 y.o. cheerful woman with severe rheumatoid arthritis and solid food dysphagia.

History of Present Illness/Complaint:

    Chief complaint is food sticking in her mid chest. She says she eats with a "quart of water" beside her. She takes a bite and a sip. She, or someone helping her, cuts up food into small pieces. She eats 3 meals/day and it takes her about 45 min-1 hour to eat which she believes is a long time. She reports things like salad as easy, and sandwiches as hard to get down. She complains of extremely dry mouth. Eating is described as effortful and painful. Pain is described in throat, esophagus, chest and stomach (rated as 3 on the EAT). She also reports choking on pills, when this happens she can become unable to breathe. She also reports occasional difficulty with feeling of water sticking (does not go down). She reports an approximate weight loss of 10 lbs over the past 2 years but does not believe this is related to swallowing problems. Her BMI is in the "normal" range. She reports coughing at times other than meals. She wakes up at night choking, and this is reported as better since her visit with and Lisinopril was changed. She has a 7-8 year history of reflux and bleeding ulcers. She sleeps with her head elevated on pillows and avoids spicy foods and takes Prilosec daily. She is on oxygen at night (2.5 L) and has CPAP for sleep apnea, but hasn't been using it.

Pertinent Past Medical History:

    ENT visit 3/0/06 revealed normal vocal fold function, pharyngeal strength appeared normal, paroxysmal laryngospasm. She is scheduled for spine surgery in 5 days for some revision fusion C7-T1 as she has developed a more kyphotic position and had increase in pain and parasthesias recently. Hypoglycemia, reactive airway disease, hypertension, tachycardia, rheumatoid arthritis. Multiple orthopedic surgeries (knees, elbow, hands). History of uterine cancer with hysterectomy, history of thyroid cancer (unknown type) with thyroidectomy, meningitis, cataract surgery. Meds: Actonel, Accolate, Synthroid, Prilosec, Celebrex, Varapamil, Zyrtec, Ditropan, Arava, iron, acidophilus, calcium citrate, Centrum silver.

Results of Clinical Evaluation:

    Patient wears a soft neck collar as prescribed over the past year due to neck pain. Normal oral mechanism examination. Articulation precise, voice quality is clear, normal resonance.

Description of Dynamic Swallow Evaluation (see Radiology Report)
Results of Dynamic Swallow

C

Figure 16–2. *(continued)* **C.** Report is generated from information included in Form. Information here does not have to be re-entered. *(continues)*

Name: **Referral:**
UCDMC #: **Birth Date:**
Exam Date: **Panel Review Date:**

As included with an esophagram, the DSS protocol is altered and only liquid contrast is offered. She has other medications as needed.

Oral transit is WNL. Mild oral residue prompts immediate spontaneous repeat swallow.

Total pharyngeal transit time (Pcl-B1) for 1cc is mildly prolonged for age @ 3.04 sec. Swallow of 20cc liquid bolus is slightly prolonged age @ 1.50 sec. due, entirely, to prolonged hypopharyngeal transit and slow PES clearing. Maximum hyoid elevation duration is, also, prolonged, perhaps as a compensatory strategy.

Pharyngeal clearing is complete. Epiglottic retroversion is absent but compensated for by a

SUMMARY:

DSS findings indicate subjective (timing) and objective (PES bar) observations that could be considered consistent with uncontrolled GER. Prolonged hypopharyngeal transit could be in response to impaired esophageal function. Delay in airway closure may increase aspiration risk, particularly of thin liquids, before maximum glottic closure is achieved although no aspiration is detected. Findings are consistent with history and complaint.

RECOMMENDATIONS:

Consider return to review videotaped exam, analysis and Panel discussion and recommendations, including early airway closure to minimize aspiration risk.

Return to Dr. _______________ for follow-up and monitoring.

Oral hygiene.

Careful behavioral GER precautions.

SIGNATURE:

Rebecca Leonard, Ph.D.
Susan McKenzie, M.S.
Alice Walker, M.S.
Cheryl White, M.S.
Jan Pryor, M.A.
Ann Sievers, R.N.
Susan Goodrich, M.S., Pediatrics

C

Figure 16-2. *(continued)*

	Name	Exam Date	Primary Diagnosis	Secondary Di	Birthdate	DOB	Ge	SSPCR	SSPES	SSHma	SSTTT
▶		6/14/2005	Cricopharyngeal Bar	achalasia of L	2/18/1921	0	m	0.02161547213	0.76	2.43	1.53
		10/11/2005	Cricopharyngeal Bar	achalasia of L	2/18/1921	0	m	0.17947103275	0.41	2.06	1.3
		6/22/2004	Cricopharyngeal Bar		11/18/1943	1	F				
		9/17/2002	Cricopharyngeal Bar		8/16/1926	1	m	0.26286116984	0.93	1.96	1.14
		10/28/2003	Cricopharyngeal Bar		7/10/1957	1	f	0.34628378378	0.24	2.12	1.5
		10/28/2003	Cricopharyngeal Bar		7/10/1957	1	f	0.43181818182	0.32	2.28	1.78
		9/17/2002	Cricopharyngeal Bar		7/28/1913	2	M	0.16463414634	0.38	1.07	2
		9/10/2002	Cricopharyngeal Bar		10/30/1915	2	F	0.08427876823	0.43	1.89	1.23
		9/10/2002	Cricopharyngeal Bar		8/16/1923	2	m	0.14102564103	0.63	3.03	2.24
		1/20/2004	Cricopharyngeal Bar		2/19/1918	2	F	0.78031383738	0.72	1.67	1.77
		7/26/2005	Cricopharyngeal Bar		12/15/1922	2	f	0.26994906621	0.17	1.23	0.85000
		10/4/2006	Cricopharyngeal Bar		8/7/1926	2	F	0.85458377239	0.25	2.14	2.1
		8/1/2006	Cricopharyngeal Bar		8/7/1926	2	F				1.2
		6/15/2004	Cricopharyngeal Bar		8/7/1926	2	F	0.56434474616	0.19	1.60	1.33
	r	2/19/2002	Cricopharyngeal Bar		1/3/1917	2	f	0.26020408163	0.72	1.50	1.5
			Cricopharyngeal Bar		1/19/1917	2	F	0.19230769231	0.27	2.12	2.98
		10/7/2003	Cricopharyngeal Bar		4/17/1912	2	f	0.20833333333	0.13	2.01	1.8
		10/24/2006	Cricopharyngeal Bar		5/26/1935	2	m	0.25398773006	0.30	2.01	1.3
		6/1/2004	Cricopharyngeal Bar		7/22/1923	2	F	0.50069156293	0.50	2.16	1.12
		11/8/2005	Cricopharyngeal Bar		5/26/1935	2	m	0.40304568528	0.15	2.50	1.47
		6/28/2005	Cricopharyngeal Bar		5/26/1935	2	m	0.56860706861	0.49	2.38	1.44
		5/24/2005	Cricopharyngeal Bar		5/26/1935	2	m				
		4/21/2005	Cricopharyngeal Bar		5/26/1935	2	m				
		4/22/2005	Cricopharyngeal Bar		5/26/1935	2	m	0.88503253796	0.55	1.64	1.45
		6/28/2005	Cricopharyngeal Bar		4/17/1912	2	f	0.03593429158	0.14	2.22	2.4
		10/7/2003	Cricopharyngeal Bar		4/17/1912	2	f	0.13913043478	0.18	2.53	1.98
		8/19/2003	Cricopharyngeal Bar		1/19/1917	2	F	0.0273381295	0.25	1.97	3.24

Figure 16–3. Once information is in the database, it can be queried to answer specific questions. Here, for example, the database is queried for patients with cricopharyngeal bar.

This capability adds insights into individual patients, but also allows us to consider groups of patients, and to investigate them in ways that allow us to predict their impairments, or their responses to certain interventions. Many of our resulting efforts are reviewed in this text.

PROS AND CONS OF OBJECTIVE MEASURES

In discussions with our peers, we sometimes hear that what we are doing is too time consuming, comprehensive, cost-prohibitive, and/or too technically difficult to be replicated in most clinical settings. This is somewhat surprising to us because our fluoroscopy evaluation, including performance of the procedure, its analysis, and report preparation, takes no more time than other comparably billed procedures, such as a language or voice evaluation. It is perhaps the case that many clinicians consider the DSS to be primarily a screening exam with limited goals, that is, to determine if a patient aspirates, and if so, to identify strategies that prevent aspiration. These are of course worthwhile objectives, and a routine component of our study, as well. Some clinicians may also be using the fluoroscopy study to make decisions about diet advancement. In our opinion, this is an objective best served by endoscopic evaluation, which permits the use of real foods and liquids (not mixed with contrast material), and does not involve radiation.

Our goal has always been to make the DSS study the most powerful diagnostic tool we can. The adherence to a uniform protocol for administration and the availability of normative data allow our approach to meet at least some of the criteria for a standardized test. This improves the power and credibility of interpretation and treatment recommendations in our own eyes, and in those of other medical professionals. For example, from the DSS we can identify and describe aspiration during fluoroscopic observations. But we can also extract information *predictive* of aspiration risk, even if no aspiration is observed during the study. Similarly, dietary recommendations based on a standardized approach to the DSS permit generalizations beyond the conditions of the fluoro suite.

We would argue, further, that there is value in elaborating swallowing impairment in a manner that permits an explanation of the mechanics of dysphagia in individual patients, allows for generalizations between and among patient groups, as well as comparisons to normal and, eventually, predicts impairment in a wide variety of pathologies. The fluoroscopy study, at best, is still a sample of a patient's swallowing capability at one point in time, and is only one piece of the information that must be considered in the management of that individual. But if certain findings can be reliably related to other variables associated with swallowing health, and if these can be used to improve treatment or minimize consequences of swallow impairment, in future patients as well as current, then they are of value. It is this kind of information that may help us not only get patients out of hospitals more quickly, but also keep them from returning with pulmonary or other complications. In our experience, it is the objective measures we collect that are most helpful to these purposes.

Once we understand patient groups well enough, we are also likely to find that some measures are of particular value for one group of patients, and others are more critical in other populations. In fact, one of our ongoing long-term objectives is to identify selected measures, even one or two , that may be of great value in individual patients. Transit times, for example, have been shown to predict aspiration pneumonia requiring repeated hospitalization in CVA patients (Johnson, McKenzie, & Sievers, 1993), whereas a measure of pharyngeal constriction predicts aspiration in other types of patients (Yip, Leonard, & Belafsky, 2006), and possibly, outcomes on other instrumental studies, such as manometry (Leonard, Belafsky, & Rees, 2006). When this kind of information is available, we can begin to apply measures selectively in individual patients, or patient populations. The task of measurement may then be expedited without loss of significant information.

To conclude this section, we return to the beginning. That is, we first became interested in acquiring objective measures from our fluoroscopy studies because of our concerns about the reliability of subjective impressions, and about the credibility of studies based solely on nonstandardized assessments. These concerns arose quickly in our setting because we were meeting regularly as a team, and trying as a group to extract both useful and accurate information from our evaluations.

In today's health care settings, it is not uncommon for clinicians to summarize studies immediately upon their completion, possibly with only brief review. In some cases, in fact, clinicians are not recording fluoroscopy studies, so that any judgments are based on a "real-time" analysis. A usual rationale offered for this practice (in inpatient settings) is that demand for patient turnover is high, and that time constraints permit nothing further. But the decisions made from the study have important, perhaps huge, consequences for individuals. If it is important to determine the competence of a patient's swallow in terms of safety and effectiveness, then it is a decision that should be made with deliberation. Presumably, we would not be subjecting patients to an invasive procedure if we did not feel the potential for valuable information was good. We would suggest again, however, that our success should be measured not simply by how many patients we discharge from hospitals, but by how many patients we discharge who are not readmitted and who are eating in a way that truly befits their capabilities, because we have made the soundest decisions possible about their care.

OBJECTIVE MEASURES

In this section of the chapter, the actual measures obtained from the dynamic study are discussed, and the rationale for their selection is presented. When available, reliability data for each measure are included in the discussion, as are gender and age differences identified in our normal populations. Reliability was initially determined for most of our measures across four individuals who made measures (using measurement criteria presented here) on a subset of swallows from 15 normal subjects. As new clinicians have become available, reliability checks have been continued, using both normal subjects and dysphagic patients in the analyses. Reliability (typically with intraclass correlation coefficients) on many of our measures has by now been established across 8 to 10 raters. Reliability has typically ranged from .90 to .98 for all measures considered, which we believe is quite acceptable. Instructions for actually making the measures is the focus of Chapter 17. Additional measurement materials are provided in the accompanying workbook and media clips.

Timing Measures

In our clinical studies, we typically obtain timing measures from, at least, the largest bolus swallowed. As noted, five of these measures represent points in *bolus transit*, which define the rate at which the bolus travels through the pharynx. Seven additional measures represent the timing of *gestures*, or structural movements, during the swallow. By tracking the bolus separately from the gestures responsible for transporting the bolus, it is possible to assess the coordination between various swallow events. In this scheme, "delay" is characterized as an increased latency between two events, as between a swallow gesture and a point of bolus transit. Swallows that require a greater than usual amount of time are then characterized as "prolonged," not delayed. A video clip labeled "DSSnormswall" is found in the media clips folder for Chapter 16. The reader is encouraged to play through this clip while reading the section on timing measures. All of the *bolus transit* and *swallow gesture* times described here are identified on the clip. *Bolus transit* measures include the following.

B1

B1 is defined as the time of the first movement of the head of the bolus past the posterior nasal spine. This measure is used to establish a zero point marking the beginning of the entry of the bolus into the pharynx. All other timing measures are compared to **B1** to determine the relative time of their occurrence during the swallow. This definition of the onset of pharyngeal transit time, **B1** in our scheme, differs from author to author (Bisch, Logemann, Rademaker, Kahrilas, & Lazarus, 1994; Curtis et al., 1984; McConnell, 1988a).

It is important to recognize that these differences in definition will likely affect comparisons across investigators. McConnel (1988a,1988b) defines the beginning of pharyngeal transit time as the moment the hyoid begins its anterior and superior movement. This is a swallow *gesture*, rather than a measure of bolus position, and thus does not describe transit. Other authors (Logemann, 1983) define the onset of pharyngeal transit relative to the mandible, for example, the time when the bolus crosses the lower or anterior rim of the mandibular ramus. In oropharyngeal cancer patients, however, the

mandibular ramus may be absent. And if a patient's head is rotated during the x-ray study, the position of the mandible will be changed relative to the midline of the pharynx, with a subsequent effect on the measured value of **B1**. The alternative we have chosen, that is, the first movement of the bolus past the posterior nasal spine, is more constantly available and readily identified in most cases. The posterior nasal spine is also a midline structure and therefore its position is less likely to be affected by rotation of the patient. If the palate is absent, the anterior border of the ramus can be used if care is taken not to allow rotation of the patient's head. The interrater reliability of our clinicians in identifying **B1** on normative studies is .99.

BV1 and BV2

BV1 and **BV2** describe transfer of the bolus from the oropharynx to the hypopharynx. The division of pharyngeal transit into multiple components is consistent with, for example, the concept of "pharyngeal transit time" as comprised of "pharyngeal delay" time and "pharyngeal response" time, as defined by Logemann (1987).

BV1

BV1 is defined as the moment that the bolus reaches the base of the vallecula. **BV1** is measured because it demarcates the boundary of the oro- and hypopharynx and, as such, marks the end of oropharyngeal transit and the beginning of hypopharyngeal transit. In patients with reasonably normal anatomy, it is easily found. This is reflected in an r value of 0.99 for **BV1** in our normative data. Patients post head and neck cancer may present with absent valleculae or valleculae severely altered in position and anatomy, however, making it impossible to measure **BV1**. **BV1** is another option to use as a reference point in the calculation of transit measures, in particular, in cases where **B1** for some reason cannot be identified.

BV2

BV2 represents the first exit of the head of the bolus from the valleculae and the beginning of hypopharyngeal transit. In larger bolus sizes, **BV1** and **BV2** are essentially indistinguishable in normal subjects, that is, the bolus does not rest in the valleculae but simply passes by it. But for a 3-cc bolus, for example, there is a significant difference between these two bolus transit points in normal subjects. By the time the bolus reaches this point, there is an increased urgency of swallow success.

BP1 and BP2

BP1 and **BP2** describe bolus movement through the PES and can be used to examine the coordination of PES opening and closing with other events.

BP1

BP1 is defined as the first entrance of the head of the bolus into the upper esophageal sphincter as the sphincter begins to open. Typically, this occurs immediately upon the opening of the pharyngoesophageal sphincter (PES) in normal subjects. The sphincter can occasionally be seen to open before the arrival of the bolus in patients who are not able to move the bolus effectively through the pharynx, however. Opening of the sphincter following its relaxation is considered to be the result of the anterior and superior movement of the hyoid bone and laryngeal structures.

BP2

BP2 is defined as the moment that the tail of the bolus clears the PES and is fully within the esophagus. This timing measurement marks both the end of pharyngeal bolus transport and, in normal subjects, the end of PES opening.

Pharyngeal Transit Times

Once bolus transit times have been identified, it is a straightforward matter to calculate pharyngeal transit times. In our scheme, three such measures are determined, including: *Total pharyngeal transit time*, which is defined as the difference between **BP2** and **B1** and represents the total time of bolus passage through the pharynx. This can be further divided into *oropharyngeal transit time* (**BV1–B1**) and *hypopharyngeal transit time* (**BP2–BV2**). Interjudge reliability for *total pharyngeal transit time* in our normative data was 0.98.

Age, Gender, and Bolus Size/Consistency Differences in Transit Times

The analysis of our 63 younger normal swallow subjects (age 18 to 65) revealed no change in pharyngeal transit time across bolus size or consistency. This finding has implications for cases in which very small or very large boluses are unmanageable. That is, if a patient is unable to propel a very small liquid bolus into the oropharynx secondary to anterior tongue and mouth abnormalities, a larger liquid bolus can be substituted for this measure and the expected time for a normal response will not be affected. In the same fashion, if a patient cannot control a large liquid bolus, or transfers the bolus to the pharynx in a piecemeal manner, timing measures made on the smaller bolus size will still accurately reflect the patient's pharyngeal transit time. In addition, if thin consistencies are difficult for the patient, then paste can be substituted and the evaluation of pharyngeal transit time should remain accurate. Our results contradict previous studies in which the subject numbers were smaller (Dodds, Stewart, & Logemann, 1990; Johnson et al., 1992).

Pharyngeal transit time did not increase significantly with increasing age in our first group of normal subjects, who ranged in age from 18 years to 65 years (Kendall, McKenzie, Leonard, Gonçalves, & Walker, 2001). This finding differs from that reported by other investigators (Cook et al., 1994; Curtis et al., 1984; Logemann, 1987; Robbins, Hamilton, Lof, & Kempster, 1992; Shaw et al., 1995). Subjects in our first group of normal subjects were chosen without regard to age, and the age distribution of the subjects is weighted more heavily toward the middle of the age range. Our findings did not change, however, when subjects were grouped by age and the means for specific age categories compared using linear regression analysis.

However, in a comparison of 62 normal subjects under 65 years to a group of 83 normal, nondysphagic subjects over 65 years, transit times were significantly different for 1-cc, 3-cc, and 20-cc bolus sizes. In general, transit times were prolonged in the elderly group. The elderly group was then further subdivided into those with no medical problems typical of an aging population (hypertension, diabetes, and osteoarthritis), and those who had one or more of these conditions. When the younger normal subjects were compared to 23 normal elderly subjects with no medical conditions, all transit times for the elderly were still significantly prolonged. We currently use values for 128 age- and gender-matched normal subjects for comparison to groups of patients (corrected for age and gender). We continue to compare individual patients, according to gender if necessary, to data for normal subjects under, and over, the age of 65 years, as appropriate (see Table 16–1).

Clinical Implications of Prolonged Bolus Transit Times

Prolonged bolus transit times have frequently been implicated in swallowing difficulty (Bisch et al., 1994; Johnson et al., 1992; Johnson & McKenzie, 1993). The longer bolus material remains in the airway, the greater the challenge to airway protective mechanisms. Previous studies in stroke victims have shown an increased risk of aspiration pneumonia in patients with prolonged pharyngeal transits as measured from a dynamic swallow study, even when no aspiration was identified on the examination (Johnson et al., 1993). In a study of elderly individuals with dysphagia with no obvious medical or surgical causes of their impairment, prolonged bolus transit times were identified in 61% of the patients (Kendall & Leonard, 2001). Delayed or prolonged pharyngeal transit time has also been shown to be associated with an increased incidence of aspiration pneumonia in several populations (Johnson et al., 1992; Johnson et al., 1993; Rademaker, Pauloski, Logemann, & Shanahan, 1994). As such, its clinical significance is well established. We typically interpret prolonged pharyngeal transit times as an indication of increased risk for aspiration and make recommendations accordingly. In some cases, however, prolonged transit times may reflect a patient's caution or fear regarding swallow safety. If so, other measures may also reflect the patient's concern, for example, hyoid displacement greater than normal (or earlier than typical), PES opening duration longer than normal.

Swallow Gesture Times

In addition to bolus transit times, we identify times when critical swallow gestures occur. Typically, these involve the onset of a structure's movement, and when it achieves maximum displacement during the swallow. In the case of the PES, we also note when it closes. The reader is encouraged to continue to move through the video clip, "DSSnormswall" to identify swallow gesture points described here. The swallow gesture times are as follows.

AEstart and AEclose (Airway Closure)

The aryepiglottic folds and the outline of the arytenoid cartilages are visible against the relative hypodensity of the pharyngeal space in the lateral projection on the x-ray. During swallowing the arytenoid cartilages are seen to elevate and approximate the down-folding epiglottis, effectively closing the supraglottic larynx and protecting the airway. During frame by frame analysis, it is possible to identify movement of these structures, in particular, when the most superior part of the arytenoid cartilages begins to elevate, and again when it makes contact with the down-folding epiglottis (Logemann, 1987). The points of onset (AEstart) and completion (AEclose) of supraglottic closure can therefore be measured. The timing of these events can then be compared to other events that occur during the swallow. In particular, it may be important to determine the relative timing of ary-epiglottic fold closure relative to bolus transit through the pharynx in patients observed to aspirate. Normally during a swallow, the arytenoid cartilages begin to move towards the epiglottis as the bolus enters the pharynx. By the time the bolus arrives at the upper esophageal sphincter (designated as **BP1**), the down-folding epiglottis is seen to approximate the arytenoid cartilages, effectively obliterating the supraglottic passage.

H1, H2, and H3 (Hyoid Displacement)

In our measurement scheme, **H1** is defined as the first superior–anterior displacement of the hyoid that results in a swallow. **H2** is marked by the first frame in which the hyoid bone has reached its maximum superior–anterior excursion during the swallow, and typically occurs in close relationship to PES opening (Cook et al., 1989; Jacob, Kahrilas, Logemann, Shah, & Ha, 1989). In our normative data, comparison of the values of **H2–B1** and **Pop–B1** (**Pop** represents the first opening of the PES during swallow) were found to be identical. **H3** indicates the first retreat of the hyoid from its maximum displacement.

The frame chosen to represent **H2** is also used when measuring the distance of maximum hyoid excursion. Reliability in defining **H1** and **H2** in normal subjects was .99 and .98, respectively. A number of authors have described the first movement of the hyoid (**H1** in our scheme) as the onset of the swallow reflex. We recently described the relationship of **H1** in our normal nonelderly and elderly subjects to a number of bolus transit points, including *B1*, *BV1*, *BV2*, *BP1*, and passing the angle of the mandible (Leonard & McKenzie, 2006).These data provide a number of options for considering the relationship between first movement of the hyoid and bolus transit and can be used to relate specific latencies to various concepts of pharyngeal swallow delay.

The onset of hyoid elevation is one of the first visible gestures in the swallow sequence and, as such, signals the onset of hypopharyngeal elevation and preparation to receive the bolus. Information about timing of the onset and maximum swallow movement of the hyoid can be especially helpful in patients whose coordination of swallowing gestures with bolus transit is in question, for example, in conditions affecting neural transmission, that is, amyotrophic lateral sclerosis, or multiple sclerosis.

Although our *r* values for **H1** and **H2** are quite good, it is nevertheless true that neither of these points may be obvious, even in normal swallowers. "Preparatory" hyoid movements are common and can complicate identification, in particular, of **H1**. It is help-ful that hyoid movement for swallow is more vigorous and stereotypic than other hyoid movements (sometimes characterized as a blur on the fluoro study), and is often preceded by a few frames of stability. In both normal and dysphagic individuals, identification of **H2** also may be problematic because the hyoid does not always move at the same rate or in a straight line to its maximum excursion. Rather, it may follow a graceful clockwise or counter-clockwise curve or figure eight, slowing significantly as it curves. The measurer must review the study carefully and fix one point in the patterned movement that best represents maximum hyoid anterior and superior displacement as **H2**. If necessary, several displacement measures can be made to determine which frame represents maximum displacement.

The point at which the hyoid returns to rest following the swallow has sometimes been used to indicate the end of the swallow. However, large variability in the measured values from our normative data for this event suggests significant behavioral overlay affecting its timing. We recommend that the return of the hyoid to a rest position be used to define the end of pharyngeal transit as a last resort, and only then with caution (McConnell, 1988a, 1988b). It is not routinely assessed in our dynamic swallow studies.

Pop, PESmax, and Pcl (PES Opening and Closing)

Pop is the time of the first frame on which the PES is open. **PESmax** represents the first time at which the PES achieves its maximum opening size. **Pcl**

is the time of the first frame on which the PES closes (usually on the tail of the bolus), marking the end of pharyngeal transit.

PES timing is of obvious importance as the culminating gesture of the swallow and the literal and figurative "bottom line" of pharyngeal transit. If the concept is not debatable, the definition of the measurement can be. Selection of a single point in time when the PES opens or closes requires selection of a precise point that can be called the PES. The location (and therefore the best place to make measures) of the PES as seen on a dynamic videofluoroscopic swallow study is unclear. It has previously been defined as a point 1.5 cm below the beginning of the tracheal air column (Kahrilas, Dodds, Dent, Logemann, & Shaker, 1988).It seems likely, however, that the position of the upper esophageal sphincter varies from subject to subject, depending on size of the individual and possibly other variables. In addition, the location of the top of the air column is often difficult to identify with precision. In our setting, acceptable reliability for precise designation of this site has not been achieved, even with quite experienced evaluators (though this has improved with improved fluoroscopy units). We have therefore chosen to define the upper esophageal sphincter as the narrowest part of the opening from the level of C3 (superior), above, to the level of C6 (inferior), below. The decision to use this definition was based on the idea, supported by experience, that the narrowest site is always the most clinically significant, that is, what limits rate of bolus passage.

Closure of the PES (**Pcl**) is almost universally used to define the end of the swallow. If hypopharyngeal tran-sit is even partially successful, **Pcl** will coincide with all or part of the bolus entering the cervical esophagus.

Em (Epiglottic Displacement)

This measure is the time of the first frame on which the epiglottis has returned to its preswallow position, marking the reopening of the supraglottic airway or return to respiratory posture following the swallow. Typically, it occurs after the closure of the PES. **Em** has been used to mark the end of pharyngeal transit (Johnson et al., 1992; Johnson & McKenzie, 1993); not surprisingly, transit times reported using this marker are longer than others reported. The measure has been particularly useful in identifying segments of the CVA population at risk for development of aspiration pneumonia (Johnson & McKenzie, 1993). Nevertheless, application of **Em** in this manner can be debated. Epiglottic return is not a critical gesture for accomplishment of pharyngeal transit and it also appears subject to behavioral interference. However, it does signal re-establishment of the pharyngeal airway, that is, a return to respiratory mode. As the calculation of **H1–Em** may reflect respiration interruption time, **Em** can be a useful measure for patients with respiratory compromise. It is included for these reasons. Reliability for this parameter on normative data was 0.99.

Swallow Gesture Durations

Once the times of various structural events have been calculated, it is possible to determine the durations between the events. The durations we obtain include the duration of maximum hyoid displacement (**H3–H2**), PES opening duration (**Pcl–Pop**), and duration of airway closure (**Em–AEc**). Our intermeasurer reliability for the value of **Pcl–Pop** was 0.92.

Age, Gender, and Bolus Size/
Consistency Differences in Swallow
Gesture Times

In contrast to *bolus transit* times, certain *swallow gesture* times in our two groups of normal subjects did vary with bolus size and consistency. PES opening time (**Pcl–Pop**) increased with increasing size of the bolus (see Table 16–1). Jacob et al. (1989) also found that the duration of PES opening increased with increasing bolus size, whereas the overall duration of the swallow remained constant. These authors interpreted this finding as indicating that the *speed* of bolus transport through the PES is increased with larger boluses. As noted previously, we did not find (in our younger normal subjects) differences in bolus transit times between the 3-cc liquid bolus and a comparably sized paste bolus (Kendall, Leonard, & McKenzie, 2001). However, we did find that, for the 3-cc liquid bolus, the hyoid remained maximally elevated longer, as compared to the paste bolus. PES opening, on the other hand, was significantly longer for the paste bolus, as compared to the liquid bolus. Our data indicated further that **EM–AEclose** also increased with bolus size, suggesting that the airway is protected longer depending on bolus size.

It is of further interest that the duration of maximum hyoid displacement (**H3–H2**) was significantly reduced in our elderly normal subjects as compared to the younger normal subjects, for the 1-cc, 3-cc, and 20-cc bolus sizes.

In contrast, there was a tendency for PES opening (**Pcl–Pop**) and airway closure (**Em–AEclose**) to be longer in the elderly normal subjects as compared to the younger subjects, but these differences were not significant. No gender differences were identified for swallow gesture times.

Clinical Implications of Swallow Gesture Times

Of these measures, duration of PES opening (**Pcl–Pop**) is perhaps of particular interest. The capability of the upper esophageal sphincter to open in a timely manner is critical to a normal swallow. An inability to do so results in incomplete or absent transit of the bolus into the esophagus. When the PES fails to open, decreased hyoid or larynx elevation or failure of cricopharyngeal relaxation may be the etiology. In addition, poor pharyngeal constriction, secondary to pharyngeal constrictor weakness or lack of tongue mobility, can impact PES opening. Whether it is a problem with timing, extent of opening, or the duration of opening, the spatial measures discussed further in this chapter can provide insight into the etiology of the dysfunction.

COORDINATION BETWEEN BOLUS TRANSIT AND SWALLOW GESTURE EVENTS

Coordination of events during the pharyngeal phase of swallowing has been considered to be reflexive, involuntary, and automatic in nature. Central mechanisms are thought to be primarily responsible for the pattern of events that propel a bolus from the oral cavity into the esophagus. Sensory feedback information and voluntary behaviors are believed secondarily to influence the sequence. Tracking of *bolus transit* separately from *swallow gesture* times permits evaluation of the coordination between and among these events. To determine normal variability in the sequencing and coordination of the swallowing gestures and points of bolus transit, we analyzed the sequence of events during swallowing of a 1-cc, a 3-cc, and a 20-cc liquid bolus in our 60 normal younger adult volunteers (Kendall, 2002). Of 180 swallows evaluated, no two swallows matched in the sequence of all the events, indicating sequence variability between subjects and within individuals depending on changes in bolus size. Variability was less during deglutition of larger bolus volumes, perhaps as a result of faster bolus transit times and less opportunity for behavioral overlay. Certain bolus and gesture timing relationships were found to exist during hypopharyngeal bolus transit that did not vary between subjects or across bolus categories. These included the following:

- The elevation of the aryepiglottic folds (**AEstart**) always began *before* opening of the pharyngeal esophageal sphincter (**Pop**).
- The sphincter always opened (**Pop**) *before* the arrival of the bolus at the sphincter (**BP1**); similarly, the sphincter closed simultaneously with or just after the tail of the bolus cleared the sphincter (**BP2**);
- Maximum hyoid to larynx approximation (**HLmax**) always occurred *after* the onset of upper esophageal sphincter opening (**Pop**);

- Maximum pharyngeal constriction (**PAmax**) always occurred *after* maximal distension of the upper esophageal sphincter (**PESmax**). Some variability in the relative timing of all other event sets analyzed by this study was found. The lack of variability in the relationships noted, however, make these useful in considerations of coordination between and among swallowing events.

For example, one timing relationship that we have investigated (Kendall, Leonard, & McKenzie, 2004) and found to be of particular clinical relevance is the timing of supraglottic closure (**AEclose**) relative to the arrival of the bolus at the upper esophageal sphincter (**BP1**). As noted, the arytenoid cartilages elevate and approximate the downfolding epiglottis (**AEclose**) during swallow, effectively closing the supraglottic larynx and protecting the airway. This mechanism may be incomplete or delayed in patients complaining of dysphagia and may lead to "penetration" of bolus material into the airway. Aspiration that occurs *during* passage of the bolus into the upper esophageal sphincter is usually the result of incomplete upper airway closure.

To evaluate the relationship of supraglottic airway closure and bolus arrival further, we analyzed the timing of these two events in our group of 60 young control subjects and also in 23 elderly control subjects (65–88 years old) without dysphagia, and without medical conditions typical of an elderly population (diabetes, hypertension, and osteoarthritis). Event timing was measured in 0.01-second intervals from videofluoroscopic studies for two liquid bolus size categories. Results of the analysis revealed that in most individuals, the arytenoid cartilages approximate the epiglottis, closing off the airway, *before* the arrival of the bolus at the pharyngoesophageal sphincter. However, in both bolus size categories, there were individuals who achieved complete supraglottic closure after the bolus had arrived at the sphincter, but *never greater than 0.1 seconds later*. No difference in the timing of supraglottic closure relative to bolus arrival at the sphincter was found between the young and the elderly subject groups. The information from this study has allowed us to objectively determine if supraglottic closure timing is delayed in patients with dysphagia and to address any delay with strategies and exercises designed specifically to correct the delay.

SPATIAL MEASURES

The acquisition of spatial (distance and area) measurements has become simpler with the digital recording of fluoroscopy studies (via digital recorder or archiving system), and techniques we currently use are described in Chapter 17. Extracting valid estimates of distance and area requires particular attention during the dynamic swallow study so that measures, and comparisons among measures, can be made for the calibration frame, the referent frame, and the frame on which the target movement is seen. Critical aspects of technique include a true lateral patient upper body position and uniform patient-to-fluoroscope arm distance, not to mention good visibility of target anatomy over the course of the exam.

Spatial measures routinely made at our facility include the following:

- **Maximum hyoid displacement**: change in hyoid position from a referent frame, **Hold**, to maximum anterior–superior displacement, **H2** (**Hold** is defined as the relationship between structures with a 1-cc bolus held in the oral cavity);
- **Pharyngeal Constriction Ratio** (PCR): a ratio of pharyngeal area measured in lateral view at its point of maximum constriction during a swallow, to pharyngeal area measured in the **Hold** posture. The ratio is referred to as the pharyngeal constriction ratio (**PCR**);
- **Maximum opening of the PES**: maximum distention of the site designated PES during swallow; and
- **Maximum approximation of the larynx and hyoid**: difference in distance between hyoid and larynx at **Hold**, and at their point of maximum approximation during the swallow.

Normative data for each of these measures, respectively, are presented in Table 16–1. The reader is again encouraged to move through the "DSSnorm-swallow" clip (in materials folder for Chapter 16) while reading this section to identify frames used in making displacement measures.

Reference Position

To measure how much a pharyngeal structure or complex of structures is displaced during swallowing, the identification of the "nondisplaced" or a reference position is obviously critical for comparison. Selecting such a position for structures of the oral cavity and pharynx has proved particularly challenging. The difficulty is related to both behavioral and conceptual issues, that is, what constitutes a "rest" position for the larynx? Conceptually, options for "rest" might include a position assumed by the patient when asked not to move, or a position at the end of a vegetative gesture, such as a sigh. In our experience, however, huge variability has been observed in these behaviors both within and between subjects. We have forgone the idea of a "rest" position, and are using a referent preparatory measure identified as "hold." In doing so, we have knowingly sacrificed the idea of measuring total range of movement because there is often displacement *to* the preparatory position. We have essentially focused on what we believe to be more meaningful and useful concepts: Range of movement related to swallow, and the identification of a reliable position to which maximum displacements can be compared. Still, behavioral interference is not eliminated, because movement for preparation for swallow varies greatly in normal and dysphagic swallowers. Nevertheless, use of the "hold" referent has enabled us to make reliable spatial measurements.

Hold — The "Reference" Position

The **Hold** position is defined by giving the subject of the study a 1-cc bolus of contrast with the instruction to hold it in the mouth before swallowing. For the purposes of the recorded swallow analysis, the frame just before any posterior movement of the bolus that results in a swallow from the hold position is defined as **Hold**. When a patient is unable to "hold" the bolus, the measure is made on the frame before onset of efforts toward oral transit.

Hyoid Displacement

Hmax. **Hmax** is defined as the distance traveled by the hyoid to the point of maximal elevation during a swallow from its position during **Hold**.

PES opening depends primarily on the elevation of the hyoid and larynx (Cook et al., 1989; Jacob et al., 1989). The anterior movement of these structures pulls open the relaxed PES, thereby creating a vacuum, or area of low pressure, at the PES site. This action, combined with gravity and pressure applied by the base of tongue and pharynx, will propel the bolus into the upper esophagus (Dodds et al., 1990; Jacob et al., 1989; McConnel, 1988b). Measurement of maximum displacement of the hyoid during swallow provides valuable insight into the forces contributing to PES opening in a given patient. Hyoid displacement also contributes to airway protection during swallow, by displacing laryngeal structures anteriorly and superiorly, under the tongue. Diminished hyoid elevation is seen in conditions that affect muscles that attach the hyoid to the mandible, for example, surgical resection of the floor of the mouth, with tissue fibrosis after radiation therapy, and neuromuscular diseases. Inability to elevate the hyoid/larynx is often accompanied by difficulties with PES opening. In fact, identification of diminished hyoid bone elevation can help distinguish failure of PES opening because of failure of cricopharyngeal relaxation from failure of PES opening because of a loss of anterior traction on the sphincter. Given the relationship between hyoid and PES, and the relative ease of identifying the hyoid on the fluoroscopic study, we feel that measurement of hyoid displacement is an important part of the dynamic swallow study interpretation.

Because **Hmax** is measured at **H2**, difficulty in identification of the precise frame of maximum displacement may lead to an inaccurate measurement of **Hmax**, as discussed earlier. Our intermeasurer reliability for **Hmax** was .95, however, suggesting that with experience it is possible to accurately estimate this point.

Hyoid to Larynx Approximation

HLhold. The distance between the hyoid, typically, the lowest portion of the hyoid body visible in the lateral view, and the inferior anterior boundary of the larynx, defined as the anterior superior border of the tracheal air column, is calculated.

HLmax. The distance between the two points is again calculated at the point of maximum approximation during the swallow, referred to has **HLmax**. The difference between **HLhold** and **HLmax** is defined as **HL**. In addition to hyoid displacement, approximation of the hyoid and larynx likely contributes to airway protection and PES opening.

Pharyngeal Area

PAhold. The area of the pharynx, that is, the two-dimensional space of the pharynx apparent in lateral view, is calculated on the **Hold** frame and is designated as **PAhold**. Our intermeasurer reliability for **PAhold** was found to be .92. Linear regression analysis of the effects of subject height and weight on pharyngeal area at the hold position in our younger group of normal subjects failed to reveal any significant differences in pharyngeal area related to these variables.

PAmax. A second measure of pharyngeal area is made when the pharynx is maximally constricted during the largest bolus swallow, and is designated as **PAmax**. As with **PAhold**, for normal subjects this measure was found to differ significantly depending on the gender of the subject (see Table 16–1). Our normative data for this parameter were collected during a 20-cc bolus swallow. Intermeasurer reliability for **Pamax** was .96.

Pamax/Pahold: Pharyngeal Constriction Ratio. A ratio of the pharyngeal area at maximum constriction to the pharyngeal area during hold is calculated. The use of a ratio minimizes gender differences noted for each of the area measurements. Although larger in the elderly normal group as compared to younger subjects, the ratio of pharyngeal area at maximum constriction and pharyngeal area at rest, referred to as the pharyngeal constriction ratio (PCR), is quite low, between 0 and 0.14 cm^2. Intermeasurer reliability for *PCR* was .95.

The posterior and downward driving force of the tongue base within the contractile chamber of the pharyngeal walls acts in concert with upper esophageal sphincter opening to ensure successful transfer of the bolus through the pharynx (Cook et al., 1989; Dodds et al., 1990; Jacob et al., 1989; McConnel,

1988a, 1988b). On the dynamic swallow study, the tongue base is seen to move posteriorly toward the posterior pharyngeal wall and combined with pharyngeal shortening (as the hypopharynx elevates) results in the obliteration or narrowing of the pharynx during the swallow. The critical role of the contractile chamber walls against which the piston must work should not escape appreciation. When the role of lingual retraction is limited because of anatomic or neurologic impairment, the compensation provided by the pharyngeal constrictors can still result in complete pharyngeal constriction. From the fluoroscopic study, some evidence pertinent to both pharyngeal constriction and tongue movement is available. Measurement of pharyngeal area represents a possibility for objectively assessing this information, in a manner that takes into account all forces accomplishing pharyngeal transit, not just the tongue.

The lateral view of the pharynx on the swallow study is a two-dimensional representation of a three-dimensional space, and we often rely on the amount of residual barium seen in the hypopharynx to define the size of the space at maximum constriction. These limitations notwithstanding, we feel that the measures provide a useful way to evaluate the "piston" action of the tongue working against the descending constriction of the pharyngeal walls. Pharyngeal area measures have the additional advantage of being relatively easy to obtain in most subjects.

When poor pharyngeal constriction is identified on the swallow study by measurement and calculation of an increased PCR, a loss of tongue mobility or bulk may be the primary etiology. If the tongue activity is relatively

normal, weakness of the pharyngeal constrictors (as is often seen in stroke victims) may be the reason. The result is usually persistent pharyngeal residue. Patients will be at an increased risk for aspiration of the residue when the glottis reopens for respiration. Strategies such as the "double swallow" or "effortful swallow," directed at clearing the residue before resuming respiration, may be recommended.

PES Distension

PESmax. The maximum opening of the PES during a swallow, **PESmax**, is measured. As discussed earlier for **Pop–Pcl**, PES is defined as the narrowest point in the opening between C3 and C6 during the swallow. Because efficient transfer of the bolus into the esophagus is dependent on adequate PES opening, some measure of PES opening is an obvious choice for inclusion in any measurement battery. As discussed previously, however, the actual location of the point designated PES is arguable. By defining the PES as the narrowest point between C3 and C6, we were able to achieve an r of 0.95 on this measure for normal subjects. (Typically, the point is between C4 and C6; in some patients with altered anatomy, however, this may vary).

Age, Gender, and Bolus Size/ Consistency Differences for Spatial Measures

Several differences in these variables were identified for spatial measures. Age differences were identified for PESmax and PCR; PESmax is reduced in the elderly, and **PCR** is increased, as compared to younger subjects (see Table 16–1). **Hmax** was reduced in elderly females, as compared to younger females, but this difference was not identified for younger and elderly males (see Table 16–1). Gender differences were also identified as significant for all displacement measures, on all bolus sizes and consistencies investigated, with the exception of **PESmax**, which did not differ significantly according to gender on any bolus considered (see Table 16–1).

Bolus size differences were noted for all displacement measures except maximum approximation of the larynx and hyoid during swallow (true for all bolus sizes). Our interpretation of this finding is that larynx to hyoid approximation (**HL**) may have more to do with airway protection, and maintaining a constant level of such during swallow, as opposed to making adjustments in size of the PES. **PESmax** did increase with increasing bolus size, presumably to accommodate the larger bolus size or in response to changes in intrabolus pressures. Increased PES opening with increasing bolus size corresponds to an increase in **Hmax** with increasing bolus sizes (in both age groups and for both males and females), and may reflect the anterior traction on the PES by the forward movement of the hyoid, as well as increased intrabolus pressures (see Table 16–1).

CLINICAL IMPLICATIONS OF IMPAIRED SPATIAL DISPLACEMENTS

Impairments in spatial displacements are an important reason for aspiration and dysphagia in many patient populations. Their calculation can provide excellent insights into causes of impairment, as well as therapeutic objectives that might be considered. Our own research, for example, has demonstrated the following:

- In a study comparing normal subjects, patients with nonobstructive cricopharyngeal bars, patients with obstructive cricopharyngeal bars and patients with Zenker's diverticuli, data suggested an association between cricopharyngeus muscle dysfunction and progressive dilation and weakness of the pharynx (Belafsky, Rees, Allen & Leonard, 2010). That is, **PAhold** increased with increasing obstruction at the level of the upper esophageal sphincter (decreased **PESmax**). Our interpretation of this finding is that, in response to prolonged obstruction at the UES, the pharynx may dilate. If so, pharyngeal constriction and clearing during swallow may be affected.
- In a subsequent study, effects of cricopharyngeal myotomy, a surgical approach to modifying obstruction at the PES, were considered for both PES opening size, **PCR** (Pharyngeal Constriction Ratio) and **PAhold**. **PESmax** was improved (increased) and **PCR** was reduced (also improved). **PAhold**, however, did not change, suggesting that dilation of the pharynx associated with long-term obstruction at the PES may be permanent (Allen, White, Leonard, & Belafsky, 2011).
- Leonard and Belafsky (2011) reported changes in various spatial

measures associated with cervical spine surgery and anterior instrumentation. Measures in two groups of patients, one <2 months from surgery, and one >2 months from surgery, were compared to normal control subjects (age- and gender-matched to patients). **PESmax** was decreased significantly in the early postsurgical group, but was improved in the late group. Other measures, including thickness of the posterior pharyngeal wall that interfered with epiglottic inversion and pharyngeal clearing, may persist and contribute to patients' continued complaints.

■ Increases in **PCR** appear to be a near-hallmark feature of swallowing in patients with myotonic muscular dystrophy (Leonard, Kendall, Johnson, & McKenzie, 2001). In some patients investigated, in fact, the pharyngeal area when maximally constricted (for a 20-cc bolus) was actually *larger* than in the **Hold** position. This suggests that pharyngeal weakness associated with this disease may become so pronounced that the presence of a large bolus causes the pharynx to distend or expand, rather than constricting to propel the bolus into the esophagus. In monitoring our myotonic muscular dystrophy patients (and others who demonstrate similar weakness), we pay particular attention to this measure in counseling patients regarding a possible transition from oral to partial or nonoral feeding.

■ **PCR** has been further shown to be associated with aspiration in a variety of patient populations (Yip, Leonard, & Belafsky, 2006). Data from 260 sequential patients undergoing dynamic swallow studies were examined for those who aspirated, and those who did not aspirate. Those patients who did aspirate (on the largest bolus swallowed) demonstrated a mean **PCR** of 0.32 cm^2, whereas those who didn't had a mean **PCR** of 0.20 cm^2 (both values were elevated, as compared to normal). Furthermore, individuals with a **PCR** greater than 0.25 cm^2 were three times more likely to aspirate, as compared to other patients. In evaluating patients, we are seriously concerned about safe swallowing in patients with **PCRs** of this value, even when we do not observe aspiration on the dynamic swallow study.

■ In a subsequent study, stroke patients (CVA) who did and did not aspirate on the largest bolus swallowed on the DSS were considered (Leonard, unpublished data). The group consisted of 300 patients. Patients with a **PCR** of 0.25 cm^2 were six times more likely to aspirate than those with values below 0.25 cm^2.

■ **PCR** may be a useful surrogate measure of pharyngeal strength. In a comparison of maximum pharyngeal pressures obtained on manometry (**PCP**), and **PCR** from a separate dynamic swallow study in the same patients, a negative correlation of −.7 was, found for the two measures (Leonard, Belafsky, & Rees, 2006). Furthermore, only two patients with a **PCR** significantly elevated from normal (for age and gender) were found to have maximum pharyngeal pressures within the normal range on manometry, and pressures for these two patients were very low, 60 and 61 mm Hg, respectively. In a subsequent study (Leonard, Rees, Belafsky, & Allen, 2011), **PCP** and **PCR** were investigated in patients undergoing simultaneous fluoroscopy and manometry studies. The correlation between the two measures, for 25 patients, was −.72. Of particular interest, no patient who had a normal **PCR** had an abnormal **PCP**; further, no patient with an abnormal **PCR** (>.25 cm^2) had normal **PCPs** (>60 mm /Hg). These results support our previous findings suggesting the potential of an objective fluoroscopic measure to predict manometric measures, when manometry is not available.

- In an investigation of elderly patients with no obvious medical or surgical cause of their dysphagia (Kendall & Leonard, 2001), 74% of patients demonstrated an elevated **PCR**. Elevated **PCR** was also found to be a factor in 75% of cases of aspiration identified in this population. Interestingly, the timing of maximum pharyngeal constriction remained appropriately coordinated with the position of the bolus in the pharynx in these same patients.

- Our comparison of younger and more elderly nondysphagic individuals revealed a large percentage of the elderly subjects with cricopharyngeal bars (31%) (Leonard, Kendall, & McKenzie, 2002). Inter-

estingly, no bars were identified in our younger group of subjects. Not surprisingly, **PESmax** was also reduced in the elderly group, as compared to the younger group. Evaluation of elderly individuals should consider the increased likelihood of apparently asymptomatic cricopharyngeal bars.

- In an investigation of factors affecting pharyngeal constriction in nonelderly and elderly normal subjects, several findings were of interest (Leonard, Kendall, & McKenzie, 2004). As described, **PCR** was elevated in the elderly, as compared to younger subjects, suggesting a reduced ability to constrict and possibly clear the pharynx during swallow. In addition, the two-dimensional pharyngeal area measured in the **Hold** position was larger in the elderly subjects, as was the distance between the larynx and the hyoid at **Hold**. The distance from the hyoid to the mandible did not differ between groups; however, the distance between the hyoid and larynx at **Hold** was significantly greater in the elderly subjects. A measure of the anterior–posterior view of the pharynx at **Hold** was also wider in the elderly subjects. These data, as well as additional information we have obtained, suggest that the pharynx in elderly subjects may be larger, or longer, as compared to younger individuals. In addition, the pharynx did not constrict as completely, and the larynx did not elevate to the same extent, in elderly subjects. These data comprise an important reference in assessing swallow in elderly dysphagic patients, in particular, in differentiating normal from abnormal in this group.

■ In an investigation of normal subjects and elderly dysphagic patients (Kendall & Leonard, 2001), it was found that maximum hyoid displacement was actually greater on smaller bolus sizes in the elderly group, as compared to individuals without dysphagia. This was interpreted as a possible compensation for the decreased duration of the hyoid at maximum displacement, and may represent a strategy that can be used with other patients.

The kinds of observations reviewed here represent just a few that can be made when large amounts of objective data become available for patients representing different disorders. In short, the use of a standardized DSS and objective measures have, in our opin-ion, allowed us to use the fluoroscopy study as a powerful diagnostic tool. It:

■ permits us to compare our patients to normal subjects according to age and gender;
■ provides an objective means of tracking changes in patients across time and treatments;
■ supplies us with a basis for characterizing dysphagia in unique patient populations;
■ allows us to go beyond the determination of aspiration versus no aspiration, or appropriate dietary recommendations, to understand the biomechanical deviations from normal deglutition that contribute to the dysphagia, and how these present a risk to patients *outside* the environment of the DSS evaluation (Table 16–2);
■ reveals information that, increasingly, we are finding can be related to other instrumental measures of swallow function; and

Table 16–2. Odds Ratios for Aspiration

	NORMS (135) (mean ± 2 sd)	PTS-NONASP (2104)	PTS-ASPIRATORS (529)	O.R. (>2 sd)
PCR (cm^2)	.07$_{(.18)}$	.16	.36	If >.25, O.R. = 5.2
Hmax (cm)	2.12$_{(1.56)}$	1.53	1.28	If <.56, O.R. = 3.0
PESmax (cm)	.86$_{(.52)}$	.87	.73	If <.34, O.R. = 2.8
TPT (secs)	1.16$_{(1.12)}$	1.56	1.81	If >2.3, O.R. = 2.8
PAhold (cm^2)	8.34$_{(6.03)}$	10.00	11.02	If >14, O.R. = 2.5

Odds Ratios for Aspiration Selected for Particular Biomechanical Measures. (Shown are values for patients who did or did not aspirate on a 20-cc liquid bolus. All diagnostic categories are included. Ratios are based on values that were more than 2 standard deviations from normal mean values for each measure. Normative data have been controlled for age and gender.)

■ is now, in our practice, a part of the repertoire of diagnostic tests routinely ordered by many physician specialists charged with evaluating and treating dysphagic patients.

In Table 16–2, odds ratios for aspiration, based on selected objective measures, are shown. Data for patients who did and did not aspirate are compared to means for an age- and gender-matched group of normal subjects ($n = 128$). Patient data were corrected for age and gender. Odds ratios were calculated for the patient groups based on values (for each measure considered) that were 2 standard deviations from the control mean. Data allow us to consider aspiration risk factors for individual patients, *even when they are not observed to aspirate during the fluoroscopy study*.

STUDY QUESTIONS

1. Which structural displacements during swallowing differ in younger and older individuals? According to gender?
2. Do pharyngeal transit times differ according to age and/or gender?
3. What subjective impressions from fluoroscopy studies have demonstrated reasonable interjudge reliability?
4. Define bolus transit at "B1," "BV1," "BV2," "BP1," and "BP2."
5. Why was the "Hold" position selected as a referent for measures of structural displacements? (as compared to a "Rest" position).
6. What are some problems in using the angle of the mandible as a marker for the onset of bolus transit?
7. What is the advantage of tracking *bolus transit* times separately from *swallow gesture* times?
8. What relationships between swallow gestures, or between swallow gestures and bolus transit, appear to be invariant in both younger and older normal individuals?
9. The measure of pharyngeal constriction, "PCR," may be a reasonable surrogate for what other instrumental measure?
10. What was unique about PES opening in the normal elderly population described?

REFERENCES

Allen, J., White, C., Leonard, R., & Belafsky, P. C. (2010). Effects of cricopharyngeus muscle surgery on the pharynx. *Laryngoscope, 120*, 1498–1503.

Bisch, E. M., Logemann, J. A., Rademaker, A. W., Kahrilas, P. J., & Lazarus, C. L. (1994). Pharyngeal effects of bolus volume viscosity, and temperature in patients with dysphagia resulting from neurologic impairment and in normal subjects. *Journal of Speech and Hearing Research, 37*, 1041–1059.

Blonsky, E. R., Logemann, J. A., Boshes, B., & Fisher, H. B. (1975). Comparison of speech and swallowing function in patients with tremor disorders and in normal geriatric patients: A cinefluorographic study. *Journal of Gerontology, 30*, 299–303.

Cook, I. J., Dodds, W. J., Dantas, R. O., Massey, B., Kern, M. K., Lang, I. M., . . . Hogan, W. J. (1989). Opening mechanisms of the human upper esophageal sphincter. *American Journal of Physiology, 257*, G748–G759.

Cook, I. J., Weltman, M. D., Wallace, K., Shaw, D. W., McKay, E., Smart, R. C., & Butler, S. P. (1994). Influence of aging on oral-pharyngeal bolus transit and clearance during swallowing: Scintigraphic study. *American Journal of Physiology, 266,* G972–G977.

Curtis, D. J., Cruess, D. F., Dachman, A. H., & Maso, E. (1984). Timing in the normal pharyngeal swallow: Prospective selection and evaluation of 16 normal asymptomatic subjects. *Investigative Radiology, 19,* 523–429.

Dantas, R. O., Kern, M. K., Massey, B. T., Dodds, W. J., Kahrilas, P. J., Brasseur, J. G., . . . Lang, I. M. (1990). Effect of swallowed bolus variables on oral and pharyngeal phases of swallowing. *American Journal of Physiology, 258,* G675–G681.

Dejaeger, E., Pelemans, W., Ponette, E., & Joosten, E. (1997). Mechanisms involved in postdeglutition retention in the elderly. *Dysphagia, 17,* 63–67.

Dodds, W. J., Man, K. M., Cook, I. J., Kahrilas, P. J., Stewart, E. T., & Kern, M. K. (1988). Influence of bolus volume on swallow-induced hyoid movement in normal subjects. *American Journal of Roentgenology, 150,* 1307–1309.

Ekberg, O., Nylander, G., Fork, F. T., Sjoberg, S., Birch-Jensen, M., & Hillarp, B. (1988). Interobserver variability in cineradiographic assessment of pharyngeal function during swallow. *Dysphagia, 3,* 46–48.

Gibson, E., & Phyland, D. (1995). Rater reliability of the modified barium swallow. *Australian Journal of Communication Disorders, 23,* 54–60.

Jacob, P., Kahrilas, P. J., Logemann, J. A., Shah, V., & Ha, T. (1989). Upper esophageal sphincter opening and modulation during swallowing, *Gastroenterology, 97,* 1469–1478.

Johnson, E. R., & McKenzie S. W. (1993). Kinematic pharyngeal transit times in myopathy: Evaluation for dysphagia. *Dysphagia, 8,* 35–40.

Johnson, E. R., McKenzie, S. W., Rosenquist, C. J., Liberman, J. S., & Sievers, A. (1992). Dysphagia following stroke: quantitative evaluation of pharyngeal transit times. *Archives of Physical Medicine and Rehabilitation, 73,* 419–423.

Johnson, E. R., McKenzie, S. W., & Sievers, A. (1994). Aspiration pneumonia in stroke. *Archives of Physical Medicine and Rehabilitation, 74,* 665.

Kahrilas, P. J., Dodds, W. J., Dent, J., Logemann, J. A., & Shaker, R. (1988). Upper esophageal sphincter function during deglutition. *Gastroenterology, 95,* 52–62.

Karnell, M. P., & Rogus, N. M. (2005). Comparison of clinician judgments and measurements of swallow response time: A preliminary report. *Journal of Speech Language and Hearing Research, 48,* 1769–1779.

Kendall, K. A. (2002). Oropharyngeal swallowing variability. *Laryngoscope, 117,* 547–551.

Kendall, K., & Leonard, R. (2001). Bolus transit and airway protection coordination in older dysphagic patients. *Laryngoscope, 111*(11 Pt. 1): 2017–2021.

Kendall, K. A., Leonard, R. J., & McKenzie S. W. (2001). Accommodation to changes in bolus viscosity in normal deglutition: A videofluoroscopic study. *Annals of Otology, Rhinology and Laryngology, 110,* 1059–1065.

Kendall, K. A., Leonard, R. J., & McKenzie S. W. (2003). Sequence variability during hypopharyngeal transit. *Dysphagia, 18,* 85–91.

Kendall, K. A., Leonard, R. J., & McKenzie S. (2004a). Airway protection: Evaluation with videofluoroscopy. *Dysphagia, 19,* 65–70.

Kendall, K. A., Leonard, R. J., & McKenzie S. (2004b). Common medical conditions in the elderly: Impact on pharyngeal bolus transit. *Dysphagia, 19,* 71–77.

Kendall, K. A., McKenzie, S., Leonard, R. J., Gonçalves, M. I., & Walker, A. (2000). Timing of events in normal swallow. *Dysphagia, 15,* 74–83.

Kuhlemeier, K. V., Yates, P., & Palmer, J. B. (1998). Intra and interrater variation in the evaluation of videofluorographic swallowing studies. *Dysphagia, 13,* 142–147.

Leonard, R., & Belafsky, P. (2011) Dysphagia following cervical spine surgery with anterior instrumentation: Evidence from fluoroscopic swallow studies. *Spine, 36,* 2217–2223.

Leonard, R., Belafsky, P. C., & Rees, C. J. (2006). Relationship between fluoroscopic and manometric measures of pharyngeal constriction: The pharyngeal constriction ratio. *Annals of Otology, Rhinology and Laryngology, 115,* 897–901.

Leonard, R. J., Kendall, K. A., Johnson, R., & McKenzie, S. (2001). Swallowing in myotonic muscular dystrophy: A videofluoroscopic study. *Archives of Physical Medicine and Rehabilitation, 82,* 979–985.

Leonard, R., Kendall, K., & McKenzie, S. (2004a). Structural displacements affecting pharyngeal constriction in nondysphagic elderly and nonelderly adults. *Dysphagia, 19,* 133–141.

Leonard, R., Kendall, K., & McKenzie S. (2004b). UES opening and cricopharyngeal bar in nondysphagic elderly and nonelderly adults. *Dysphagia, 19,* 182–191.

Leonard, R. J., Kendall, K. A., McKenzie, S., Gonçalves, M. I., & Walker, A. (2000). Structural displacement in normal swallowing: A videofluoroscopic study. *Dysphagia, 15,* 146–152.

Leonard, R., Rees, C., Belafsky, P., & Allen, J. (2011). Fluoroscopic surrogate for pharyngeal strength: The pharyngeal constriction ratio (PCR). *Dysphagia, 26,* 13–17.

Logemann, J. (1983). *Evaluation and treatment of swallowing disorders.* San Diego, CA: College-Hill Press.

Logemann, J. A., Boshes, B., Blonsky, E. R., & Fisher, H. B. (1977). Speech and swallowing evaluation in the differential diagnosis of neurologic disease. *Neuro-logia, Neurocirugia, and Psiquiatria, 18*(2–3 Suppl.), 71–78.

McConnel, F. M. S. (1988a). Analysis of pressure generation and bolus transit during pharyngeal swallowing. *Laryngoscope, 98,* 71–78.

McConnel, F. M. S. (1988b). Timing of major events of pharyngeal swallowing. *Archives of Otolaryngology-Head and Neck Surgery, 114,* 1413–1418.

McCullough, G., Wertz, R. T., Rosenbek, J. C., Mills, R. H., Webb, W. G., & Ross, K. B. (2001). Inter-and intrajudge reliability for videofluoroscopic swallowing evaluation measures. *Dysphagia, 16,* 110–118.

Perlman, A. L., Booth, B. M., & Grayhack, J. P. (1994). A study of interrater reliability when using videofluoroscopy as an assessment of swallowing. *Dysphagia, 13,* 223–227.

Rademaker, A. W., Pauloski, B. R., Logemann, J. A., & Shanahan, T. K. (1994). Oropharyngeal swallow efficiency as a representative measure of swallowing function. *Journal of Speech and Hearing Research, 37,* 314–325.

Robbins, J., Hamilton, J. W., Lof, G. L., & Kempster G. B. (1992). Oropharyngeal swallowing in normal adults of different ages. *Gastroenterology, 103,* 823–829.

Scott, A., Perry, A., & Bench, J. (1998). A study of interrater reliability when using videofluoroscopy as an assessment of swallowing. *Dysphagia, 13,* 223–227.

Shaw, D. W., Cook, I. J., Gabb, M., Holloway, R. H., Simula, M. E., & Panagopoulos, V., & Dent, J. (1995). Influence of normal aging on oral-pharyngeal and upper esophageal sphincter function during swallowing. *American Journal of Physiology, 268*(3 Pt 1), G389–G396.

Yip, H., Leonard, R., & Belafsky, P. (2008). Can a fluoroscopic estimation of pharyngeal constriction predict aspiration? *Otolaryngology-Head and Neck Surgery, 135*(2), 215–217.

17

Dynamic Swallow Study
Measurement Techniques

Rebecca Leonard

TIMING AND DISPLACEMENT MEASURES

The measures described in this chapter represent our current best thoughts about what types of data are usefully obtained from the dynamic swallow study (DSS). They reflect our "borrowings" from other clinicians and investigators, as well as many of our own conventions, and over time have proven useful to us in assessing our patients (Crary, Butler, & Baldwin, 1994; Dejaeger, Pelemans, Ponette, & Joosten, 1997; Dengel, Robbins, & Rosenbek, 1991; Logemann, Kahrilas, Begelman, Dodds, & Pauloski, 1989; Perlman, VanDaele, & Otterbacher, 1995). But we also believe strongly that a great way to study swallowing, normal and disordered, is to try to "measure" it. The dynamic swallow study affords a unique opportunity to do this, to sample and quantify at least some events that are critical to the complex swallow sequence. It is in the inter-est of the study not only as an excellent diagnostic and treatment planning tool, but also as a tool for learning, that this chapter is included.

Once familiar with the strategies used, readers will be able to make their own measurements from the sample swallow studies included in the Chapter 17 materials folder, and to compare their results with ours. Other materials are included in the workbook accompanying this text. The video tutorial, "DSS:OBJECTIVE MEASURES," will facilitate the mechanics of displacement measurement. You can observe a measurement being made, and then try it yourself. For readers who are currently involved in performing and analyzing studies, comparisons to the scheme used in our setting may be of interest. For readers who have not had extensive experience with the dynamic swallowing study, the materials provided should represent an in-depth introduction to the value and potential of this assessment tool, as well as to a number of issues that befuddle both clinicians and investigators working in this area.

HARDWARE AND SOFTWARE

Timing Measures

We will assume that, at this point in time, most clinicians performing fluoroscopic swallow studies are working with digital media. However, whether review of studies takes place on a computer, or on some other device, for example, digital recorder, videorecorder, the features described here are critical for calculating the time between two events. Intervals can be calculated simply (if tediously) by determining the number of frames between them, recognizing that each frame is equal to 1/30th of a second (if the study is filmed at that rate). Alternatively, timing information can be superimposed on the recorded media, eliminating the need to manually convert frames to sec.

Our DSS studies are currently recorded on our institution's video archiving system (Image Stream Medical Inc., Little, MA). The studies recorded can be reviewed directly, but are typically downloaded to clinicians' desktops for the purpose of extracting measures. Timing information in hundredths of a second is recorded on each study from a timing generator interfaced between the x-ray unit and the recording device during filming of the study. Several timing generators serve this purpose. One used at our Center is the Horita Video Stopwatch VS-50 (Horita, Mission Vijeo, CA). The cable coming from the fluoro unit (same one usually attached to the VCR, DVR or archiving unit) is attached to the "video in" port

of the Stopwatch. A second cable is then attached to the "video out" port on the back of the timing device. The other end of this cable is connected to the "video in" port of the recording device (Figure 17–1). By interfacing the timer between the fluoro and the recorder in this manner, timing information can be superimposed on the recording.

The user has the option of where to position the timing information on the monitor, and of adjusting the size and color of the numeric display. The ability to place the time signal in different positions, that is, all four corners of the screen, is a desirable feature in whatever generator is used. If timing information can only be positioned in one location on the screen, it may obscure events or landmarks in the x-ray study that are critical to visualize.

With the timing generator activated, timing information will appear on the monitor. Because timing information will appear on every frame recorded, it is not necessary to start every swallow attempted by a patient at time "0." Our typical practice is to turn on the timer when we begin recording, and to leave it on throughout the study. All timing measures are then calculated from whatever time marks the beginning of an event, to the time that marks the end of the event.

Once the study is recorded, there are several options for playback. Media saved as .mov or .avi files work quite well with **QuickTime** (for PC or Mac computers, respectively, and available from www.apple.com) and **GOM Player** (http://www.gomplayer.com). Both (free) software programs allow the user to stop each frame, advance or reverse one frame at a time, and play back in slow motion. All of these features are critical to determining times between actual swallow events. View-

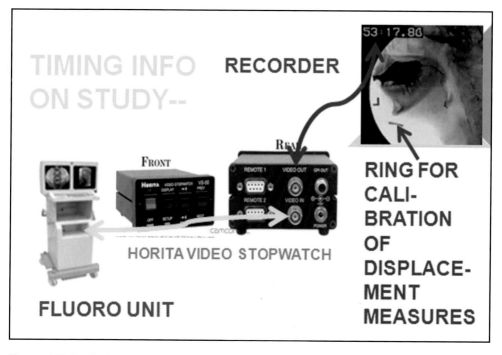

Figure 17-1. Timing information is superimposed on recorded study in the manner shown.

ing the study in this manner, we attempt to identify and note the times described in Table 17–1, all but one of which are made from the lateral view x-ray. Typically, we acquire these times, at least, for the largest bolus swallowed. As previously described, both *bolus transit* and *swallow gesture* times are noted.

Once the timing events have been determined, it is also possible to calculate durations of critical swallow gesture events during the swallow, for example, how long the upper esophagus remains open, how long the hyoid remains maximally displaced. For some populations, these values may be of particular interest. For example, patients who are typically described as "deconditioned," that is, have experienced a prolonged period of inactivity, or experience early and serious fatigue, often demonstrate reductions in duration (as well as in reduced displacements and

prolonged times) not necessarily seen in other populations. In our scheme, the following bolus times and swallow gesture durations are considered of particular interest:

Oropharyngeal transit time: duration of bolus transit through the oropharynx, from the posterior nasal spine (*B1*) to the time of bolus exit from the valleculae (*BV2*).

Hypopharyngeal transit time: duration of bolus transit through the hypopharynx, from the time the bolus head exits the valleculae (*BV2*) to the time of bolus tail clearance of the PES (*BP2*).

Total pharyngeal transit time: sum of oropharyngeal and hypopharyngeal transit times (*BP2–B1*).

PES opening duration: time from PES opening to PES closing (**Pcl–Pop**).

Table 17-1. Timing Measures Presented for Both *Bolus Transit* and *Swallow Gesture* Events During Swallow. Exact order may vary depending on characteristics of bolus and on individual impairment to normal swallow.

B1	Onset of bolus transit through the pharynx. In our studies, this time represents the "zero" point to which all later events during the swallow are compared. It is defined as the first movement of the bolus past the posterior nasal spine that leads to a swallow. If the bolus is large, its head may extend beyond the posterior nasal spine at "Hold." If a portion of bolus material falls in or toward the valleculae early, this is regarded as valving failure or inadequate instruction/attention and is considered a part of oropharyngeal transit, that is, B1 would start with the early bolus loss. OPT would likely be prolonged in this case, and the explanation for it (inability to contain the bolus orally, inattention, etc.) would be included in the narrative.
AEs	Start of arytenoid-epiglottis approximation to close the supraglottic airway.
H1	First onset of hyoid displacement that leads to a swallow. The hyoid sometimes moves around prior to the swallow. Try to be certain you identify H1 as the *first movement that leads to the swallow*. The nature of this movement is typically quite distinctive, so rapid and abrupt that it is blurred/hard to recognize in the fluoro study. In some patients, the hyoid is elevated at "Hold," possibly in response to expected difficulty. This can be noted in the narrative and may explain hyoid displacement that appears reduced during the swallow.
BV1	Bolus head arrival at the base of the valleculae.
BV2	Exit of bolus head from the valleculae (apparent with small bolus sizes; with larger sizes, BV1 and BV2 are typically the same because the bolus does not stay in the valleculae or is flowing laterally.)
AEc	Arytenoid-epiglottis approximation indicating supraglottic airway closure is maximally achieved.
H2	Hyoid arrival at maximum displacement (typically, anterior and superior). In some cases, the hyoid may pause at this point; if not, it may take checking several spots to know which represents the maximum displacement from Hold.
Pop	First opening of the lumen at the PES during swallow (defined as the narrowest point between C4 and C6).
BP1	Head of bolus enters PES. If it doesn't, this is noted in the narrative.
PES max	PES achieves maximum opening during the swallow.
H3	Hyoid begins to retract from maximum displacement.
HLmax	Hyoid and larynx achieve maximum approximation during the swallow.
PA max	Pharyngeal chamber is maximally obliterated/constricted during the swallow.
BP2	Tail of bolus clears PES. If it doesn't, this is noted in the narrative.
Pcl	PES closes. If it doesn't, no time is recorded for this event. In normal swallowers, Pcl and BP2 are typically the same.
Em	Epiglottis returns to its upright position; supraglottic airway opens.

Airway closure duration: time supraglottic airway remains closed during the swallow (**Em–AEc**).

Hyoid maximum duration: duration of maximum hyoid displacement (**H3–H2**).

We would suggest that even one or two timing measures may be particularly helpful in evaluating an individual patient. For example, normative data available for total pharyngeal transit times permit the clinician to determine whether a seemingly prolonged swallow is truly long and, if so, to consider the aspiration risk posed by the finding. Another measure that is frequently of interest to us is the interval between PESop (opening of the PES) and AEcl (closing of the airway). Typically, normal swallowers *close* the airway before the upper esophagus *opens*. Given the need for protecting the airway from bolus material, the order of these events is quite expected. Even among our normal subjects, however, opening of the upper esophagus was [infrequently] noted to occur before complete closure of the airway, but the delay was never more than .1 sec. If a longer delay is identified in a patient, it provides good evidence that strategies aimed at earlier airway protection are indicated, assuming the absence of a mechanical impairment that prevents airway closure.

BOLUS TRANSIT AND SWALLOW GESTURE TIMES

Calculating Times and Durations

Included with this chapter is a media clip entitled "DEMOSwallow." It is from a 53-year-old male with a primary complaint of solid food dysphagia. With the clip open in QuickTime (or GOM Player) go through the study and decide which times correspond to the *bolus transit* and *swallow gesture* times previously described. **Be sure to play back and forth through the clip several times when you are trying to identify precise times**. It can be difficult trying to do this frame by frame until you've watched the action a few times. The timing events, and the times we decided on, are presented here, in the order of their occurrence on the clip (go down first column, then second, then third). Incidentally, the average measurement error across 5 to 7 judges approximated .06 seconds for timing measures. Furthermore, reliability across judges for all timing measures was at least .90, and often greater than .95. This means that, if you are within a frame or 2 (each frame = .03 secs) of our values, you are making judgments quite similar to ours. Below are our values for the 20-cc bolus:

B1	—53.18.79	**BP1**	—53.19.43
AEs	—53.18.79	**PESm**	—53.19.69
H1	—53.19.33	**HLm**	—53.19.73
BV1	—53.19.33	**H3**	—3.19.79
BV2	—53.19.33	**PAm**	—53.19.89
AEc	—53.19.39	**BP2**	—53.20.03
Pop	—53.19.43	**Pcl**	—53.20.03
H2	—53.19.64	**Em**	—53.20.19
Pop	—53.19.43		

Once you decide on the times, you can also calculate durations between events (in seconds). Here are some examples, including our calculations:

Oropharyngeal transit time:
(*BV2–B1*)—.54 secs

Hypopharyngeal transit time:
(*BP2–BV2*)—.70 secs

Total transit time:
(*BP2–B1*)—1.24 secs

PES opening duration:
(*Pcl–Pop*)—.66 secs

If you compare the values obtained to the normative data (under 65 yrs) presented in Chapter 16, you will be able to determine how this patient compares. In general, his times and durations are prolonged as compared to the normal population, although they are within 2 s.d. of the means for these values. Transit time is prolonged primarily due to prolonged oropharyngeal transit. The patient does have a PES bar with slight jet (reflecting increased flow rate through the PES).

For all transit times currently in use, our reliability across several judges is greater than .90. The average deviation from the mean across judges is on the order of .06 seconds for all timing measures, which is about two frames (each time you advance 1 frame on tape or disk, you are advancing .03 seconds). If your measures are within a click or two of ours (within .06 seconds), your values added to ours would likely produce comparable reliability results.

Displacement Measures

The displacement measures that we routinely obtain, most from the lateral view x-ray, include: (1) maximum displacement of the hyoid during swallow (**Hmax**); (2) maximum opening of the PES during swallow (**PESmax**); (3) maximum approximation of the hyoid and larynx during the swallow (**HL**); and (4) a measure of pharyngeal constriction (**PCR**). From the A/P view, we also obtain a measure of maximum PES opening (**A/P–PESmax**) (Table 17–2). With the exception of maximum **PES** openings, the displacement measures are made from two images, one representing the structure at rest, or in a stable position that can be reliably achieved on a repeat study, and another representing the structure at its point of maximum displacement or constriction during the swallow. The pseudo-rest position we use is obtained with a 1-cc bolus held in the oral cavity, a position we refer to as "**Hold**."

In our setting, displacement measures are an integral part of both assessment and treatment of patients. They are of course useful in understanding the mechanics of oral-pharyngeal dysphagia. But these data are also the basis of many treatment recommendations. Measures of **PESmax** may direct us to limit bolus sizes (as it is volume dependent) or to other intervention, for example, Shaker exercise, dilation, myotomy designed to increase opening of the upper esophageal sphincter. Limitations in **Hmax** or **HL** may lead to behavioral techniques that have shown promise in increasing displacement, for example, EMST (Expiratory Muscle Strength Training), or possibly, to hyoid-laryngeal suspension surgery. If **PCR** is increased, and this is related primarily to pharyngeal muscle involvement, then strategies that optimize residual structures that may be more intact, for example, tongue, may be attempted. If involvement is unilateral, then identification of the more intact side may be important. In some cases, for example, Zenker's diverticulum, measuring the depth of the diverticu-

Table 17–2. Images Required for Displacement Measures

1cc Hold:	Identifies a pre-swallow frame "referent" to which movement of structures during the swallow can be compared. In our scheme, "**Hold**" is defined as the position of structures with a 1-cc bolus held in the oral cavity. A frame from the imaging study representing **Hold** is identified and saved. This will serve as the **Hold** referent for the 1-cc swallow, and for all subsequent swallows (i.e., 3-cc, 20-cc).
Hold: Hyoid	Hyoid position relative to the 3rd and 4th vertebrae is marked in the **Hold** frame and saved. This position of the hyoid will be compared to its maximally elevated position during the swallow.
Hmax	Hyoid position maximally elevated (at time H2) relative to the 3rd and 4th cervical vertebrae is identified and saved. The difference between the hyoid in this position and in the **Hold:Hyoid** position defines maximum hyoid displacement during the swallow.
PESmax	The greatest expansion during swallow of the site designated PES (narrowest opening in lateral view of upper esophagus at maximum distension between, typically, C4 and C6).
HLhold	The distance between the hyoid and larynx at **Hold** is measured.
HLmax	The distance between the hyoid and larynx at the point of their maximum approximation during the swallow is measured. The difference in this distance and the distance between the 2 structures at **Hold** defines maximum approximation of the hyoid and larynx during the swallow (**HL**)
PAhold	The boundaries of the pharynx before swallow are outlined in the **Hold** frame and this area is calculated for later comparison to the pharynx maximally constricted.
PAmax	The boundaries of the pharynx when it is maximally constricted are outlined, and this area is calculated and noted. The ratio of **PAmax** to **PAhold** is referred to as the Pharyngeal Constriction Ratio (**PCR**).

lum provides the surgeon with insight into whether an external or internal surgical approach is indicated. In short, as with other objective measures, displacement information influences not only our understanding of dysphagia, but also, our attempts to treat it.

Tools and Techniques for Displacement Measures

All displacement measures are currently obtained with a software tool called **Universal Desktop Ruler** (UDR) (http://www.avp.soft, available for $30.00). Hyoid displacement requires overlaying two images, one presenting the hyoid at "Hold," and the other representing its maximum anterior/superior displacement during the study. For this measure, we use **ImageJ** (available free at (rsbweb.nih.gov/ij) and **UDR**. In the following images, each measure will be illustrated. As with timing measures, **QuickTime** (or other appropriate media player) is used to identify frames of interest. We would suggest the reader download the necessary programs (a free trial version of **UDR** can be downloaded; other programs (QuickTime, ImageJ) are free and all will work on PC or Mac running Windows via Bootcamp). Using the **"DSS:OJBECTIVE MEASURES"** media clip (*a tutorial for displacement measures*) included in materials for this chapter, the reader can try making all the measures, and compare values obtained to ours.

As noted previously, displacement measures are referenced to two positions: (1) In a pseudo-rest position, referred to as "**Hold.**" This is the position of structures with a 1cc bolus held in the oral cavity; and (2) at their points of maximum displacement or constriction during the swallow.

Prior to measuring displacements, the number of pixels (which is what your monitor is divided into) must be converted into a known value (cm). We refer to this process as "calibration," and it is described here and in Figure 17–2.

CALIBRATE

1. Place ring or coin of known diameter on patient's mid-chin for lateral view; reposition to neck for filming in anterior-posterior view. (Measure is obtained with patient holding a 1-cc liquid bolus in the oral cavity.) See Figures 17–2 and 17–3.

2. **UDR's** "MEASURING SCALE" is selected (Figure 17–4). Then a line is extended along the diameter of the ring (the automatic "magnify" feature of **UDR** is helpful in identifying boundaries at each end of the ring.) When the line is completed, right clicking on the mouse will indicate the number of pixels selected. In the opened dialog box, the user enters the number of centimeters represented by the ring, thus converting pixels into a measurement unit. Re-drawing the line, using **UDR's** "DISTANCE MEASURING" tool, allows the user to

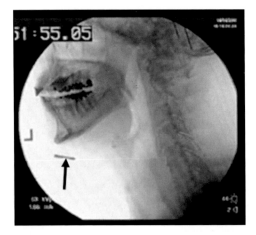

Figure 17–2. Ring of known diameter is positioned in midline of chin. Known diameter is 1.9 cm. A coin or other radiopaque object could also be used.

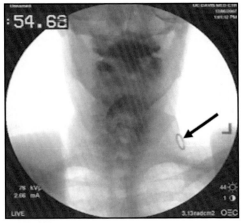

Figure 17–3. In A-P view, ring is positioned at approximate level of PES (UES).

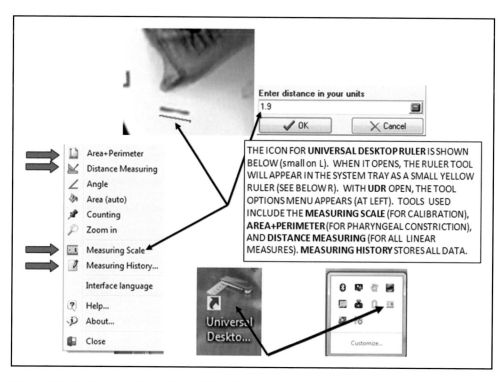

Figure 17–4. The icon for **Universal Desktop Ruler** is shown.

check accuracy of the first measure entered. That is, when the second line is drawn along the ring and measured, the value should be very close to 1.9 cm.

The icon for **Universal Desktop Ruler** is shown in Figure 17–4. When opened (by clicking on it), the tool will appear in the system tray at the bottom right of the computer screen as a small yellow ruler, also shown above. With UDR open, the tool options menu appears (at left in the figure). Tools used include MEASURING SCALE (for calibration), AREA+PERIMETER (for pharyngeal constriction) and DISTANCE MEASURING (for all linear measures). MEASURING HISTORY records all measures made, allowing measures to be printed, manually recorded, or cop-

ied and pasted into another program, such as Microsoft Excel.

DISPLACEMENT MEASURES AT "HOLD"

Instructions are as follows:

1. Identify a frame that reveals the 1-cc bolus being held in the oral cavity. Measurements taken at this point will provide a reference point for three measures of maximum displacement/constriction, including hyoid, hyoid to larynx and the pharyngeal constriction ratio (**PCR**); see Figures 17–5A through 17–5D. This area will be measured again when the pharynx is maximally constricted during the swallow. In both cases, evidence of air space or residual bolus material is

A. PHARYNGEAL AREA AT HOLD (CM²) -- USE RULER TOOL'S AREA+PERIMETER TO OUTLINE PHARYNX.

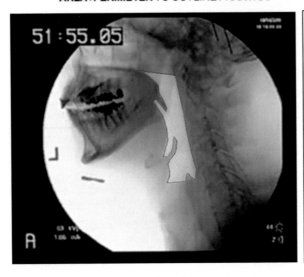

EXTEND A LINE FROM THE POSTERIOR NASAL SPINE TO PHARYNGEAL WALL AT TUBERCLE OF ATLAS, ALONG POSTERIOR PHARYNGEAL WALL, TO (AND JUST OVER) ARYTENOID (**DON'T ENTER LARYNGEAL VESTIBULE**), STRAIGHT ACROSS TO EPIGLOTTIS, SUPERIORLY ALONG BASE OF TONGUE AND SOFT PALATE UNTIL DRAWING CLOSES ON ITSELF AT STARTING POINT.

IF TONGUE IS NOT TOUCHING VELUM DURING MAXIMUM CONSTRICTION, USE SHORTEST DISTANCE BETWEEN TWO AND THEN COMPLETE AREA.

B. HYOID-LARYNX AT HOLD -- USE RULER TOOL'S **DISTANCE MEASURING** TO DEFINE DISTANCE.

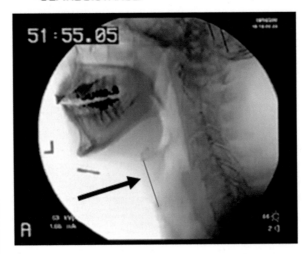

USE **DISTANCE MEASURING** TO MEASURE DISTANCE FROM INFERIOR POINT OF HYOID TO TOP OF TRACHEAL AIR COLUMN (IN CM). THIS VALUE WILL BE COMPARED TO VALUE MEASURED AT POINT WHEN TWO STRUCTURES ARE MAXIMALLY APPROXIMATED.

Figure 17-5. A. Measure of pharyngeal area at hold. **B.** Distance between top of hyoid and bottom of larynx (top of tracheal air column) at "**Hold.**" *(continues)*

C. HYOID AT HOLD. COPY THIS FRAME IN QUICKTIME (OR WITH **MWSNAP**) FOR LATER COMPARISON TO HYOID MAXIMALLY DISPLACED (THIS MEASURE WILL BE MADE IN IMAGEJ.)

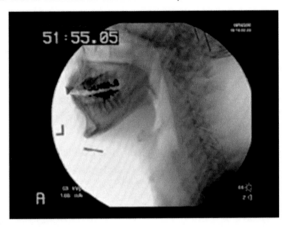

WHEN YOU COPY THIS FRAME, IT IS STORED IN THE **SYSTEM CLIPBOARD** AND CAN BE OPENED IN **IMAGEJ**. SEE BELOW:

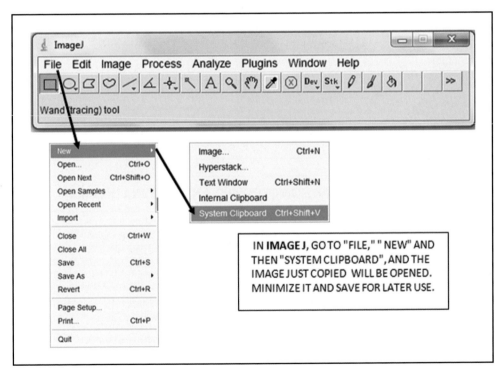

Figure 17–5. *(continued)* **C.** Image illustrating position of hyoid at "Hold" position. **D.** Image of hyoid at "Hold" is opened in ImageJ. Enter ImageJ and click on FILE, NEW and SYSTEM CLIPBOARD. Image will appear and can be minimized for later use.

included in the area measurement. The ratio of the area maximally constricted (**PAmax**) to the area with the 1cc bolus held in the oral cavity (**PAhold**) is defined as the Pharyngeal Constriction Ratio (**PCR**).

DISPLACEMENT MEASURES AT MAXIMUM POINTS OF DISPLACEMENT/CONSTRICTION

2. Identify frames for 20-cc (or other) swallow that represent structures maximally displaced, constricted, or open (Figures 17–6A through 17–6D). The final displacement measure in lateral view is **Hmax**. In QuickTime, find and copy image of hyoid at maximum displacement. Again click on FILE, NEW, and SYSTEM CLIPBOARD to open image just copied. Then maximize image of hyoid at "**Hold**" (previously minimized in system tray) and place two images side by side, as illustrated in Figure 17–7A.

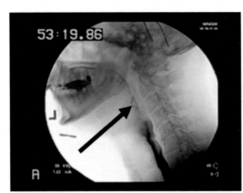

A. PHARYNX AT POINT OF MAXIMUM CONSTRICTION.

USE UDR AND **AREA+PERIMETER** TO MEASURE PHARYNGEAL AREA AT POINT OF MAXIMUM CONSTRICTION. **INCLUDE ANY RESIDUAL AREA AND BOLUS RESIDUE.** IF MORE THAN ONE AREA IS PRESENT, MEASURE BOTH AND ADD. THIS NUMBER WILL BE NUMERATOR IN PHARYNGEAL CONSTRICTION RATIO (**PCR**). DENOMINATOR IS AREA MEASURE CALCULATED ON "HOLD" FRAME (PAmax/PAhold= **PCR**)

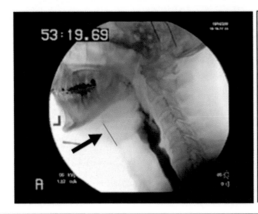

B. MAXIMUM APPROXIMATION OF HYOID AND LARYNX (HLmax)

MEASURE DISTANCE FROM HYOID TO LARYNX AT POINT OF MAXIMUM APPROXIMATION (USE SAME LANDMARKS ON HYOID AND LARYNX AS USED TO MEASURE DISTANCE IN "HOLD" POSITION.) TYPICALLY, MEASURING FROM BOTTOM OF ANTERIOR HYOID TO TOP OF TRACHEAL AIR COLUMN IS OPTIMAL. DIFFERENCE BETWEEN THIS VALUE AND VALUE BETWEEN STRUCTURES MEASURED AT "HOLD" IS **HL**.

Figure 17–6. A. Pharyngeal area is outlined at point of maximum constriction. **B.** Distance between hyoid and larynx is measured at point of maximum approximation. Difference between **HLhold** and **HLmax** is **HL**. *(continues)*

C. MAXIMUM PHARYNGOESOPHAGEAL SEGMENT OPENING (PES)

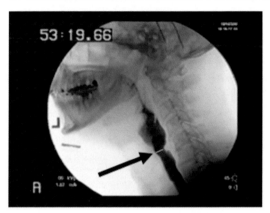

PHARYNGOESOPHOAGEAL OPENING IS DEFINED AS NARROWEST POINT BETWEEN C4-C6 WHEN THIS AREA IS MAXIMALLY DISTENDED DURING SWALLOW (**PESmax**). THIS PATIENT HAS A SMALL CRICOPHARYNGEAL BAR, MAKING IDENTIFICATION EASIER. USE DISTANCE MEASURING TO DETERMINE (CAN ALSO DO THIS IN A/P VIEW). *Be careful to measure only the lumen of the opening..not the walls!*

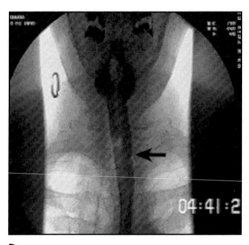

Figure 17–6. *(continued)* **C.** Maximum distension of upper esophageal sphincter during swallow. **D.** Maximum opening of the upper esophageal sphincter (**PESmax**) can also be made in the anterior-posterior view (**A/P–PESmax**).

D

The line tool in ImageJ (at arrow in Figure 17–7A) is then used to extend, on both images, a straight line along the anterior border of C2-C4 (cervical vertebrae 2 and 4) (Figure 17–7B). Once the line is drawn, enter "EDIT" and click on "DRAW." This will fix the lines on the vertebrae. When images are overlaid, this will enable the landmarks to be visible. Use the pencil tool (also shown in Figure 17–7B) to outline the anterior portion of the hyoid in both images.

Once these steps are completed, the rectangle tool in ImageJ (shown at arrow

in Figure 17–7C) is used to extend a box around a portion of the image on the L (either image can be used) that shows both the hyoid and the vertebra that have been outlined. See Figure 17–7C.

For pasting, follow these steps:

1. Highlight the image on the R in the figure by clicking on it.
2. Then enter "EDIT" and "PASTE CONTROL." Set "Paste Control" to "BLEND," as shown in Figure 17–7D. Once the segment on the L has been copied, enter EDIT and

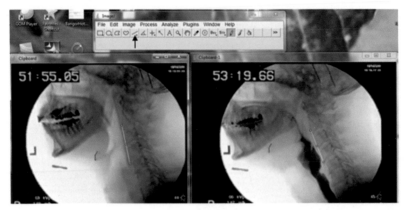

D. MAXIMUM HYOID DISPLACEMENT (Hmax)

FOR THIS MEASURE, TWO IMAGES ARE SUPERIMPOSED AND DIFFERENCE BETWEEN HYOID AT "HOLD" AND MAXIMALLY DISPLACED IS CALCULATED. OPEN **IMAGE J** TO MAKE THE MEASURE:

A

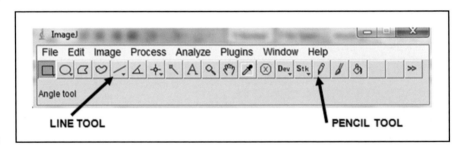

B

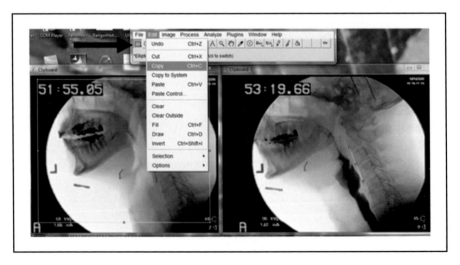

C

Figure 17–7. A. Hyoid at "Hold" and maximally displaced are identified, copied, and ultimately placed side by side in ImageJ. **B.** Line tool (L) and pencil tool (R) are used to outline hyoid and vertebra in both images. **C.** Rectangular box is extended (from top left to bottom right) around relevant portions of image and the segment selected is copied. *(continues)*

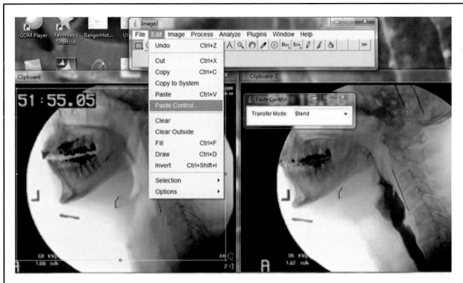

A. "COPY" RECTANGULAR SELECTION AND SET "PASTE CONTROL" TO "BLEND."

D

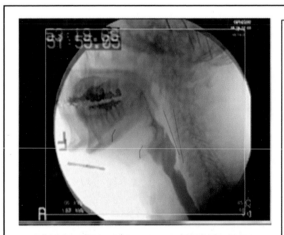

B. PASTE L IMAGE ON R, AS SHOWN ABOVE.
NOTE THAT LINES ON VERTEBRA DO NOT
ALIGN! ALIGNMENT WILL REQUIRE
ROTATING ONE OF THE IMAGES.

IMAGES ARE SUPERIMPOSED, BUT VERTEBRAE ARE NOT ALIGNED. ONE IMAGE MUST BE ROTATED TO ALIGN VERTEBRAE. IN THIS CASE, WE WILL ROTATE IMAGE ILLUSTRATING HYOID MAXIMALLY DISPLACED. TO ROTATE:

A. REMOVE SUPERIMPOSED IMAGE BY CLICKING *OUTSIDE* THE YELLOW RECTANGLE.*

B. HIGHLIGHT IMAGE ILLUSTRATING HYOID MAXIMALLY DISPLACED.

ALWAYS "UNDO" BY CLICKING OUTSIDE RECTANGULAR SELECTION. SIMILARLY, ALWAYS HIGHLIGHT (BY CLICKING ON) IMAGE YOU ARE EITHER COPYING FROM, OR TO.

E

Figure 17–7. *(continued)* **D.** Enter "EDIT" and "PASTE CONTROL." Set "Paste Control" to "BLEND." **E.** L and R images are overlaid. *(continues)*

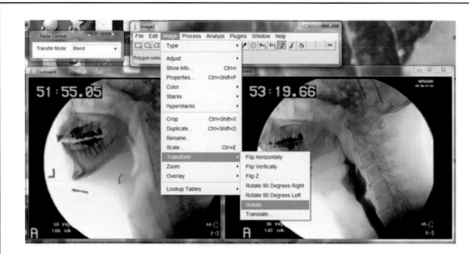

C. ENTER "IMAGE," SELECT **"TRANSFORM"** AND THEN **"ROTATE."**

F

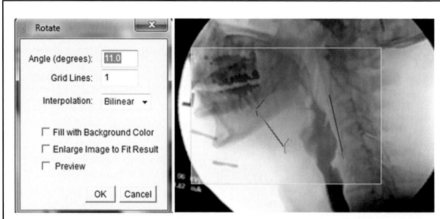

D. ENTER A VALUE (AT "ANGLE") FOR HOW MUCH YOU NEED TO ROTATE TO ALIGN THE LINES. IN THIS CASE, ROTATION OF THE "HYOID MAXIMALLY DISPLACED" IMAGE BY 11° IS SELECTED AND THE IMAGE IS ROTATED. THE RECTANGULAR SELECTION IS THEN RE-PASTED. IT IS APPARENT IN THE FIGURE THAT THE VERTEBRAE ARE NOW ALIGNED (BLACK LINES ON VERTEBRAE APPEAR AS ONE). NOW UDR'S **DISTANCE MEASURING** CAN BE USED TO MEASURE THE DIFFERENCE BETWEEN THE HYOID AT "HOLD," AND MAXIMALLY DISPLACED (UDR MEASURE SHOWN IN RED). **IN MANY CASES, IMAGES WILL NOT REQUIRE ALIGNMENT, BUT IF NOT, ALIGNING THEM IS CRITICAL TO ACCURATE MEASUREMENT. NOTE THAT LINES INDICATING VERTEBRA AND HYOID ON EACH IMAGE ARE CLEARLY VISIBLE EVEN WHEN 2 IMAGES ARE SUPERIMPOSED.**

G

Figure 17-7. *(continued)* **F.** With the image on the R again highlighted, enter IMAGE in the ImageJ toolbar, then go to TRANSFORM and ROTATE. **G.** Image is rotated and segment is again pasted. This time, the vertebrae align, and **UDR** is used to measure the distance between common points on the hyoids shown.

PASTE CONTROL; by "Transfer Mode," select BLEND. Then highlight the image on the R (by clicking on it) and select PASTE. Images will be overlaid, as shown in Figure 17–7E. Once the rectangular selection is copied, it can be pasted. Click and drag the pasted segment to align the vertebrae. It is apparent that the vertebrae lines do not align. To correct this, one of the images needs to be rotated. To rotate the image, refer to Figures 17–7F and 17–7G.

The hyoid measure is perhaps the most difficult measure to make but, with practice, it becomes straightforward. In our experience, a complete set of timing and displacement measures, as illustrated in this chapter, including entering data in a spreadsheet or database and generating a report, may require 30 minutes of clinical time. Just making a set of measures for one swallow may take no more than 5 or 10 minutes. Our experience suggests the effort, in terms of benefit to both clinician and patient, is worth this expenditure, and is in fact quite reasonable for patients with complex oral-pharyngeal dysphagia. Even one or two measures on individual patients, however, may elucidate their dysphagia and contribute significantly to treatment planning. We hope that ongoing efforts to expedite the process will translate into its widespread use in dysphagia practice.

STUDY QUESTIONS

1. How is "PESmax" defined? Where is it measured?
2. What is "PCR?" How is it measured?
3. How is airway closure time defined?
4. Why is a ring of known diameter placed on the patient's chin during the DSS? Does the location of the ring ever need to change? Why?
5. What equipment is required to make timing measurements from a fluoro study?
6. What does "Hold" refer to? How is it used in making displacement measures?
7. When might it be of particular interest to measure PES opening size from the anterior/posterior view?
8. Think of three ways objective measures may be used in treatment planning.
9. When are BV1 and BV2 likely to be the same?
10. Can you describe how maximum hyoid displacement is measured using IMAGEJ?
11. How is approximation of the larynx to the hyoid measured?
12. Explain why it might be useful to track *bolus transit times* separately from *swallow gesture times*.

REFERENCES

Crary, M., Butler, M., & Baldwin, B. (1994). Objective distance measurements from videofluorographic swallow studies using computer interactive analysis: Technical note. *Dysphagia, 9*, 116–119.

Dejaeger, E., Pelemans, W., Ponette, E., & Joosten, E. (1997). Mechanisms involved in postdeglutition retention in the elderly. *Dysphagia, 12*, 63–67.

Dengel, G., Robbins, J., & Rosenbek, J.(1991). Image processing in swallowing and speech research. *Dysphagia, 6*, 30–39.

Kay-Pentax, 2 Bridgewater Lane, Lincoln Park, NJ. Swallowing Workstation.

Logemann, J., Kahrilas, P., Begelman, J., Dodds, W., & Pauloski, B. (1989). Interactive computer program for biomechanical analysis of videoradiographic studies of swallowing. *American Journal of Roentgenology, 153,* 277–280.

Perlman, A., VanDaele, D., & Otterbacher, M. (1995). Quantitative assessment of hyoid bone displacement from video images during swallowing. *Journal of Speech and Hearing Research, 38,* 579–585.

18

The Treatment Plan

Rebecca Leonard
Katherine A. Kendall
Susan McKenzie
Susan J. Goodrich

Patients referred to the dysphagia team are evaluated and then presented at a weekly team meeting. At the team presentation, relevant information from the patient's medical history/chart review, results of current physical examinations or clinical evaluations, findings on bedside or clinical swallow evaluations, and results of videofluoroscopic study are discussed. If related exams have been completed (i.e., esophagram, manometry, endoscopy), these are considered as well. Patients' medical records, pertinent test results, and related information are available for review by team members who were not part of the patient's clinical evaluation. The goal is to identify risk factors to safe and effective swallowing, as well as potential for oral eating. The information is assimilated by members of the team, who then summarize and prioritize team recommendations. Typically, the speech pathology mem-

bers of the team assume responsibility for presenting patients and preparing reports. In this chapter, we discuss how recommendations are translated into a treatment plan, and review the major categories of therapies that are recommended for individual patients. In addition, record-keeping details that permit the simultaneous generation of a written report and entry of information into a dysphagia data-base are described.

PRELIMINARY CONSIDERATIONS

As noted, the goal for each patient is to determine both risks and potential for oral eating, and to then develop a treatment plan appropriate to these considerations. Presented in Figure 18–1 is a flow chart that illustrates the review process. Some of the information is of course based on our diagnostic tests, but other insights are also critical, for

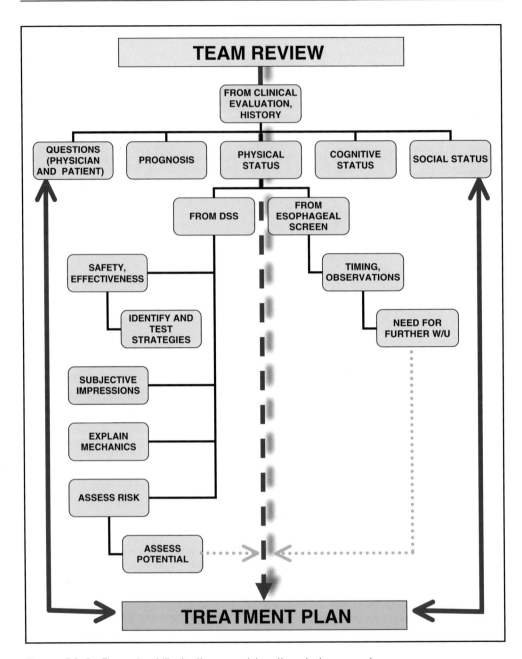

Figure 18–1. Flow chart illustrating considerations in team review.

example, the patient's *prognosis* for recovery. One patient may be hospitalized, but nearing release to home or a care facility. Another may be seriously impaired at the time of evaluation, but be expected to recover, perhaps fairly rapidly, to a normal or near-normal level of function. Other individuals may have progressive conditions likely to produce further deterioration in swallow function. Understanding prognosis is a key element of treatment planning. Other factors related to the patient's *medical* and *physical* status will also influence treatment planning. For example, recommendations for a fragile patient with poor pulmonary status are likely to differ from those for a patient with similar swallowing difficulties who can tolerate some degree of aspiration.

Recommendations must also take into account *the patient's social or living situation* and *cognitive status.* The impact of treatment recommendations on human resources (caregivers and their capabilities), as well as on technical resources (obtaining and preparing particular food types) must be considered. If recommendations involve the patient's independent participation in feeding, i.e. use of strategies, maneuvers, then appropriate cognitive and physical skills are imperative. The team makes every effort to provide preliminary recommendations and precautions for safe feeding as soon as sufficient information is available. In some instances, however, *additional diagnostic studies* are required before a treatment plan can be finalized. Such studies may be necessary to establish a medical diagnosis, when this is in question, or to further elaborate or treat a problem that has been identified. *In infants and young children, special studies* are frequently required before interpretations of findings, and treatment recommendations, can be completed. Some of these were discussed at greater length in Chapter 9. Commonly requested studies, however, include neurodevelopmental assessment and communication skills evaluation. In infants, pulmonary workup is often needed to determine the adequacy of respiratory support for swallowing.

Initial team recommendations may also include a *referral* of the patient to other medical specialists for further evaluation. For example, if there are concerns about esophageal function in swallowing that have not been addressed, or about the possibility of serious gastroesophageal reflux disease, referral to gastroenterology or specialist in esophagology is indicated. Questions about neuromotor integrity or sensation that have not been previously raised warrant referral to neurology. Issues regarding laryngeal function are most often considered prior to the team evaluation; if not, an otolaryngology referral is generated. Similarly, concerns about dentition or oral hygiene may warrant a dental evaluation. In our experience, the advantage of having a network of specialists who act as an extended part of the dysphagia team is extremely useful. These specialists are familiar with team functions and objectives, have had experience with patients with similar problems, and are typically willing to see patients as expediently as possible. Finally, team meetings in our setting begin with a presentation of the *referring professional's concerns and questions*, as well as the *patient's questions or complaints*, and a successful review typically will have answered these inquiries or, at least, made substantial progress in answering them.

TREATMENT PLAN

Dysphagia team recommendations directly related to the management and treatment of dysphagia fall into several categories. For our purposes, treatments can be classified as behavioral, medical, or surgical. Examples of these treatments, and the indications for prescribing them in individual patients, or particular groups of patients, are discussed next.

BEHAVIORAL THERAPIES

A therapist specializing in oropharyngeal swallowing disorders, most often a speech-language pathologist, provides behavioral therapy to patients suffering from dysphagia. Physical therapists and occupational therapists may also provide swallowing therapy, and/or other therapies of value. For example, a physical therapist may be consulted when there are concerns about a patient's head/neck or body posture in support of respiration and swallowing, or about appropriate seating during eating. Occupational therapists may become involved in rehabilitation of motor skills required for a particular function related to eating, as in the use of feeding utensils or adaptive devices used for this purpose. In some instances, nursing professionals also participate in swallowing therapy. In hospitals and other care facilities, the combined efforts of the swallowing-disorder therapist and nurses charged with a patient's care may be used to "mass" patient trials with various therapeutic strategies, and to monitor a patient's response to these strategies.

In general, behavioral therapies are recommended when the strength, endurance, and/or mobility of structures involved in swallowing are diminished, and when diagnostic probes have indicated that swallowing may be facilitated, or made safer, by bolus manipulation, postural compensations, facilitative maneuvers, or adaptive devices. Behavioral therapies are also recommended when it is believed that a more appropriate initiation or timing of certain swallowing events may be induced by selective stimulation of particular structures or systems. Summaries of the rationale and objectives for each of these interventions, and examples of each, are presented here.

A number of systematic reviews evaluating the efficacy of selected strategies, in adults and in pediatric populations, are currently available and should be of value to clinicians considering their use (Arvedson, Schooling, & Frymark, 2010a, 2010b; Ashford, McCabe, Wheeler-Hegland, Frymark, Mullen, et al., 2009; Clark, Lazarus, Arvedson, Schooling, & Frymark, 2009; Foley, Teasell, Salter, Kruger, & Martino, 2008; McCabe, Ashford, Wheeler-Hegland, Frymark, Mullen, et al., 2009). Readers are encouraged to investigate these and other publications that offer critiques of therapies utilized in dysphagia treatment, in particular, prior to using them in their own clinical practice.

Improving Strength/Mobility/ Endurance of Structures

Related to the model of swallowing discussed in earlier chapters, exercise is directed to improving the effectiveness of valves and chambers involved in swallowing (i.e., lip seal, breath holding, pharyngeal constriction). Indications for therapy directed to improving the strength, range of motion, endurance, and agility of the gestures involved include clear evidence of weakness or limited movement of the mandible, lips, tongue, pharynx, larynx, or pharyngoesophageal segment Specific examples of this type of problem include failure to contain bolus material in the mouth related to an inability to maintain lip closure, or failure to protect the airway related to an inability to elevate the larynx or close laryngeal valves. Such findings are typical of certain patient populations, for example, patients treated with radiation therapy for head and neck cancer, or patients with muscle weakness secondary to neurogenic disease. Poor structural mobility and muscular weakness should be documented by the physical examination and confirmed with diagnostic studies such as the dynamic swallow study (DSS). Specific exercises should be aimed at improving the capabilities of residual swallowing gestures, and/or those with the most compensatory potential.

A number of swallowing exercise programs have shown promise in recent years. One described by Shaker et al. (1997) demonstrated increased pharyngoesophageal (PES) opening in normal elderly adults and in a group of nonoral patients with dysphagia with abnormal PES function (Shaker et al., 2002). The specific exercise involves lying on the back and elevating the head sufficiently to observe the toes without moving the shoulders. Both sustained head elevation and repetitive elevations are used. The authors reported that normal elderly adults who did the exercise three times a day for a period of 6 weeks demonstrated significant increases in PES opening, as well as the anterior excursion of the larynx, as compared to a sham exercise group. The patient group demonstrated similar findings and was also noted to show improvement in self-assessment of function. Recently, the same exercise

has shown promise in increasing thyrohyoid muscle shortening, an action that contributes to both PES opening and airway protection during swallow (Mepani, Antonik, Massey, Kern, Logemann, et al., 2009). In our experience, not all patients are able to perform the exercise recommended, and Easterling, Grande, Kern, Sears, and Shaker (2005) have reported a fairly high noncompliance in a group of nondysphagic elderly adults. When this type of therapy is indicated, however, we routinely include this exercise in our home protocol for patients who are able to perform it.

Another exercise demonstrating promise is one first described by Robbins, Gangnon, Theis, Kays, and Hind (2005). This exercise requires the placement of a pressure sensitive bulb (Iowa Oral Performance Instrument) into the oral cavity between the tongue and palate. The goal is to compress the bulb as completely as possible with the tongue. In the study noted, normal elderly adults completed the resistance training over an 8-week period. Both swallowing pressures and isometric pressures were significantly increased at the end of the exercise period, and the authors recommend the use of lingual resistance exercise in patient populations with lingual weakness and swallowing disability, in particular, in patients whose difficulties are related to age-related conditions. Of particular interest in this study was the finding of increased lingual volume after completion of the training, as documented by magnetic resonance imaging (MRI) before and after therapy. Addition of muscle mass is the goal of many strength training programs traditionally directed to limb and trunk muscles, but evidence of vascular and tissue changes in swallow structures with exercise is just beginning to emerge. Tongue strengthening exercises have also been used with some success in dysphagic head and neck cancer patients (Lazarus, 2006; Sullivan, Hind, & Roecker, 2001). Another exercise that has been described is referred to as the "Masako" maneuver (Fujiu & Logemann, 1996). The maneuver involves swallowing with the tongue held between the teeth; the intent is to strengthen tongue-pharynx contact. To our knowledge, reports on the effectiveness of the strategy in a large number of patients have not been described (Doeltgen, Macrae, & Huckabee, 2011). At least one recent report suggests no pre- and post-differences in normal adults undergoing a 4-week exercise program with the maneuver (Oh, Park, Cha, Woo, & Kim, 2012).

Therapy directed to respiratory muscles should also be considered in treatment planning for patients with dysphagia. Silverman et al. (2006) reported increases in expiratory muscle strength in patients with idiopathic Parkinson's disease following a specific respiratory muscle training program. The authors suggest that such training leads to improved respiratory driving forces necessary not only for cough and speech, but also for swallowing. In patients with tracheostomy, for example, it has been demonstrated that occlusion of the tracheostomy tube results in improved swallow timing, as opposed to swallows with the tube unoccluded (Gross, Mahlmann, & Grayhack, 2003). The inference is that the increased subglottal pressures associated with occlusion of the tube facilitate swallow.

Sapienza and Wheeler (2006) note that expiratory muscle strength training (EMST) potentially benefits both airway protection and swallow-related behaviors such as hyoid and laryngeal elevation. Electromyography has revealed increased activation of anterior suprahyoid muscles during EMST (Wheeler, Chiara, & Sapienza, 2007). Troche, Okun, Rosenbek, Musson, Fernandez, et al. (2010) demonstrated improved airway safety, in the form of reduced scores on the Penetration-Aspiration Scale, in Parkinson's patients undergoing four weeks of similar training. Improvements in both cough and pulmonary function with EMST have also been reported for Parkinson's patients who demonstrated penetration and/or aspiration on fluoroscopic swallow studies (Pitts, Bolser, Rosenbek, Troche, Okun, & Sapienza, 2009).

Of additional interest is evidence that exercise directed to one function or system of the upper aerodigestive tract may produce cross-system benefits. For example, patients with Parkinson's disease and dysphagia underwent fluoroscopic studies of swallowing before and after undergoing a program of Lee Silverman Voice Therapy (LSVT/LOUD) (El Sharkawai et al., 2002). Goals of the therapy were to improve vocal loudness, in part by retraining patients' perceptions of their own loudness levels. Although no specific efforts were directed to swallowing, the authors reported a 51% reduction in the number of oropharyngeal swallow abnormalities observed post-treatment, including reductions in oral and pharyngeal transit times, improved ability to form a bolus, and reduced pharyngeal residue postswallow.

These studies demonstrate the potential of exercise in treating dysphagia, and provide objective evidence substantiating tools used by dysphagia (as well as speech and voice) clinicians for many years. In addition, recent evidence from studies in animals (primarily) and in stroke patients suggest that exercise therapies lead to changes in brain function or cortical reorganization, as well as to changes in blood flow and muscle volume/composition (Barbay et al., 2006; Behan, Moeser, Thomas, Russell, Wang, Leverson, & Conno, 2012; Carnaby-Mann, Crary, Schmalfuss, & Amdur, 2012; Gobbo & O'Mara, 2005; Kleim, Jones, & Schallert, 2003; Nudo, 2003, 2005, 2007; Nudo & Friel, 1999; Ogura, Matsuyama, Goto, Nakamura, Koyano, 2012). These intriguing findings demand additional inquiry, as do questions regarding which therapies may be indicated for which patients, and how best to deliver these therapies. For example:

- Should an exercise simulate the dynamics of the impaired function as closely as possible, that is, be task specific, or is more general, nonspecific, training directed to strengthening involved structures equally useful? Current thinking widely supports the use of the former, that is, exercise that simulates the impaired function as closely as possible (Cerny & Burton, 2001). But a case might be made that any exercise that strengthens pertinent muscle groups is likely to produce some benefits. Sapienza and Wheeler (2006) note, for example, that if a patient is aspirating, effortful swallow training may not be indicated. Rather, a nonswallowing exercise that is safe, and that promotes improved strength, coordination, or endurance of muscles involved in swallowing,

is a useful substitute. Robbins (2011) discusses potential neuromotor bases for therapies that may subserve multiple functions of the oral cavity, pharynx and larynx, that is, breathing, eating and speaking, and suggests that our emerging understanding of these may eventually contribute to expanded or novel treatments directed to their mutual rehabilitation, as well as to prevention of their functional decline with aging.

- Related to the first question, what is the role of dynamic versus static muscle training, or isometric (muscle length stays the same) versus isotonic (muscle tension is constant)? Again, dynamic exercises are more likely to simulate target functions involved in swallowing. Stathopoulos and Duchan (2006) suggest, however, that static exercises designed to improve neuromuscular support for the function may be a useful or necessary prelude to dynamic training. And both the Robbins et al. (2005) and Shaker et al. (2002) studies incorporated static training exercises that improved particular aspects of function, tongue pressures, and PES opening, respectively, that are critical to effective swallow.

- What are the best delivery methods for exercise programs? That is, how many repetitions of the exercise, how many times per day, over how many weeks, constitutes the best approach, and should this protocol be tailored with respect to patient group? In general, available evidence supports the use of multiple repetitions of sets of exercises, several times a day, over a period of several weeks. However, precise combinations likely to be more beneficial than others, and under what circumstances, have not been elaborated. Similarly, little information is available regarding the permanence of exercise effects, or the necessary requirements for maintaining any beneficial gains of exercise.

■ Finally, what is "fatigue," what role should it play in designing training programs, and is it more or less important in certain types of patients? Are there some types of patients, in fact, for whom exercise is contraindicated? Interestingly, exercises have been shown to be effective even in some populations with degenerative diseases, such as spinal muscle atrophy and Duchenne's muscular dystrophy (Koessler et al., 2001). But exercise that exacerbates fatigue may not be advisable in particular patients. Investigators are beginning to explore these and related questions, and it is likely that significant gains in our understanding of exercise physiology and its applications in dysphagia therapy will be forthcoming in the next few years.

Obviously, no behavioral therapeusis is appropriate until disease processes resulting in neural, muscular, or connective tissue changes have been ruled out or identified and managed. The etiology of the impairment dictates the principles and goals of therapy. Because etiologies of specific impairments vary widely between and even within patient groups, the dysphagia therapist will need to carefully question the referring physician or dentist for information regarding the basis for the impairment, and the potential for improvement. These specialists should also caution against some exercises, if necessary. In burn patients, for example, therapeutic approaches must consider scar tissue or regenerating superficial tissues, which are quite fragile. In cancer patients, bony structures may have been removed or weakened, muscle tissue may have been removed or altered by radiation, and muscular attachments may be very different from normal. Exercises undertaken without regard to these possibilities may result, for example, in breaking a weakened bone. Understanding the limitations and alterations unique to a particular patient is critical to designing and implementing appropriate therapy. If the dysphagia therapist is to provide optimally safe and effective therapy, familiarity with principles of exercise therapy will also be of value, even required (Clark, 2003; Stathopoulos & Duchan, 2006). In some instances, multiple behavioral therapies, that is, strengthening exercises and movement therapy, or behavioral therapy combined and coordinated with surgical or prosthetic treatments, can interact to facilitate the success of all therapies. Again, it is incumbent on the dysphagia therapist to recognize the need for, understand the advantages of, and work within the framework of multiple treatment modalities when appropriate.

As noted previously, work to improve the strength, mobility, endurance, and agility of the oral, pharyngeal, and laryngeal structures cannot be done without a stable platform (head/neck and upper body postural stability) from or against which the head, jaw, lips, tongue, palate, and larynx can move. If neck or torso stability is questionable or unsupportive, consultation with occupational or physical therapists is indicated. Collaborative efforts will help to develop a strengthening program and/or compensatory postural support strategies that will allow work on mandibular, labial, lingual, palatal, and laryngeal gestures.

Performance Feedback Tools

If sensory mechanisms have been affected, alternative or improved sources of feedback will need to be identified or established if patients are to receive the fullest benefit of exercise therapies for deglutition. A number of devices that provide feedback regarding various physiologic events may help serve this purpose. As discussed in Chapter 11, visual feedback provided by a flexible fiberoptic nasopharyngoscope attached to a video camera (alternatively, a scope with a camera in its tip) and monitor can provide excellent information to patient and clinician regarding a number of physiologic events or maneuvers which are otherwise difficult to observe (i.e., pharyngeal constriction, laryngeal elevation, and vocal-fold adduction).

Other commercially available systems provide immediate visual feedback regarding muscle function. Computer-assisted EMG biofeedback systems with surface electrodes present visual evidence of the presence and amplitude of the electrical activity of muscle units close to the electrode. As an objective indication of muscle effort in the area of the electrode, such information may be a very useful clinical tool. There are some limitations to use of EMG in the head and neck, however. For example, surface electrodes cannot be targeted at a particular muscle. Wire or needle electrodes must be used if this is desired. In addition, an increase of effort in a muscle, or group of muscles, does not signal a successful movement of a structure(s) directed to swallow. Accomplishment of the goal gesture(s) must be assessed by some other means. This is of particular concern when the gesture in question, for example, PES opening, cannot be easily visualized by the patient or clinician.

Another commercially available feedback device is the Iowa Oral Performance Instrument (IOPI) (Blaise Medical, Inc., Hendersonville, TN). The system, used by Robbins et al. (2005) in the study cited earlier, consists of a pressure transducer connected to a battery-operated display unit. The IOPI measures pressure produced by squeezing a small bulb placed on the tongue (a small bulb for hand-squeezing strength is included) and can be used to develop strength or endurance of squeezing. Normative data are presented in the manual that accompanies the device. When the IOPI intraoral bulb is used to develop tongue strength or endurance, it may be helpful to isolate effort to the tongue by supporting or stabilizing the mandible. The IOPI strengthens lingual muscle groups that accomplish elevation against the palate in a gently rounded shape. Thus, it may strengthen the lingual configuration required to hold the bolus on the mid tongue during oral preparation for swallow. The intraoral bulbs are small and require a normal or near-normal lingual bulk, however, limiting its use in glossectomy patients. A dental laboratory may be able to custom make bulbs for patients postoral cancer or with orofacial anomalies whose tongues do not fill the oral cavity. The bulb can be moved around in the mouth and may be used to strengthen specific tongue sites as long as the bulb and the tongue can be seen (to ensure the exercise is being done correctly). Although there are no norms for this kind of task, the patient's performance on successive trials can be compared. Unfortunately, the bulb can be tolerated only in the oral cavity and, in some patients, not at all sites in the oral cavity.

The Therabite (Therabite Corporation, 3415 West Chester Pike, Suite 302, Newtown Square, PA 19073; 1993) is an excellent tool for feedback regarding range of mandibular opening. It can be used to develop masseter strength in different positions, but gives no feedback regarding strength or effort. Our own experience with Therabite in increasing mandibular opening in patients postoral cancer has been very positive.

External Stimulation

Transcutaneous Electrical Stimulation. In addition to specific exercise regimens, there are a number of externally implemented techniques to facilitate stretching of muscles, connective tissue, and scars, including the application of temperature, massage, and ultrasound. Recently, transcutaneous electrical stimulation has been used to treat a wide variety of dysphagic impairments. This stimulation can take different forms, for example, be activated continuously (Freed, Freed, Chatburn, & Christian, 2001) or only during swallow attempts (Leelamanit, Limsakul, & Geater, 2002), and vary according to

specific frequency-intensity-duration patterns. One intent of stimulation has been to enhance contraction of muscles involved in swallowing, in particular, by increasing the number of motor action potentials supplied to the muscle or muscles involved. To date, the effects of therapies incorporating transcutaneous electrical stimulation have produced mixed results (Beom, Kim, & Han, 2011; Carnaby-Mann & Crary, 2008; Blumenfeld, Hahn, Lepage, Leonard, & Belafsky, 2006; Freed, Freed, Chatburn, & Christian, 2001; Heck, Doeltgen, & Huckabee, 2012; Humbert et al., 2006; Ludlow, Humbert, Saxon, Poletto, Sonies, & Crujido, 2007). In particular, it is not clear whether electrical stimulation improves over more traditional therapy strategies that are delivered according to the same protocol of frequency/intensity as that associated with stimulation (see Carnaby-Mann & Crary, 2007; Clark, Lazarus, Arvedson, Schooling, & Frymark, 2009; Humbert, Michou, Macrae, & Crujido, 2012; Ludlow, 2010).

A recent report by Furuta, Takemura, Tsujita, and Oku (2012) described increased frequency of swallowing in normal subjects with surface electrodes delivering an "interferential current" to tissues of the neck. This form of transcutaneous stimulation differs from traditional techniques by utilizing two high frequencies for stimulation that, as the name implies, interfere with each other. The combination produces a different, lower, frequency, that is, the "interferential" frequency. Purportedly, the resulting stimuli produce less discomfort than the use of a single lower frequency stimulus, enabling greater or deeper levels of stimulation. The potential of interferential stimulation in dysphagia therapy will likely be elaborated with additional investigation.

Muscle Stimulation. Other stimulation techniques involve electrode placements directly into targeted muscles. Though more invasive, these techniques offer more potential for directly affecting muscle activity. Kagaya, Baba, Saitoh, Okada, Yokoyama, et al. (2011), for example, have provided preliminary evidence of greater movements in the hyoid and laryngeal elevator muscles with implanted, as compared to surface, electrodes. Ludlow et al. (2000) reported the use of electrodes implanted in the thyroarytenoid muscle in dogs. Intermittent stimulation was provided to the muscle over periods of up to 8 months, and appeared to produce changes in muscle function consistent with improved airway protection. Burnett, Mann, Cornell, and Ludlow (2003) described the use of electrical stimulation applied via hooked-wire electrodes into the geniohyoid, mylohyoid, and thyrohyoid muscles of nondysphagic subjects. Interestingly, bilateral stimulation of the mylohyoid and/or thyrohyoid with subjects at rest produced approximately half of the laryngeal elevation typically observed during a swallow. Burnett, Mann, Stocklosa, and Ludlow (2005) reported an electrical stimulation device that can be self-triggered. That is, when a subject initiates a swallow, defined by the authors as the onset of thyrohyoid activity leading to a swallow, a button can be pushed that delivers electrical stimulation to the suprahyoid muscles. To date, this technique has not been shown to alter muscle activation patterns, but it does represent an interesting concept that deserves further inquiry.

Neural Stimulation. The use of cortical stimulation techniques to facilitate swallowing, in particular, with stroke patients, has received significant attention in the last few years. Repetitive Transcranial Magnetic Stimulation (rTMS) and Transcranial Direct Current Stimulation (tDCS), the techniques most often described, involve the superficial application of low levels of electrical current to the brain. The stimulation can change the polarity of neurons in the area of application. Purportedly, if cortical areas of the unaffected hemisphere representing the pharynx can be expanded (assuming intact brainstem and peripheral structures) swallowing recovery may be facilitated. Cortical stimulation may be paired with other swallowing techniques, that is, exercise, maneuvers, to maximize therapy efforts. Although in their infancy as therapeutic techniques, early reports of their potential have been promising (Gow, Rothwell, Hobson, & Hamdy, 2004; Hummel, Celnik, Giraux, Floel, et al., 2005; Khedr, Abo-Elfetoh, & Rothwell, 2009; Kumar, Wagner, Frain, Zhu, et al., 2011; Schlaug, Renga & Nair, 2008).

No exercises, especially stretches, should cause pain. Patients, especially aggressive patients, should be counseled regarding potential injury when doing stretching exercises. Frequency and intensity of exercise sessions will depend on patient tolerance, and also on the specific goals of treatment. That is, strength exercises may be more taxing than exercises designed to improve endurance, leading to more rapid patient fatigue and, of necessity, briefer sessions. Therapy strategies and exercises that are directed to mobility/strength/endurance impairments are summarized in Table 18–1.

Table 18–1. Exercises for Improving Movement, Strength, and Endurance of Swallowing Gestures

Impairment	Indications	Goal	Tasks May Include
Limited control, agility or ROM of neck rotation, extension and flexion	Neck mobility is important in development of compensatory strategies to facilitate oral transit, airway protection or PES opening.	Range,control, agility adequate for needed task	Obtain consult from Physical Therapy. Depending on need, tasks may focus on development of agility of movement as well as control And ROM.
Trismus	Before trismus can be addressed therapeutically, etiology must be identified by a physician or dentist. When mandibular opening is inadequate for eating or oral hygiene, and a disease process has been ruled out or treated, therapy may be appropriate.	Adequate opening for feeding route (spoon, fork, cup, or biting), for denture or palatal prosthesis placement and for oral hygiene.	Maintain mandible-maxilla alignment while increasing passive and active range of mandible opening. Can be done with a variety of props, from simple to sophisticated. For example, stacked tongue blades placed between the molars can facilitate maintenance of maximal opening. During stretch, the patient can relax, bite gently, then attempt further opening and insert another tongue blade in the stack (while it is in place). Movements should be made slowly. Maximum stretch should be maintained ≥15 seconds. The Therabite (Atos Medical, Horby, Sweden) is a more sophisticated device, especially useful for marked trismus or when alignment of mandible and maxilla is difficult to maintain. The cost, of course, is greater.
Weakness or absence of mandibular support/ control	Absence of or asymmetry in achievement or maintenance of mandible-maxilla approximation, or inadequate mandibular stability to support lingual work against the palate for bolus control, mastication or speech.	Symmetric mandible-maxilla approximation supportive of potentials for posture, oral nutrition/hydration and speech	Establish optimal alignment passively or actively, and present exercises graded for endurance. Slowly diminish support (if that is necessary) and increase time position is sustained. Increase strength and control using graded resistance and biting/munching tasks to strengthen muscles of mandibular closure and opening. Mandibular lateral and A/P ROM may be addressed depending on potential.

Impairment	Indications	Goal	Tasks May Include
Weakness or absence of buccal tone	Inability to prevent food from falling into the buccal sulci in a patient with potential for oral preparation and oral transit.	Increased buccal tone.	Isometric tightening of the buccal area or squeezing of soft objects between the cheek and teeth/gums or from the buccal sulcus to the molar surface. Both oral opening and object size can be graded during squeezing tasks. Maintain mandible alignment throughout.
Diminished labial opening	Inadequate opening for eating, speech, or oral hygiene (also diminishes mandible opening).	Adequate labial opening size for eating. Adequate change of shape for speech.	Tasks depend on etiology (scarring, resection of muscle, muscle weakness) and may include passive stretching and exercises to increase range and strength of lateral commissure movement. Maintain mandible alignment throughout.
Partial or complete absence or weakness of labial strength and/or ability to close	Inability to maintain labial closure in a variety of mandibular positions, including rest, with oral incontinence for saliva, liquid, food, or air during labial pressure consonants.	Oral continence for saliva management, eating/drinking and speech.	Establish closure passively or actively, and present exercises graded for maintenance then endurance: Slowly diminish support (if that is necessary) and increase time position is sustained. Increase strength at selected sites using squeezing and holding tasks with and without resistance. Develop agility for desired range using tasks graded for speed and accuracy. Maintain mandible alignment throughout.
Unilateral partial or complete lingual weakness or missing lateral lingual tissue	Diminished or absent ability to form, hold or manipulate the bolus with bolus loss into the lingual sulcus of the weak side. Consonant and mild vowel distortions.	Posterior bolus retention-release control for airway protection. Bolus and airflow control (minimize lateral "leaks") and lingual shaping range and agility	Maximize lingual symmetry at rest and in a variety of non-speech and speech gestures. Maximize posterior lingual-palatal valve strength and agility and lingual lateralization and lateral lingual elevation (for cupping)on the weak side with passive, then active ROM tasks, resistance to lateral and elevation gestures. Squeezing and lingual manipulation tasks may be appropriate. Palatal prosthesis may facilitate therapy.

continues

Table 18-1. *continued*

Impairment	Indications	Goal	Tasks May Include
Bilateral anterior lingual weakness or missing anterior lingual tissue	Diminished or absent ability to form, hold or manipulate the bolus with bolus loss into the anterior lingual sulcus. Anterior consonant and vowel distortions.	Bolus and airflow control and lingual shaping range and agility.	Establish target lingual non-speech and speech positions passively or actively, and present exercises graded for maintenance then endurance: Slowly diminish support (if that is necessary) and increase time position is sustained. Increase strength at selected sites using squeezing and holding tasks with and without resistance. Develop agility for desired range using tasks graded for speed and accuracy. Maintain mandible alignment throughout. Palatal prosthesis may facilitate therapy.
Bilateral posterior lingual weakness or missing posterior lingual tissue	Diminished or absent ability to form, hold or manipulate the bolus with bolus loss into the oropharynx. Posterior consonant and vowel distortions.	Strength and agility of bolus retention-release and transfer to the pharynx. Improved palatal contact for speech sound production.	Establish target lingual-palatal contact passively or actively, and present exercises graded for maintenance then endurance: Slowly diminish support (if that is necessary) and increase time position is sustained. If sqeezing tasks are used, object must be anchored. Palatal prosthesis may facilitate therapy.
Bilateral lingual weakness	Diminished or absent ability to form, hold, transfer, or manipulate the bolus with bolus loss into the oropharynx, and the lingual sulci	Oral transit with minimum loss into the sulci and maximum coordination with initiation of swallow gestures.	Address sequentially as above.

Impairment	Indications	Goal	Tasks May Include
Absent tongue	Inability to form a bolus. Inability to transfer a bolus without compensatory strategies. Severely distorted speech sounds	Development of compensatory mandibular, labial and head/neck movement strategies.	Develop ROM and agility of movements needed for compensations that take advantage of gravity. Consider mandibular or maxillary shaping prosthesis.
Unilateral or complete weakness or missing tissue of the palate	Velopharyngeal incompetence for speech and oral and/ or oropharyngeal transit. Diminished ability to transfer the bolus through the posterior oral cavity or oropharynx.	Adequate velopharyngeal closure if tissue is adequate. Effective obturation if tissue is inadequate.	Feedback for velopharyngeal closure can be elusive. There is some commercially available, inexpensive equipment, e.g., SeeScape. Sustained blowing against resistance may strengthen closure, as long as tongue facilitation is ruled out. Endoscopic feedback may be helpful for some patients. Excercises may be helpful even with obturation. Obturation may actually recruit improved compensatory participation in closure from the lateral and posterior pharyngeal walls.
Unilateral, bilateral, or regional failure of pharyngeal constriction	Poor pharyngeal transit in the affected area increasing risk of aspiration of pharyngeal residue after the swallow.	Improved bolus compression	Maximize lingual retraction range and strength, laryngeal elevation and supraglottic closure and pharyngeal constrictor participation. Provide resistance by holding the tongue forward manually and retract the tongue against this resistance. Maximize extent of externally visible signs of laryngeal elevation. Practice effortful swallow and "hawking" of secretions for expectoration.

continues

Table 18–1. *continued*

Impairment	Indications	Goal	Tasks May Include
Incomplete glottic closure	Increased risk of aspiration during maximum closure for swallow. Inadequate vocal quality and loudness	Improved glottic closure	Attempt to establish conditions resulting in improved vocal fold approximation while avoiding using pitch, positional, compression and respiratory support strategies. Increase endurance with tasks graded for time, pitch, onset, loudness, position, and respiratory support.
Incomplete supraglottic closure	Increased risk of supraglottic penetration prior to closure for swallow and aspiration of this residue when respiration is resumed. May contribute to incomplete hypopharyngeal clearing.	Improved supraglottic closure	Habituate early and effortful laryngeal closure and elevation for swallow. Maximize extent and sustained time of externally visible signs of laryngeal elevation.
Inadequate PES opening for swallow	Incomplete pharyngeal transit with increased risk of aspiration of pharyngeal residue after the swallow	Maximum PES opening.	Once the muscles of the PES have relaxed, PES opening is influenced by elevation of the laryngeal/hyoid complex and by intra-bolus pressures. Therapeutic approaches to optimizing PES opening thus include maximizing extent and timing of hyoid/laryngeal elevation and the effects of pharyngeal compression of the bolus.

BOLUS MANIPULATION

Therapeutic probing during bedside/ clinical or videofluoroscopic evaluations may suggest that a patient can manage particular types or amounts of food materials safely and efficiently, but have difficulty with others. Therapeutic strategies directed at elaborating the patient's potential for improved swallowing by manipulating bolus materials, and at establishing the patient's facility with these selected materials, are described here. Strategies are tailored to an individual patient, as there are few if any data establishing the value of particular strategies with particular patient groups.

Bolus characteristics can be manipulated to compensate for timing/coordination or constriction/patency impairments of the oral and/or pharyngeal chamber or of the lingual-palatal, velopharyngeal, laryngeal, or PES valve. Characteristics of the bolus that lend themselves to manipulation include: (1) *Properties that maximize sensory feedback about the bolus and its position*, and (2) *Properties that affect bolus deformability and/or bolus flow in response to gravity or compression.* For simplicity, the properties are presented here somewhat separately, but, in fact, bolus properties combine, heightening some properties and minimizing others.

Properties That Maximize Sensory Feedback About the Bolus and Its Position

Properties that maximize sensory feedback include temperature, taste, size, and texture. Swallow initiation has been reported to be facilitated with cold instrument stimulation of the faucial pillars (Lazzara, Lazarus, & Logemann, 1986). There is some evidence that a cold bolus may stimulate swallow initiation for some populations (Kagel & Leopold, 1992); and some patients report that thermal characteristics of the bolus affect their dysphagia (Martin, 1994). On the other hand, Bisch, Logemann, Rademaker, Kahrilas, and Lazarus (1994), investigating post-CVA and neurologically impaired patients, did not find significant effects on transit times or durations with a chilled bolus. Temperature is known to affect esophageal function (Meyer & Castell, 1983). We routinely include chilled bolus presentation in evaluation of patients with suspected neural or neuromuscular etiologies.

Common potentially irritating taste characteristics of the bolus may facilitate swallow initiation in some populations (Logemann, Pauloski, Colangelo, Lazarus, Fujiu, Kahrilas, et al., 1995; Palmer, McCulloch, Jaffe, Neel, 2005). Palmer et al. (2005), for example, reported that a sour bolus produced stronger muscle contractions in mylohyoid, geniohyoid, and anterior belly of the digastricus muscles than a water bolus in normal individuals. Pelletier and Lawless (2003) noted that citrus acid and citric acid-sucrose boluses produced more dry swallows and decreased both aspiration and penetration in neurogenic patients as compared to a water bolus, possibly because of increased gustatory and trigeminal stimulation of the brainstem. However, we have been reluctant to apply this strategy in most patient populations, fearing the potentially noxious effects of bolus materials used should they penetrate the laryngeal, tracheal, and nasal airways and the lungs.

Irritating tastes may be safer and still useful when introduced in tiny, dilute amounts to the lips or anterior oral cavity where they will stimulate saliva that must be swallowed. Size, viscosity, and texture of the bolus may add to tactile feedback. For patients who are able, mastication may lead more easily to swallow. When patients are not able to masticate, simply manipulating the bolus briefly may facilitate swallow initiation. Carbonation increases the "texture" of liquids and is known to improve esophageal clearing (Wong & Johnson, 1983). Carbonation has also been reported to shorten pharyngeal transit times and reduce both aspiration and amount of residue (Bulow, Olson, & Ekberg, 2003). Alternating thermal, taste, and texture characteristics during therapeutic feeding or a meal may keep the interest of the swallower, supporting vigilance regarding swallow.

Finally, manipulation of bolus placement to maximize available sensory capabilities is a valuable compensatory maneuver for patients with sensory impairment. If a sensory deficit is unilateral, for example, bolus material on the more intact side may facilitate swallow.

Properties That Affect Bolus Deformability and Flow in Response to Gravity or Compression

Bolus viscosity is a powerful tool and manipulation of it may represent the most popular compensatory strategy. We use the term, "viscosity," but the properties of bolus materials are complex. From a rheological science perspective, thickened foods and beverages are classified as complex fluids. Unlike simple fluids, for example, oil, or water, the flow behavior of these bolus types cannot be adequately described by single values for viscosity and density alone. For example, the viscosity of a starch- or gum-thickened drink depends on time under flow, and the final "steady-state" viscosity value depends on the shear rate, or how fast the material flows. An appropriate selection of parameters to describe the properties of a complex fluid during swallowing requires a fluid mechanical analysis of the swallowing process itself.

Clinically, viscosity is referred to in common categories: liquid, thick liquid, puree, soft solid, and so on. However, viscosity characteristics exist as a continuum from water (least) to (for example) hard candy (most), The National Dysphagia Diet (described in Chapter 10) specifies centiPoise (cP) ranges for thick nectar-like, honey-like, and spoon-thick liquids, but the range even for each of these categories is also broad, with significant viscosity differences within each. Other factors that influence viscosity are related to the patient, for example, saliva production, mucosal integrity, or ability to prepare a bolus to some uniform consistency prior to swallowing it. In short, specification of "viscosity" is complex. For the clinician charged with treating dysphagic patients, it is important to understand the complexity of the issue, and to recognize that viscosity tolerance range is likely to be compressed in dysphagic patients, even those who are eating orally, as compared to normal. Understanding the unique mechanics of swallow impairment in individual patients is particularly critical to identifying bolus materials most likely to be managed safely and effectively. The discussion of bolus manipulation that follows is from this perspective, that is, involves matching bolus materials to a patient's specific *mechanical* impairment.

Thin liquids are easily deformed and move very readily in response to gravity and compression. Adequate transit relies less on strength of constriction, patency of the chambers, and mucosal/salivary facilitation, and more on agility and coordination to control the bolus, time its transit through the pharynx and protect the airway. Thin liquids, that is, water, being almost completely deformable, will pass most easily through narrow sites in transit (e.g., a stricture, an incompletely opened PES, or an incompletely closed airway).

As viscosity of the bolus increases, it moves more slowly in response to gravity or compression. A more viscous bolus, thus, requires less agility and control and is more forgiving when timing of swallow and coordination of transit with gestures is impaired. However, with increases in viscosity, adequate transit becomes more reliant on strength of constriction and mucosal/salivary facilitation. As the bolus becomes less deformable, it is less likely to pass through narrow sites in transit, and may lodge above them instead. Thus, a liquid may be aspirated, but a less deformable bolus may obstruct the airway. The most viscous consistencies require adequate mastication and salivary mixing prior to initiating oral or pharyngeal transit.

Patients with dysphagia, as mentioned, are unlikely to tolerate a full range of bolus viscosities, but may be able to eat orally by compressing the range (see Chapter 10 for examples.). When viscosity is being considered in treatment planning, it is important to keep these principles in mind:

Bolus size affects bolus flow in response to gravity or compression. Large liquid bolus sizes may be compensatory for incomplete oral or pharyngeal constriction and decrease work per meal, but may be risky if laryngeal function is compromised. Small bolus sizes increase swallows/work per meal, but are less reliant on competent laryngeal function to protect the airway. Choice of bolus size may also be influenced by mechanical factors. For example, PES opening is volume dependent, that is, increases with increased in bolus volume. A patient with limited opening may therefore have greater success with smaller bolus sizes.

Placement of the bolus at a particular site on the tongue or in the oropharynx can take advantage of the swallower's anatomic and motoric strengths or, as noted before, greater sensory integrity, while avoiding his weaknesses.

POSTURAL COMPENSATIONS

Postural manipulation is indicated when it appears that a patient can either redirect bolus material in a manner that improves swallowing efficiency (i.e., amount of bolus attempted that actually makes it to the esophagus), improves protection of the airway, or both. Changes in head/neck and upper body position, first described by Logemann (1983), can have a powerful effect on bolus flow through the oral and pharyngeal chambers. Tilting the upper body or the head changes the impact of gravity on the bolus and, in some cases on poorly supported anatomy. In addition, capital flexion, extension, or rotation change the size and shape of the pharyngeal chamber and may impact PES opening. Positional changes do not necessarily have to be dramatic to be effective. In our practice, positions are frequently combined to facilitate safe oral and pharyngeal transit.

Position Strategies That Exploit Gravity

Tilting the Upper Body

Effective use of upper body tilting requires that the cervical spine remain in neutral relation to the thoracic spine and the shoulders. If neutral position is not maintained, the effects of upper body tilting may be lost. If the upper body is tilted laterally or posteriorly, bolus flow will be biased to the "downhill" side, diverting it (to a point) away from the airway. Upper body tilting is useful when bolus transit and the sequence of pharyngeal swallow gestures are discoordinated, when pharyngeal constriction is incomplete, or pharyngeal transit is prolonged. The degree of "tilt" will impact (depending on bolus viscosity) bolus transit time and the size of bolus tolerated without overflow into the airway. When postural support of the anterior pharyngeal wall structures (the tongue and hyoid/laryngeal complex) is poor, as is the case in some anatomic, neurologic, or neuromuscular conditions, the pharyngeal airway may be improved when the upper body is tilted anteriorly.

Tilting the Head

If the head is tilted laterally, bolus flow through the oral chamber will be biased to the downhill side. If only the head is tilted, the site of bolus entry to the pharynx is affected (it would enter on the "downhill" side), but not the course the bolus takes through the pharynx.

Lateral head tilting may be useful when lingual movement, sensation, or anatomy is unilaterally impaired. Tilting the head anteriorly (*capital flexion*) will keep the bolus in the anterior oral cavity unless it is actively transferred by compression. Thus, neck flexion requires purposeful initiation of pharyngeal transit/bolus entry to the pharynx, and may be useful when linguapalatal valving is impaired. Capital flexion also minimizes the likelihood that oral residue will fall into the pharynx after the swallow. On the other hand, tilting the head posteriorly (*capital extension*) facilitates oral transit of consistencies that will flow with gravity. Safe use requires adequate laryngeal airway protection. Because extension can *at times* be an obstacle to pharyngeal transit, it is usually used in sequence with flexion (extend-flex). An example of a patient with partial tongue resection using the extension strategy to bypass the oral cavity is included in the materials folder for Chapter 18 (Pt. Strategy 1 video clip). A variation of position strategies is illustrated in Strategy 2a and 2b. Strategy 2a illustrates an infant having difficulty extracting bolus material through a nipple; in Strategy 2b, the feeder provides jaw support, which helps stabilize the oral cavity and facilitates the baby's management of the nipple. In our experience with infants, this kind of strategy, and identifying a nipple that allows the baby to control flow (neither too fast nor too effortful), is often quite successful.

Positions That Impact Pharyngeal Chamber Shape and Function

Capital flexion, extension, and rotation change the shape of the pharyngeal chamber, thus impacting bolus flow. *Capital flexion* alters the oropharyngeal space such that airway protection is facilitated for some patients (Logemann, 1983). An example of a patient with supracricoid laryngectomy and only the arytenoid-epiglottis valve available for airway protection is seen using this strategy in the Strategy 3 video clip (materials folder for Chapter 18). In our experience, *capital extension* narrows the pharynx, closes the valleculae, and impacts mobility of the hyoid/larynx complex. Some patients with poor oral capabilities but good ability to protect the airway may benefit from this posture. *Capital rotation* diverts the bolus toward the opposite side and can be very useful when pharyngeal constriction is incomplete, sometimes even when the impairment appears symmetric, but certainly when constriction and PES opening are asymmetric (Logemann, Kahrilas, Kobara, & Vakil, 1989). Because it diverts the bolus to one side of the pharynx or the other (around the epiglottis in some patients), capital rotation may also be useful for patients with incomplete vallecular clearing, especially for a more viscous bolus. In our experience, when capital rotation is used to compensate for asymmetric pharyngeal wall function, the direction of most facilitative rotation is not completely predictable. In other words, in some patients, pharyngeal transit is facilitated by rotation away from the affected side.

FACILITATIVE MANEUVERS

This category of therapeutic strategy refers to physiologic postures or gestures that have been demonstrated to improve swallowing efficiency or safety, and that a patient can learn to use for these purposes. Such maneuvers differ from strategies discussed earlier in this chapter. Other categories of compensatory strategies (bolus manipulation, positional changes) can to some extent be imposed on the swallower by a feeder. Facilitative maneuvers require sophisticated and active participation by the swallower, good muscular kinesthetic and proprioceptive sense, movement control, and ability to understand, learn, and apply the strategy during the swallow. For some patients, considerable time and effort will be required to develop the strategies to the point of habituation. Thus, facilitative maneuvers are appropriate when less labor-intensive maneuvers fail. Some maneuvers are very familiar. Often patients who perceive their dysphagia are seen to apply these strategies spontaneously: generally increased effort (during a single swallow or by repeating swallows), jaw thrust, and expectoration of pharyngeal residue. Other maneuvers are likely to be unfamiliar and more difficult to learn. These involve altering the extent and/or timing of laryngeal behaviors for swallow, with the goals of providing improved laryngeal closure for airway protection and/or improved PES opening for pharyngeal clearing.

Maneuvers that attempt to recruit increased effort are probably the simplest to learn and habituate. For these maneuvers, the patient is instructed to "swallow as hard as you can, squeezing all your swallow muscles harder" or "after you swallow, swallow once (or twice or more)." At least one study has reported increased duration of tongue base contact and increased pharyngeal pressures with *effortful swallow* (Lazarus, Logemann, Song, Rademaker, & Kahrilas, 2002). Other authors reported no change in hypopharyngeal intrabolus pressure with increased effort, however (Bulow, Olson, & Ekberg, 2003). Hiss and Huckabee (2005), using manometry, reported a later onset of swallow but increased pharyngeal pressures on effortful swallows. These authors suggest, thus, that effortful swallow may be more appropriate for patients with weak pharyngeal constriction than those with prolonged pharyngeal transit times. In normal subjects, effortful swallow has been associated with increased durations of hyoid displacement, PES opening and laryngeal vestibule closure (Hind, Nicosia, Roecker, Carnes, & Robbins, 2001). In 8 patients with pharyngeal dysfunction, effortful swallow was associated with reduced depth of bolus penetration into the larynx, but penetration was not prevented by the gesture (Bulow, Olsson, & Ekberg, 2001).

Maneuvers with the goal of providing improved airway protection include the frequently described *supraglottic* and *super supraglottic* maneuvers. These maneuvers seek to develop closure of the airway prior to bolus entry into the hypopharynx and to maintain closure throughout hypopharyngeal transit. These strategies are appropriately offered to patients whose airway closure timing is delayed relative to bolus position in the pharynx for neurologic (i.e., CVA) or anatomic (i.e., supraglottic laryngectomy) reasons and to patients whose *supraglottic* and *glottic* closure is incomplete. On lateral videofluoroscopy, delayed glottic closure is identified by aspiration prior to the swallow, as actual glottic closure cannot be seen

in this view. Observation requires an anterior–posterior view of the larynx and vocal folds or, preferably, endoscopic examination of the larynx. It is possible to observe the approximation of the epiglottis and arytenoid, that is, supraglottic structures, and to assess the competency of this gesture.

For the *supraglottic* maneuver, the patient voluntarily initiates airway closure before oral transit begins and reopens the airway after the swallow, releasing the breath audibly to blow any residual off the folds. The instruction may be: "Put the bolus in your mouth, hold your breath, and keep holding it as you swallow. When the swallow is done, let your breath go in a sudden, audible breath." We typically do not instruct the patient to cough, because, in energetic and diligent patients this instruction has appeared to contribute to vocal abuse with characteristic vocal fold changes. However, the power of effective "hawk-spit" is illustrated in Strategy 4 (materials folder, Chapter 18) by a patient with a pill stuck in the valleculae.

For the *"super" supraglottic* maneuver, the patient voluntarily and with effort initiates airway closure before oral transit begins. Effortful closure, such as is achieved when "bearing down" or fixing the upper body for heavy lifting, usually elicits supraglottic laryngeal constriction, thus supplementing glottic airway protection. The instructions are as above, with the addition of this significant effort. Both supraglottic and super-supraglottic maneuvers can be extended to include more than one swallow at a time as long as pulmonary function supports holding the breath for longer than one swallow. Instructions would be: "Hold your breath hard, keep holding your breath while you drink as much as you want from this cup, stop drinking, then let your breath go suddenly and audibly."

Another strategy involving submental and neck musculature is the *Mendelsohn maneuver* (Jacob, Kahrilas, Logemann, Shah, & Ha, 1989). The behavior targeted is elevation of the larynx for a prolonged period. The maneuver has been demonstrated to increase both displacement and duration of hyoid movement during swallow (Kahrilas, Logemann, Krugler & Flanagan, 1991; Wheeler-Hagland, Rosenbek, & Sapienza, 2008), and to prolong PES opening (Boden, Hallgren, & Hedstrom, 2011). Other authors have reported differences in the timing/duration of additional swallow events with the Mendelsohn maneuver (Kahrilas, Logemann, Krugler, & Flanagan, 1991; Lazarus, Logemann, & Gibbons, 1993; McCullough, Kamarunas, Mann, Schmidley, Robbins, & Crary, 2012). The maneuver is appropriately applied when videofluoroscopy reveals: (1) slowed transit of the bolus through the pharynx and PES, so that the PES closes before the bolus has been completely transferred; and (2) incomplete PES opening, so that transit through the PES itself is slowed and it closes before the bolus has been completely transferred. The success of this maneuver in increasing or prolonging PES opening *cannot be* assessed clinically, even using techniques such as EMG feedback regarding activity of the hyoid elevators. Teaching involves identification of maximal hyoid/larynx elevation and then prolongation of this position during swallow.

An additional maneuver that has sometimes been effective, in our experience, is voluntary *mandibular advance-ment*. In patients with limited PES opening but good control of oral structures, this maneuver has been observed on fluoroscopy to apparently facilitate increased opening of the PES. The patient is instructed to jut the jaw forward at the same time swallow is initiated. A video clip illustrating this maneuver is included in the materials folder for Chapter 18 (Strategy 5).

FACILITATIVE DEVICES

Facilitative devices modify the delivery of bolus material into the swallowing tract or change the shape of the tract in a manner that positively impacts swallowing efficiency and/or safety. For example, a syringe and catheter allow placement and delivery of the bolus to particular areas of the oral or pharyngeal cavities (see an example in the materials folder for Chapter 18, Strategy 6). These instruments may be useful in bypassing certain structures incapable of adequately directing or propelling the bolus to the pharynx, or in facilitating movements conducive to bolus management.

Devices as simple as a modified spoon or a mandibular sling may allow management of food materials previously prohibited. In children, a variety of different nipples may aid and modify the delivery of liquid to the oral cavity. Different sizes and shapes of cups and bowls can also facilitate feeding and swallowing in both children and adults.

A palatal augmentation appliance, or palatal prosthesis, is sometimes useful in reshaping the oral cavity in a manner that facilitates bolus manipulation. For example, lowering of a particular area of the palate, such as the palatal vault, or certain portions of posterior or lateral palate, may improve tongue-to-palate contact for mashing or sealing a bolus, or for propelling the bolus posteriorly (Logemann, 1983). Palatal appliances are indicated in some patients with dysphagia with restricted lingual mass or motility because of either surgical ablation or neuromuscular impairment (Logemann, Kahrilas, Hurst, Davis, & Krugler, 1989; Wheeler, Logemann, & Rosen, 1980). If nasal regurgitation is present because of structural or neuromuscular impairment of the velopharyngeal port, the prosthesis may be extended to become a palatal lift or obturator. In rare instances, as in a patient with total glossectomy, a mandibular prosthesis may be of value in shunting bolus materials safely into the pharynx (Gillis & Leonard, 1983).

There is some evidence in studies of velopharyngeal dysfunction for speech that prosthetic appliances in the oral cavity (i.e., palatal lift appliances), may stimulate muscle activity (Blakely, 1960, 1964, 1969; Blakely & Porter, 1971; Weiss, 1971; Wong & Weiss, 1972). For the most part, the available reports appear largely anecdotal. In fact, in one study (Shelton, Lindquist, Arndt, Elbert, & Youngstrom, 1971), objective measures were acquired before and after prosthesis reduction, with no significant changes noted for oral or nasal sound pressure level, nasal air pressure, articulation proficiency, or in pharyngeal wall movement as seen on cine-fluorography.

In our clinical experience, however, it has occasionally been possible to reduce the size of a prosthetic appliance. It has been presumed that the reductions were possible because of improved or increased muscle function in residual tissues, or even because of an increase in the bulk of residual tissues. Somewhat similarly, in the larynx, it has been our impression that augmentation of a fixed vocal fold on a temporary basis may have produced improved compensatory activity in the intact vocal fold, and perhaps prevented the development of less desirable compensatory behaviors, such as false-fold constriction/medialization. These clinical impressions are intriguing, and suggest a potential for prosthetic appliances (or augmentative substances) that has not been fully explored.

Improved Initiation and Timing of Swallowing Events by Selective Stimulation

Implicit in some stimulation techniques is the belief that certain sensorineural thresholds critical to swallowing have been impaired and that these can be influenced, in particular, heightened, in a manner that impacts positively on the initiation, timing, and/or completeness of swallow and various swallowing events.

Primary to sensory cueing is orientation, that is, alerting the patient to the task. Reduction of noise, light, and other distractions, selective positioning, and verbal cuing may all enhance the patient's level of alertness. Verbal cues are general, such as the patient's name, or instructive, such as "swallow," "close your lips," or "chew," and may be accompanied by visual cues or demonstration. Children may benefit from additional orientation techniques. Rosenthal, Sheppard, and Lotze (1995) suggest prefeeding preparation may include rituals, attendance to state, including fatigue, readiness/playtime activities, and prosthesis placement. Morris and Klein (1987) have noted that a "ready state" may be enhanced by such factors as soothing music. Sensory cues involving taste or smell can also be used to heighten alertness. During the feeding task itself, pacing of bolus delivery is suggested as a technique to help improve breath control and stamina (Rosenthal, Sheppard, & Lotze, 1995). The usefulness of a particular technique or cue will vary depending on each patient's individual needs and abilities, and may require revision during the rehabilitative process, depending on goals and progress.

Direct stimulation of oral-pharyngeal structures prior to introduction of a bolus has also been used in attempts to facilitate swallowing. For example, rubbing or massaging the gums provides sensory input that may serve to "alert" and "orient" oral structures. Alexander (1987) suggests such preliminary preparation of cheek, lip, and tongue musculature using tactile/pressure input and muscular elongation. Graded pressure stimuli, firm to light touch, can also be applied to various muscles and muscle groups in preparation for functional activities. Special brushes used to stroke the lips, tongue, and gums will provide further oral stimulation and, possibly, facilitate function. Use of an exaggerated suck in the oral stage of swallow has also been described as useful for facilitating the initiation of pharyngeal swallow (Logemann, 1997). Recent evidence suggests that both oral and trunk/limb tactile/kinesthetic stimulation in pre-term infants may facilitate development of oral feeding skills (Fucile, Gisel, McFarland, & Lau, 2011, 2012).

Other types of mechanical stimulation have also been considered. Fujiu, Toleikis, Logemann, and Larson (1994) experimented with mechanical tapping, Sinclair (1970) with heavy and light stimulation of the posterior faucial pillars, and Kaatzke-McDonald, Post, and Davis (1996) with single and repetitive touch. Power et al. (2004) used a vibratory stimulus at 5 Hz presented to the faucial pillars and described *inhibition* of corticobulbar projections and *lengthened* swallow response times. Conversely, stimulation with a lower frequency stimulus (0.2 Hz) in the same study appeared to increase corticobulbar excitability, with no observed alterations in swallow initiation latency, pointing to the need for understanding specific effects of various stimuli on brain activity and swallow function *prior* to their wide clinical use.

Thermal stimulation, or icing, of the anterior faucial pillars by touching or stroking them with a chilled laryngeal (00) mirror has been shown in some studies to increase the speed of initiation of the pharyngeal swallow and improve timing of subsequent swallowing events (Kaatzke-McDonald, Post, & Davis, 1996; Lazzara, Lazarus, & Logemann, 1986). Other authors have demonstrated no substantial effect with this technique, however (Ali, Laundl, Wallace, deCarle, & Cook, 1996; Rosenbek, Robbins, Fishback, & Levine, 1991). Rosenbek et al. (1991) reported some immediate effects in CVA patients exposed to thermal stimulation, but no residual effects at one-month post-treatment. Martin (1994) reported thermal stimulation to be most effective when combined with other input modalities, including cognitive stimulation and the presence of a bolus.

Kaatzke-McDonald et al. (1996) reported an increase in swallow latency (rather than the desired decrease) with cold stimulation, and no changes with touch or chemical (glucose, saline) stimulation. Knauer, Castell, Dalton, Nowak, and Castell (1990) reported no changes in resting pressure of the upper esophageal sphincter or swallow coordination using both thermal stimulation and a variety of pharmacological agents.

Of additional interest are recent studies demonstrating changes in cortical behavior with electrical stimulation which has been used either to increase muscular contractions directly by increasing motor input to involved muscles (as described previously), or to influence sensory input to reflex arcs associated with swallowing. Hamdy, Azia, Rothwell, Hobson, and Thompson (1998) reported that electrical stimulation of the pharynx (5 Hz) produced changes in the size of cortical motor representation involved in swallow. Interestingly, the increased size was bilateral but asymmetric, and appeared to be associated with a decrease in the size of esophageal cortical representation. In a subsequent study, Fraser et al. (2002) monitored the effects of pharyngeal stimulation with transcranial magnetic stimulation in acute onset, hemispheric stroke patients. The authors identified increases in cortical pharyngeal representation and excitability, in particular, in the undamaged hemisphere, with 5-Hz stimulation for a period of 10 minutes. The changes were reportedly associated with improved swallowing function, as well. On the other hand, stimulation with other frequencies resulted in inhibition of pharyngeal excitability and longer delays in swallow initiation, as defined by the authors. Such studies not only demonstrate both positive and adverse effects of stimulation on cortical and brainstem structures, but help provide a sound basis for rehabilitation efforts incorporating stimulation techniques in selected populations.

COMPUTER APPLICATIONS IN BEHAVIORAL THERAPIES

Increasingly, computerized applications, or "apps," are available for both clinician and patient use. In some cases, these can provide feedback regarding performance. In others, more comprehensive treatment tools are available. Though the digital devices that run these applications may not be within every patient's budget, the applications themselves are often quite reasonable, even free. One that was developed at our Center is called the *iSwallow*. The application works on Macintosh iPad, iPod, or iPhone platforms, and can be downloaded free at http://www.ucd voice.org/iSwallow/. This particular application includes media clips demonstrating various exercises (as well as other maneuvers/strategies), and allows the clinician to assign particular activities to individual patients, and then alert the patient when it is time (at home, during the day) to perform the exercise, as well as to track the actual practice activity.

MEDICAL THERAPIES

Medical therapies designed specifically for the treatment of dysphagia of any cause have not been developed. Rather, therapies designed to treat the underlying medical condition resulting in dysphagia are the mainstay of medical therapy. The need to identify the etiology of the dysphagia becomes all the more important so that appropriate treatment can be instituted.

Neuromuscular Disease

When a neuromuscular disease is the etiology of the dysphagia, whether or not the medical therapy appropriate for treating the condition has been maximized must be ascertained. For any patient with dysphagia, a review of other medications prescribed for the patient will help determine if any of them may contribute to dysphagia. Many drugs affect the cholinergic nervous system and are known to have an effect on swallowing (see Chapter 2). Occasionally, the same drugs prescribed to treat the neuromuscular disease may have a deleterious effect on swallowing. A balance between therapeutic benefit and side effects must be achieved.

Gastroesophageal Reflux

Gastroesophageal reflux may contribute to the swallowing difficulties of an individual patient, and to certain patient populations (i.e., asthma [Babb, Notarangelo, & Smith, 1970; Duclone, VanDevenne, & Jovin, 1987], scleroderma, gastroparesis). Patients who demonstrate a cricopharyngeal bar on the dynamic swallow study are also at risk for reflux. In all such cases, an antireflux regimen is indicated. Reflux precautions should also apply in any patient who has been identified by the swallow team evaluation to be at risk

for aspiration, for example, a patient with glottic incompetence.

In our practice, antireflux recommendations begin with behavior modifications. Patients are advised not to eat before bedtime. The last meal of the day should be at least 3 hours and preferably 4 hours before the patient assumes a supine position. No bedtime snacks are allowed. Digestion and gastric emptying will have adequate time to be completed while the patient is upright and gravity aids in minimizing the increased risk of reflux that exists during this period. Once the patient does go to bed, it is recommended that the head of the bed be elevated by 4 to 6 inches. The effect of gravity is therefore never completely removed. Patients are advised to use blocks under the front feet of the bed. This is more effective than trying to elevate the head with the use of pillows alone, as with this method patients will often assume a more supine position during sleep. Prior to going to bed, it is recommended that the patient take an antacid medication. This will neutralize any residual acid in the stomach and diminish the irritation to the upper aerodigestive tract should the patient experience reflux during the night.

Throughout the day, but especially at the evening meal, it is recommended that certain foods be avoided. These are foods thought to increase gastric acidity or to lower the lower esophageal sphincter resting tone. In addition, foods that result in a diuresis, such as caffeine-containing beverages, are to be avoided to prevent dehydration. Our list includes coffee, tea, peppermint, chocolate, citrus fruits, and alcohol. Meals high in fat content are known to increase the risk of reflux and a low fat diet in general is recommended. Patients are also advised not to use tobacco.

If behavior modification alone is not adequate to control reflux symptoms, specific medications can be added to the regimen. H2-blockers, such as cimetidine and ranitidine, are a standard therapy and can now be purchased over the counter. Our own preference is to have patients take these medications at a dose proven to be effective. Thus, medications are prescribed for them with specific recommendations for the dose and schedule believed to be most appropriate for their condition. When symptoms persist despite the use of H2-blockers, proton-pump inhibitors, such as omeprazole and lansoprazole, can be prescribed. These medications are more powerful than the H2-blockers in terms of decreasing gastric acid production and they are extremely well tolerated. Typically, proton pump inhibitors are prescribed for a period of 2 to 3 months. Once the symptoms of gastric reflux have been controlled for this period of time, the proton pump inhibitors will be replaced by H2-blockers. If the patient tolerates this change, they can be maintained longterm on the H2-blockers, if indicated. Occasionally, medications that increase the rate of gastric emptying such as metaclopramide and cisipride are helpful in the control of reflux disease and can be prescribed along with proton pump inhibitors in patients where reflux has been very difficult to control.

Xerostomia

Xerostomia impedes bolus lubrication and bolus flow and is deleterious to oral mucosal and dental health and esophageal GER defense (Zide, 1990). Poor bolus flow results in bolus residue on the surfaces on the tongue and palate, in the crevices and on the walls of the pharynx, placing the patient at risk for aspiration after the swallow. Predictably, in a swallower with xerostomia, residue is likely to increase with viscosity of the bolus, increasing the risk of aspiration of a potentially obstructive bolus. Treatment of xerostomia includes maximizing hydration, limiting mouth-breathing, minimizing use of products that would contribute to xerostomia (including many medications, mouthwashes, and toothpastes containing alcohol) or favor increased oral bacterial growth. We also recommend maximizing general hydration and oral hygiene, using one or a combination of over-the-counter products or the prescription drug pilocarpine. Patients with xerostomia need to avoid potentially irritating foods (acidic and pepper-hot) because of oral sensitivity or GERD. Strategies to wet the bolus carefully during oral preparation prior to initiation of oral transit can improve completeness of oral and pharyngeal transit. Certain factors (i.e., Sjögren's syndrome and related autoimmune conditions, radiation effects, medications that dry mucosal tissues or decrease salivary flow, iron or vitamin (B12) deficiency), predispose patients to xerostomia and are therefore important to identify during evaluation.

SURGICAL THERAPIES

Although many forms of dysphagia respond to nonoperative therapy, selected conditions may benefit from surgical therapy. To identify these lesions and conditions, a thorough understanding of the physiology of swallowing is necessary (see Chapters 1 and 2). Successful swallow depends on the normal functioning of a number of structures acting as sphincters or valves that sequentially close and open to permit bolus material into the upper esophagus. Other structures, including the oral cavity, pharynx, and esophagus, must expand and compress to first propel and then clear bolus material as it moves through the aerodigestive tract. Dysphagia secondary to structural or anatomic abnormalities that result in incompetence should lead the clinician to consider surgical correction. Careful evaluation of individual cases must be performed to ensure that the defect lends itself to surgical correction. In cases where structural integrity of the oral cavity and pharynx have not been compromised, but muscular weakness is the etiology of the dysphagia, surgery can occasionally improve the condition by repositioning structures into an arrangement more favorable for weakened muscle contraction.

The first sphincter function in swallow is comprised of the lips and oral musculature. Oral-labial incompetence results in drooling and poor bolus preparation. Both the clinical and dynamic swallow study may reveal loss of the test bolus onto the chin and difficulty with bolus positioning within the oral cavity. Surgical therapies designed to release contractures that prevent oral closure or are designed to recreate an intact obicularis oris muscle can improve dysphagia caused by this type of defect (Morris, Bardach, Jones, Christiansen, & Gray, 1995).

During oral preparation of the bolus, the soft palate contacts the base of the tongue to create the oral-pharyngeal valve, which prevents the bolus from entering the pharynx prematurely. Defects of the soft palate, as in the case of a cleft palate or an oropharyngeal cancer resection, can prevent closure of the valve and may allow early entry of the bolus into the pharynx. The soft palate elevates during the pharyngeal phase of the swallow to become a key element of the nasopharyngeal sphincter. Nasal regurgitation, therefore, is another consequence of a soft palate defect. Both early pharyngeal penetration and nasal regurgitation can be identified during a dynamic swallow study. Soft palate tissue defects and soft palate muscular weakness may be surgically repaired with local flaps such as a superiorly based pharyngeal flap (Stepnick & Hayden, 1994). Palatal obturators are also an option for correction of palatal soft tissue defects or muscle weakness and should be considered along with surgical therapy.

The tongue plays a major role in bolus preparation and is a key element of the oropharyngeal valving mechanism. It also creates the primary driving forces in oral and pharyngeal bolus propulsion. Adequate tongue mobility is crucial for these functions, especially for pharyngeal bolus propulsion. When the tongue is tethered anteriorly or laterally, such as after a floor of the mouth cancer resection, a dynamic swallow study may suggest poor pharyngeal contraction as the tongue's restricted mobility precludes adequate contact with the posterior pharyngeal wall during the pharyngeal phase of the swallow. In some cases, reconstruction at the time of resection may include procedures designed to minimize tethering. In others, secondary surgical therapy may be indicated to improve mobility. A tissue defect of the tongue base results in the loss of tongue bulk, and like mobility impairment, may be apparent in poor pharyngeal constriction on the dynamic swallow study. It is important to clinically differentiate problems related to loss of bulk, as opposed to loss of mobility. Tongue bulk defects may improve with surgical replacement of lost tissue with local, regional, or free tissue flaps (Anthony, Singer, & Mathes, 1994; Bodin, Lind, & Arnander, 1994; Harries, 1996; Pauloski, Logemann, Fox, & Colangelo, 1995; Wolff, Dinemann, & Hoffmeister, 1995).

Defects of glottic valving, such as occur with vocal fold paralyses, result in poor vocal fold closure during deglutition. Aspiration of the bolus during the pharyngeal phase of the swallow, as the bolus passes by the elevated larynx, can typically be detected on the dynamic swallow study. Several surgical alternatives are available for the correction of vocal fold paralyses and other causes of glottic incompetence (Carroll, Rosen, & Soose, 2011). However, it must be kept in mind that vocal fold medialization may not always be successful in eliminating aspiration (Yip, Kendall, & Leonard, 2005).

Once the bolus has been prepared to be swallowed and has been propelled into the pharynx by the base of the tongue, the upper esophageal sphincter must open to allow passage of the bolus into the upper esophagus. The process involves relaxation of the cricopharyngeus muscle followed by the active anterior/superior displacements of the hyoid and larynx that actually open the PES. Factors that affect relaxation, or produce fibrosis of the muscle, as well as factors that limit hyoid and larynx displacements, may all result in impaired opening, that is, cricopharyngeal dysfunction. Cricopharyngeal achalasia, defined as a failure of the cricopharyngeus m. to relax, may result from neuromuscular disease (McKenna & Dedo, 1992; St. Guily, Petrie, Bokowy, Angelard, & Chaussade, 1994) or gastroesophageal reflux (St. Guily, Moine, Perie, Bokowy, Angelard, et al., 1995). The cricopharyngeus muscle or PES may also fail to open for other reasons, for example, fibrosis related to radiation. On the dynamic swallow study, cricopharyngeal dysfunction may appear as a "cricopharyngeal bar" or by decreased diameter of the maximum upper esophageal opening (UES). The fluoro study cannot differentiate between failed relaxation and other causes of dysfunction. And neither the dynamic swallow study nor upper esophageal sphincter manometry have consistently predicted patients who will benefit from surgery (McKenna & Dedo, 1992; Shaw et al., 1996). On the other hand, there is evidence to suggest that cricopharyngeal myotomy can correct failure of cricopharyngeal relaxation as evaluated with manometry (Ellis, 1995; Schmitz, Bitonti, & Lemke, 1996).

A study of 20 patients treated at our center by cricopharygeal myotomy for cricopharyngeal dysfunction used videofluoroscopic swallow studies before and after repair to evaluate patients. Prior to myotomy, the mean PES opening size for a 3-cc bolus was 0.30 cm ± 0.17, which was 57% of the mean of 60 normal controls (0.52 cm ± 0.15) ($p < 0.001$). After repair, the mean PES opening for the same bolus size improved to 0.51 cm ± 0.16 ($p < 0.0001$).

The PES opening size in patients who had undergone repair was comparable to that of the normal controls ($p > 0.05$) (Yip, Kendall, & Leonard, 2005). Our Center has also described pharyngeal dilation with prolonged obstruction at the UES related to cricopharyngeal bar or Zenker's diverticulum (Belafsky, Rees, Allen, & Leonard, 2010). Pharyngeal dilation, or an enlarged pharynx at rest, may interfere with complete clearance of bolus material from the pharynx during swallow. A recent study of cricopharyngeal myotomy performed in 54 patients (Allen, White, Leonard, & Belafsky, 2011) revealed that, although both UES opening and pharyngeal constriction were improved, the pharynx remained dilated. At our institution, this evidence has led to more aggressive treatment of cricopharyngeal bar in some patients.

Other procedures that are currently being tested or for which there are limited data available also appear to hold promise for patients with limited PES opening. As noted, in some cases, the opening size is not limited solely (or perhaps at all) by inability of the cricopharyngeus m. to relax, but to other mechanical factors that preclude the active opening of the PES. For example, patients with weak or ineffective pharyngeal constriction, and/or with limited anterior-superior movement of the hyoid-larynx complex may be unable to open the PES or propel bolus material through it, even if the cricopharyngeus m. relaxes. Belafsky (2010) has described a "swallow expansion device" that will permit an individual to *manually* open the PES by pulling on a surgically-implanted device that advances the cricoid cartilage during swallow. This device is currently in the development stages but may eventually offer potential for oral eating to selected patients who have little or none (see "Swallowing Expansion Device [SED]—Fluoroscopy" and "Swallowing Expansion Device [SED]—Endoscopy" in the Media Clips folder accompanying this chapter).

Another strategy for improving PES opening is dilation (or dilatation), often, serial dilations. Dilation involves the use of a catheter with an inflatable balloon placed through the PES to, in effect, "stretch" it. Belafsky (2012) has developed a "double-balloon" dilator that more closely approximates the actual opening orifice, allowing greater opening diameters to be achieved. An example of the procedure is included in the Media Clip folder (see "Double Balloon Dilation").

PES relaxation is no more important to successful swallow than elevation of the hyoid/larynx complex. If these structures are not able to exert pull on the upper esophagus by their superior and anterior displacement, even a relaxed PES may not open. It is often difficult to distinguish patients who fail to relax the PES from those who fail to elevate the hyoid/larynx complex. The underlying pathology of the dysphagia and the clinical presentation of the patient are currently the best distinguishing features of these two patient groups. Patients with fibrosis of the suprahyoid muscles following head and neck radiation, previously removed suprahyoid muscles, or weakened suprahyoid muscles following stroke may be unable to elevate the hyoid. The dynamic swallow study in these cases is likely to demonstrate diminished hyoid bone elevation and poor larynx-to-hyoid approximation in addition to failure of the PES to open. Surgical therapy to correct this problem has not been performed extensively. The largest experience with surgery to elevate the hyoid and larynx has been in patients with obstructive sleep apnea in which the surgery is done to permanently enlarge the upper airway (McBride & Ergun, 1994; Riley, Powell, & Guilleminault, 1994; Sher, Schechtman, & Piccirillo, 1996). Anecdotal experience with surgical correction of poor hyoid and laryngeal elevation in dysphagia has been successful, however (Kendall, Leonard, & McKenzie, unpublished data). Patients who appear to be optimal candidates for the procedure are those who demonstrate an inability to close the laryngeal vestibule during swallow, but who do have normal, for example, nonradiated, anterior neck tissue.

Esophageal achalasia and strictures are often treated with esophageal dilations. The swallow study does not routinely include an evaluation of the entire esophagus but the A/P screen previously described is often helpful in identifying proximal strictures in patients after laryngectomy. The finding of a narrowing that does not change during bolus passage is suggestive of a stricture. The definitive diagnosis is made on endoscopy, which can be immediately followed by dilation.

Dysphagia is often multifactorial. Surgical therapy may be able to correct part of the problem but often other difficulties will persist. Patients need to be counseled about the limitations of surgery so that their expectations will be realistic. An immediate return to normal swallow is unusual. Progress after surgery is more likely to be gradual, and a period of postoperative swallow therapy may be required to realize the fullest benefit from surgery.

TREATMENT IMPLEMENTATION AND FOLLOW-UP

When an appropriate treatment plan has been finalized for a patient, it is the task of the dysphagia team to communicate the plan to the patient and all relevant caregivers. The report accompanying the plan will include summaries of the patient's medical and feeding history, and descriptions of procedures performed as a part of dysphagia assessment. Objective measures from the patient's performance on the dynamic swallow study are compared to available normative data, and summarized in terms of oral, pharyngeal, laryngeal, and esophageal function. Any pertinent additional observations are noted, and a summary statement of the patient's current capabilities and impairments is offered (see Figures 18–2A through D and Figure 18–3).

The summary of findings from the clinical and radiographic evaluations should include conclusions that the referring professional may not be able to draw independently, that is, what do the findings suggest about the etiology and severity of the impairment, its impact on nutrition and respiratory health, and prognosis for improvement. For example, research from our own institution indicates that, in post-CVA patients, a pharyngeal transit time between 3 and 5 seconds is associated with a 48% increased risk of developing aspiration pneumonia (Johnson, McKenzie, Rosenquist, Lieberman, & Sievers, 1992). Such information, when

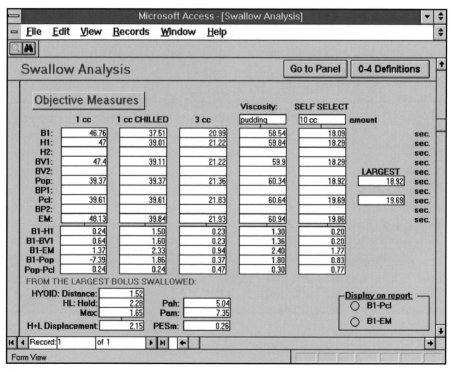

A

B

Figure 18–2. A. Information entered into patient information form of database (Microsoft Access). **B.** Timing and displacement data from DSS entered into objective measures form (database calculates values). Subjective impressions can also be entered. *(continues)*

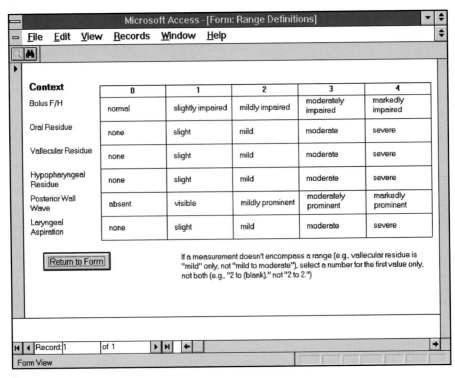

Figure 18-2. *(continued)* **C.** Observations for oral function, pharyngeal function, and laryngeal function are included. Pharyngeal function section is illustrated. **D.** Additional observations.

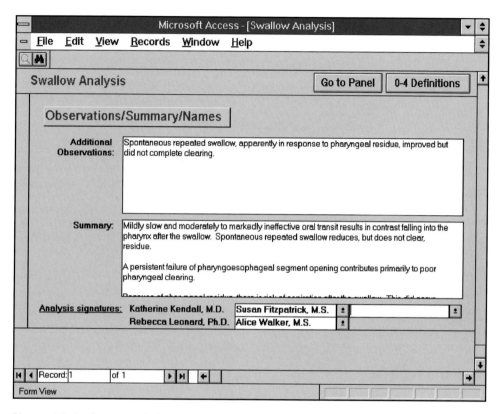

Figure 18–3. Summary information is entered.

available, is included in the summary as an indication of the potential impact of the dysphagia on the patient's respiratory health. In another case, a major feature of the dysphagia might be poor hypopharyngeal clearing. An appropriate summary would categorize the severity of the impairment, suggest its etiology in terms of pharyngeal function (weak pharyngeal constriction, inadequate hyoid/laryngeal elevation, poor PES opening), and remark on the increased risk of aspiration following the swallow. With the summary complete, recommendations from the team are enumerated. Presented in Table 18–2 are items our own team considers in determining each patient's risk and potential for oral eating.

It is extremely important that the plan be disseminated not just to caregivers in the patient's immediate environment, but to all those who are likely to be a part of the patient's life until, at least, re-evaluation is planned. If there are timing variables in the plan, that is, it has been recommended that the patient be on a liquid diet for a particular amount of time, then be advanced to a different diet, and so on, it will be critical to note the starting date of the plan in such a way that this information is not lost if the patient is moving from one setting to another. Members of the team who should be contacted in the event of a question regarding the treatment plan also need to be clearly indicated in the written version of the

Table 18–2. UCDavis: Potential and Risk for Oral Intake

Pt. Name _____ *MR#* _____ *Date* _____ **TOTAL:** _____

Diagnosis _____ *EAT* _____ *FOIS* _____

PROGNOSIS FOR ORAL EATING:

0. Stable   1. Improvement Expected   2. Decline Expected

DISEASE/CONDITION IMPACT ON EATING/DEGLUTITION:

1. Unclear/NA   1. Minimal/Mild   2. Moderate   3. Severe

PHYSICAL STATUS:

Positioning for Meals

1. Upright/Sitting   1. Assisted/Upright for Meals   2. Positioning Difficult

Oral Control

0. WNL   1. Reduced   2. Impaired

Oral Care   Dentition

0. WNL   1. Poor Oral Hygiene   0. WNL   1. Edentulous/Missing Teeth

Pulmonary Status

0. WNL   1. Sedentary/Min. Exercise   2. Hx Aspiration   3. Known Lung
                                             Pneumonia(s)   Disease

Nutritional Status   Eating Method

0. WNL   1. Malnourished/Obese   0. Oral   1. Some Oral/Tube   2. Non-oral

Aerodigestive Tissue Health

0. WNL   1. Dryness/Thick Secretions   2. Sensory Impairment   3. Markedly Altered
                                                                      (res., rad., fibrosis)

COGNITIVE STATUS:

0. Understands/Follows   1. Understands/Follows   2. Unable to Understand/
                                   with Assistance   Follow

SOCIAL STATUS:

0. Independent   1. Assisted with Good Support   2. Assisted with No/
                                                                  Marginal Support

FLUORO FINDINGS (15 to 20-cc bolus):

Bolus Mgmt (fluoro):   0. Full Range   1. Limited (1 to 3-cc)

Aspiration/Penetration   0. No asp/pen.   1. Asp/pen controlled with strategies
                                2. Asp not well-controlled

TPT (secs)	0. WNL	1. >1 sd	2. >2 sd
Hmax (cm)	0. WNL	1. <1 sd	2. <2 sd
PESmax (cm)	0. WNL	1. <1 sd	2. <2 sd
HL (cm)	0. WNL	1. <1 sd	2. <2 sd
PCR (cm^2)	0. WNL	1. >1 sd	2. >2 sd
PAhold (cm^2)	0. WNL	1. >1 sd	2. >2 sd

plan. In our setting, copies of the plan will be included in the patient's medical record, but will also be posted at bedside, included in hospital discharge plans, and provided to the patient's primary care and referring physicians. If a final report is not yet available prior to discharge, then oral or handwritten summaries are used. A particularly valuable practice is to encourage the patient, family members, and available caregivers to meet with one or more members of the team to review findings from the evaluation and to discuss the treatment plan at length. This investment in time and communication is typically educational for all participants and helps to ensure optimal implementation of the plan.

Recommendations for follow-up are included in the report, but it is the responsibility of the patient's referring physician to monitor the patient and determine the need for follow-up visits or re-evaluation. Few generalizations are possible regarding the timing of reevaluation, because this must be tailored to an individual patient. However, it is often dependent on meeting certain objectives or completing other treatments. For example, it may be recommended that a head and neck cancer patient return for re-evaluation when strategies for airway protection have been learned in therapy and can be consistently performed. Upon demonstration of this capability, changes in diet can be considered. In a patient recovering from stroke, on the other hand, timing of follow-up may be more related to a change in the patient's general condition, in particular, if the patient is more aware, or alert, or cognitively intact, then changes in diet may be appropriate. In other instances, it may be recom-

mended that a patient return for follow-up when other therapies have been completed. For example, a head and neck cancer patient who is undergoing postoperative radiation may need to return at the end of this treatment. Or a patient with myasthenia gravis may be asked to return when medical therapy for the condition is stabilized. Patients with feeding tubes need to be monitored, in particular, if it is likely/possible that they may be able to resume total oral eating. Whatever the individual circumstances, it is important that any changes from the treatment plan in effect be monitored carefully by the patient's caregivers, and that reevaluation be initiated when there is reason to suspect that the patient's capabilities have altered, for better or worse, in a way that raises new questions about the safety and efficiency of swallowing/food management.

In a busy clinical practice, it is easy to be so overwhelmed with the day to day problems of individual patients that there may be little provocation for retrospection about groups of patients. However, if we are to benefit from more than just repetition (i.e., performing dysphagia assessments on a large number of patients), it is necessary to build time into the schedule for scrutiny and critical review. One practice that has proved useful to our team is to periodically ask a question of ourselves, for example, how often have we observed a pseudovalleculae in laryngectomized patients, and are there similarities in these patients' surgical reconstructions, or how many of our head and neck cancer patients were swallowing without difficulty within 6 months of postoperative radiation therapy, and how many of these underwent dysphagia therapy? One or two team members typically assume responsibility for researching our records for relevant data, which are then presented in preliminary form to the team. The group discussions generated by these exercises have led to a better understanding of swallowing, particular patient populations, and surgical and medical variables that influence swallowing, and have even generated more formal research projects. Our approach to assessment and treatment is subject to continual change as a consequence of such retrospective review, hopefully in ways that advance our care of patients.

RECORD KEEPING

Our team evaluates and treats several hundred patients each year, and our disordered populations include neurogenic, head and neck cancer, pediatric and adult, and patients who are otherwise healthy with vague complaints of swallowing difficulty. In many cases, we follow patients over time and across multiple treatments. One tool that we have found of great value in managing the amount of "paperwork" generated by the team practice is the use of a computerized system that enables us to input patient information data, which can then be used for multiple purposes. The system, based on Microsoft's "Access" program for PC computers, required some time to learn, set up, and implement. In addition, forms for data input that would be applicable for all patients, allow us to input everything from case history interview information to measures made of dynamic swallow studies, and satisfy the various diverse interests of team members also required

repeated efforts. However, as appropriate input parameters and output report forms were finalized, the advantages of a database approach to record-keeping became quite clear. At this point, we are able to enter information about a patient once, use it in multiple reports, and revise only data that need updating when the patient is seen for follow-up. We are also able to query the database to identify patients who meet particular criteria, for example, all patients with vocal-fold paralyses seen from 2004 to 2007 who aspirated liquids but did well on other bolus consistencies. This capability has expedited our clinical work, particularly the time spent away from patients, and has also made the critical review process previously described much more comprehensive and expedient. Our ability to assess treatment outcomes in specific patient groups, or according to specific treatment variables, for example, has benefited greatly from this approach.

EVALUATING EFFECTS OF TIME/TREATMENT

As noted, many patients are followed over time and treatments by our team. It is imperative that we have good, that is, valid, reliable, assessment tools not only to diagnose dysphagia, but also to track change in our patients. An excellent way to do this is to examine *biomechanical* measures of swallow before and after treatments, or across time. The dynamic swallow study (DSS) has proven to be an integral part of our repertoire in treatment evaluation, allowing us to quantify changes in bolus transit times, swallow gesture times, and structural displacements associated with our interventions in a standardized manner. We have used this tool to assess effects of behavioral therapies, medical management strategies, and various surgeries. We have also used the DSS to help monitor changes in patients with, for example, degenerative conditions that may eventually require them to consider nonoral methods of eating. Manometry is a related biomechanical tool used to document changes in swallowing pressures associated with time or treatment (discussed in Chapter 13).

Other observations from fluoroscopy studies do not provide quantitative data pertinent to bolus transit timing or swallow gesture displacements, but do provide insights into swallowing function, including, simply, the presence of aspiration or penetration. Aspiration may be seen on an initial study and be absent on a subsequent study. The Penetration-Aspiration Scale is an ordinal scale that provides a more objective rating of these subjective observations, including the extent of bolus entry into the airway, and the patient's ability to respond/clear this stimulus (Rosenbek, Robbins, Roecker, Coyle, & Wood, 1996).

Additional evidence of the effects of time/treatment may be based on other types of *imaging studies*. For example, a chest x-ray that helped document aspiration pneumonia also provides evidence of lung recovery. Endoscopy of the pharynx, larynx (see Chapter 11), and/or the esophagus (see Chapter 13) is another imaging tool that can be used to monitor a patient's progress with behavioral, medical or surgical interventions. *Laboratory studies* are frequently a part of treatment assessment. For example, a CBC (complete blood count) can establish or rule out an infectious or inflammatory disease, and a

nutritional evaluation may include the determination of serum protein and albumin levels (see Chapter 10) important to improved nutrition. *Special studies* include pH testing to monitor the effects of medication or surgery on reflux events (see Chapter 6), and scintigraphy, used to determine percent of bolus material aspirated.

Many other criteria can be included in assessing outcomes. *Clinical evidence* of a patient's ability to move from nonoral to oral feeding, reductions in time required for oral feeding, or in restrictions necessary for oral eating, are examples of extremely useful variables to consider in assessment. Stable weight or weight gain, normal temperatures, and improved ability to manage saliva are similarly useful as signs of a patient's improving condition. Measures that incorporate patients' own appraisals of their eating or swallowing abilities are increasingly recognized as important. These might be classified as *self-assessment* tools. One that was developed at our institution and is used routinely is the EAT-10 (Belafsky, Mouadeb, Rees, Pryor, Postma, Allen, & Leonard, 2008). The American Speech-Language Hearing Association has developed the NOMS (National Outcomes Measurement System) that includes a section on dysphagia and assesses patients' functional progress and satisfaction with their progress (American Speech-Language-Hearing Association, http://www.asha.org). Two additional survey tools that have undergone extensive development are the SWAL-QOL (swallowing quality of life) and SWAL-CARE (swallowing quality of care) (McHorney, Bricker, Kramer, Rosenbek, Robbins, Chignell, Logemann, & Clarke, 2000; McHorney,

Bricker, Robbins, Kramer, & Rosenbek, 2000; McHorney, Robbins, Lomax, Rosenbek, Chignell, Kramer, & Bricker, 2002). These instruments are designed for patients with oropharyngeal dysphagia, and involve the completion of a set of questions pertinent to social, psychological, and cultural domains of swallowing/eating function, and to patients' perceptions of the quality of care received for their dysphagia. In a recent study (McHorney, Martin-Harris, Robbins, & Rosenbek, 2006), associations between the two survey tools and results of videofluoroscopy studies were examined in 386 patients. The Penetration Aspiration Scale previously referenced was used to evaluate the fluoroscopy studies. Interestingly, though not surprising to clinicians, relationships between the surveys and the Penetration Aspiration Scale were generally weak. The authors suggest this reflects evidence not only of a generally recognized lack of covariance between patient-based measures of function and clinician-based measures, but also, the need to consider both in evaluating treatment effects. This is a point well-taken, in our opinion. No single test, study, or opinion is likely to adequately and accurately assess changes with time or treatment.

THE TEAM APPROACH

Nowhere is the advantage of a multidisciplinary approach to dysphagia assessment more obvious than in the team-developed treatment plan. Etiologies of dysphagia cross many disease and disorder categories. The bodily systems that contribute to, or are affected by, dysphagia are extensive in number, and

complex. Potential treatments range from medical, to surgical, to behavioral. And the implications of dysphagia for an individual's physical, mental, and social well-being can be enormous. An effective treatment plan must reflect this understanding of the dysphagia gestalt, and this requires, in our opinion, as many relevant and thoughtful specialty resources as we can bring to bear. The likelihood of failing to recognize salient features of either the patient or the disorder is minimized, and the likelihood of developing an appropriate model for treatment is maximized. To some extent, of course, the effectiveness of a team is determined by the relative strengths of each member, and by the interprofessional dynamics present in team activities. But the opportunity to share expertise, to formulate objectives for treatment that reflect each specialist's concerns and knowledge base, and to then collectively prioritize the components of the plan, is well worth the effort required to establish a team and to maintain whatever diligence is necessary to ensure that it functions effectively as a team.

STUDY QUESTIONS

1. What factors, beyond the results of instrumental evaluations, should be considered in making treatment recommendations for a patient?
2. What are some of the indications for recommending exercises designed to improve strength or mobility of structures?
3. Would respiratory exercises ever be considered appropriate for a patient with dysphagia? Under what circumstances?

4. What is the "IOPI"? The Shaker exercise? What are they designed to do? Is there evidence to support their effectiveness?

5. How might electrical stimulation affect a muscle? What is meant by "selective stimulation"?

6. What characteristics of a bolus might be manipulated to facilitate swallow?

7. What are "postural compensations," and how might they facilitate swallow?

8. Do "facilitative maneuvers" require more from a patient than other strategies? Why? What are some of these maneuvers, and why/when would each be implemented?

9. What behavioral recommendations to patients are typically included in reflux management?

10. What might be useful treatments in managing xerostomia?

11. Which of the following might benefit from a surgical procedure? What kind of procedure(s)?
    a. Oral closure defects.
    b. Velopharyngeal valve failure.
    c. Reduced pharyngoesophageal opening size.
    d. Esophageal stricture.

12. What types of assessment tools might be useful in determining the effects of time or treatment?

REFERENCES

Alexander, R. (1987). Oral-motor treatment for infants and young children with cerebral palsy. In E. Mysak (Ed.), *Seminars in speech and language* (pp. 87–100). New York, NY: Thieme.

Ali, G., Laundl, T., Wallace, K., deCarle, D., & Cook, I. (1996). Influence of cold stimulation on the normal pharyngeal swallow response. *Dysphagia, 11*, 2–8.

Allen, J., White, C. J., Leonard, R., & Belafsky, P. C. (2011). Effects of cricopharyngeus muscle surgery on the pharynx. *Laryngoscope, 120*, 1498–1503.

Anthony, J. P., Singer, M. I., & Mathes, S. J. (1994). Pharyngoesophageal reconstruction using the tubed free radial forearm flap. *Clinics in Plastic Surgery, 21*, 137–147.

Arvedson, J., Clark, H., Lazarus, C., Schooling, T., & Frymark, T. (2010a). Evidence-based systematic review: Effects of oral motor interventions on feeding and swallowing in preterm infants. *American Journal of Speech-Language Pathology, 19*, 321–340.

Arvedson, J., Clark, H., Lazarus, C., Schooling, T., & Frymark, T. (2010b). The effects of oral-motor exercises on swallowing in children: An evidence-based systematic review. *Developmental Medicine and Child Neurology, 52*, 1000–1013.

Ashford, J., McCabe, D., Wheeler-Hegland, K., Frymark, T., Mullen, R., Musson, N., . . . Hammond, C. S. (2009). Evidence-based systematic review: Oropharyngeal dysphagia behavioral treatments. Part III—impact of dysphagia treatments on populations with neurological disorders. *Journal Rehabilitation Research Development, 46*, 185–194.

Babb, R. R., Notarangelo, J., & Smith, V. W. (1970). Wheezing: A clue to gastroesophageal reflux. *American Journal of Gastroenterology, 53*, 230–233.

Barbay, S., Plautz, E. J., Friel, K. M., Frost, S. B., Dancause, N., Stowe, A. M., & Nudo, R. J. (2006). Behavioral and neurophysiological effects of delayed training following a small ischemic infarct in primary motor cortex of squirrel monkeys. *Experimental Brain Research, 169*, 106–116.

Behan, M., Moeser, A. E., Thomas, C. F., Russell, J. A., Wang, H., Leverson, G. E., & Connor, N. P. (2012). The effect of tongue exercise on serotonergic input to the hypoglossal nucleus in young and old rats. *Journal of Speech Language and Hearing Research, 55*, 919–929.

Belafsky, P. C. (2010). Manual control of the upper esophageal sphincter. *Laryngoscope, Supplement 1,* S1–S16.

Belafsky, P. C., Mouadeb, D. A., Rees, C. J., Pryor, J. C., Postma, G. N., Allen, J., & Leonard, R. J. (2008). Validity and reliability of the Eating Assessment Tool (EAT-10). *Annals of Otology, Rhinology, and Laryngology, 117,* 919–924.

Benninger, M. S., Crumley, R. L., Ford, C. N., Gould, W. J., Hanson, D. G., Ossoff, R. H., & Sataloff, R. T. (1994). Evaluation and treatment of the unilateral paralyzed vocal fold. *Otolaryngology-Head and Neck Surgery, 111,* 497–508.

Beom, J., Kim, S. J., & Han, T. R. (2011). Electrical stimulation of the suprahyoid muscles in brain-injured patients with dysphagia: A pilot study. *Annals of Rehabilitation Medicine, 35,* 322–327.

Bisch, E. M., Logemann, J. A., Rademaker, A. W., Kahrilas, P. J., & Lazarus. C. L. (1994). Pharyngeal effects of bolus volume, viscosity, and temperature in patients with dysphagia resulting from neurologic impairment and in normal subjects. *Journal of Speech and Hearing Research, 37,* 1041–1049.

Blakely, R. W. (1960). Temporary speech prostheses as an aid in speech therapy. *Cleft Palate Bulletin, 10,* 63–65.

Blakely, R. W. (1964). The complementary use of speech prostheses and pharyngeal flaps in palatal insufficiency. *Cleft Palate Journal, 2,* 194–198.

Blakely, R. W. (1969). The rationale for a temporary speech prosthesis in palatal insufficiency. *British Journal of Disorders of Communication, 4,* 134–139.

Blakely, R., & Porter, D. (1971). Unexpected reduction and removal of an obturator in a patient with palate paralysis. *British Journal of Disorders of Communication, 6,* 33–36.

Blumenfeld, L., Hahn, Y., Lepage, A., Leonard, R., & Belafsky, P. C. (2006). Transcutaneous electrical stimulation versus traditional dysphagia therapy: A non-concurrent cohort study. *Otolaryngology-Head and Neck Surgery, 135,* 754–757.

Bodén, K., Hallgren, A., & Witt Hedström, H. (2006). Effects of three different swallow maneuvers analyzed by videomanometry. *Acta Radiologica, 47,* 628–633.

Bodin, I. K., Lind, M. G., & Arnander, C. (1994). Free radial forearm flap reconstruction in surgery of the oral cavity and pharynx: Surgical complications, impairment of speech and swallowing. *Clinics in Otolaryngology, 19,* 28–34.

Bulow, M., Olsson, R., & Ekberg, O. (2003). Videoradiographic analysis of how carbonated thin liquids and thickened liquids affect the physiology of swallowing in subjects with aspiration on thin liquids. *Acta Radiologica, 44,* 366–372.

Burkhead, L. M., Sapienza, C. M., & Rosenbek, J. (2007). Strength-training exercise in dysphagia rehabilitation: Principles, procedures, and directions for future research. *Dysphagia, 22,* 251–265.

Burnett, T. A., Mann, E. A., Cornell, S. A., & Ludlow, C. L. (2003). Laryngeal elevation achieved by neuromuscular stimulation at rest. *Journal of Applied Physiology, 94,* 128–134.

Burnett, T. A., Mann, E. A., Stocklosa, J. B., &, Ludlow, C. L. (2005). Self-triggered functional electrical stimulation during swallowing. *Journal of Neurophysiology, 94,* 4011–4018.

Carnaby-Mann, G., & Crary, M. A. (2007). Examining the evidence on neuromuscular electrical stimulation for swallowing: A meta-analysis. *Archives of Otolaryngology-Head and Neck Surgery, 133,* 564–571.

Carnaby-Mann, G., & Crary, M. A. (2008). Adjunctive neuromuscular electrical stimulation for treatment-refractory dysphagia. *Annals of Otology Rhinology and Laryngology, 117,* 279–287.

Carnaby-Mann, G., Crary, M. A., Schmalfuss, I., & Amdur, R. (2012, June 17). Effects of Mendelsohn maneuver on measures of swallowing duration post stroke. *Dysphagia.* (Epub ahead of print)

Carroll, T., Rosen, C., & Soose, R. J. (2011). Unilateral vocal fold paralysis and treatment. Available at eMedicine.medscape.com/article/863779.

Cerny, F., & Burton, H. (2001). *Exercise physiology for health care professionals.* Champaigne, IL: Human Kinetics.

Clark, H. M. (2003). Neuromuscular treatments for speech and swallowing: a tutorial. *American Journal of Speech-Language Pathology, 12,* 400–415.

Clark, H., Lazarus, C., Arvedson, J. Schooling, T., & Frymark, T. (2009). Evidence-based systematic review: Effect of neuromuscular electrical stimulation on swallowing and neural activation. *American Journal of Speech-Language Pathology, 18,* 361–375.

Cook, I. J., Dodds, W. J., Dantas, R. O., Massey, B., Kern, M. K., Lang, I. M., . . . Hogan, W. J. (1989). Opening mechanism of the human upper esophageal sphincter. *American Journal of Physiology, 257,* G748–G759.

Doeltgen, S. H., Macrae, P., & Huckabee, M. L. (2011). Pharyngeal pressure generation during tongue-hold swallows across age groups. *American Journal of Speech-Language Pathology, 20,* 124–130.

Duclone, A., Van Devenne, A., & Jovin, H. (1987). Gastroesophageal reflux in patients with asthma and chronic bronchitis. *American Review of Respiratory Disease, 135,* 327–332.

Easterling, C., Grande, B., Kern, M., Sears, K., & Shaker, R. (2005). Attaining and maintaining isometric and isokinetic goals of the Shaker exercise. *Dysphag*ia, *20,* 133–138.

Ellis, F. H. (1995). Pharyngoesophageal (Zenker's) diverticulum. *Advances in Surgery, 28,* 171–189.

El Sharkawi, A., Ramig, L., Logemann J. A., Pauloski, B. R., Rademaker, A. W., Smith, . . . Werner, C. (2002). Swallowing and voice effects of Lee Silverman Voice Treatment: A pilot study. *Journal of Neurology, Neurosurgery and Psychiatry, 72,* 31–36.

Foley, N., Teasell, R., Salter, K., Kruger, E., & Martino, R. (2008). Dysphagia treatment post stroke: A systematic review of randomized controlled trials. *Age and Ageing, 37,* 258–264.

Fraser, C., Power, M., Hamdy, S., Rothwell, J., Hobday, D., Hollander, I., . . . Thompson, D. (2002). Driving plasticity in human adult motor cortex is associated with improved motor function after brain injury. *Neuron, 30,* 831–840.

Freed, M. L., Freed, L., Chatburn, R. L., & Christian, M. (2001). Electrical stimulation for swallowing disorders caused by stroke. *Respiratory Care, 46,* 466–474.

Fucile, S., Gisel, E. G., McFarland, D. H., & Lau, C. (2011). Oral and non-oral sensorimotor interventions enhance oral feeding performance in preterm infants. *Developmental Medicine and Child Neurology, 53,* 829–835.

Fucile, S., Gisel, E. G., McFarland, D. H., & Lau, C. (2012). Oral and nonoral sensorimotor interventions facilitate suck-swallow-respiration functions and their coordination in preterm infants. *Early Human Development, 88,* 345–350.

Fujiu, M., & Logemann, J. A. (1996). Effect of a tongue-holding maneuver on posterior pharyngeal wall movement during deglutition. *American Journal of Speech Language Pathology, 5,* 23–30.

Fujiu, M., Toleikis, R., Logemann, J. A., & Larson, C. R. (1994). Glossopharyngeal evoked potential in normal subjects following mechanical stimulation of the anterior faucial pillar. *Electroencephalography and Clinical Neurophysiology, 92,* 183–195.

Furuta, T., Takemura, M., Tsujita, J., & Oku, Y. (2012). Interferential electric stimulation applied to the neck increases swallowing frequency. *Dysphagia, 27,* 94–100.

Gillis, R., & Leonard, R. (1983). Prosthetic treatment for speech and swallowing in patients with total glossectomy. *Journal of Prosthetic Dentistry, 50,* 808–814.

Gobbo, O. L., & O'Mara, S. M. (2005). Exercise, but not environmental enrichment, improves learning after kainic acid-induced hippocampal neurodegeneration in association with an increase in brain-derived neurotrophic factor. *Behavioural Brain Research, 159,* 21–26.

Gow, D., Rothwell, J., Hobson, A., Thompson, D., & Hamdy, S. (2004). Induction of long-term plasticity in human swallowing cortex following repetitive cortical stimulation. *Clinics in Neurophysiology, 115,* 1044–1051.

Gross, R. D., Mahlmann, J., & Grayhack, J. P. (2003). Physiologic effects of open and closed tracheostomy tubes on the pharyngeal swallow. *Annals of Otology, Rhinology and Laryngology, 112,* 143–152.

Hamdy, S., Aziz, Q., Rothwell, J. C., Hobson, A., & Thompson, D. G. (1998). Sensorimotor modulation of human cortical swallowing pathways. *Journal of Physiology, 506,* 857–866.

Harries, M. L. (1996). Unilateral vocal fold paralysis: A review of the current methods of surgical rehabilitation. *Journal of Laryngology and Otology, 110,* 11–16.

Heck, F. M., Doeltgen, S. H., & Huckabee, M. L. (2012, March 5). Effects of submental neuromuscular electrical stimulation on pharyngeal pressure generation. *Archives of Physical Medicine Rehabilitation,* Mar. 5, (Epub ahead of print)

Hind, J. A., Nicosia, M. A., Roecker, E. B., Carnes, M. L, & Robbins, J. (2001). Comparison of effortful and noneffortful swallows in healthy middle-aged and older adults. *Archives of Physical Medicine Rehabilitation, 55,* M634–M640.

Hiss, S. G., & Huckabee, M. L. (2005). Timing of pharyngeal and upper esophageal sphincter pressures as a function of normal and effortful swallowing in young healthy adults. *Dysphagia, 20,* 149–156.

Huckabee, M. L. (2007). Maximizing rehabilitative efforts for dysphagia recovery: SEMG biofeedback monitoring. *Kay Elemetrics: Swallowing application notes.* Pinehurst, NJ: KayPentax.

Humbert, I. A., Michou, E., Macrae, P. R., & Crujido, L. (2012) Electrical stimulation and swallowing: how much do we know? *Seminars in Speech and Language, 33,* 203–216.

Humbert, I. A., Poletto, C. J., Saxon, K. G., Kearny, P. R., Crujido, L., Wright-Harp, W., . . . Ludlow C. L. (2006). The effect of surface electrical stimulation on hyolaryngeal movement in normal individuals at rest and during swallowing. *Journal of Applied Physiology, 101,* 1657–1663.

Hummel, F., Celnik, P., Giraux, P., Floel, A., Wu, W. H., Gerloff, C., & Cohen, L. G. (2005). Effects of non-invasive cortical stimulation on skilled motor function in chronic stroke. *Brain, 128,* 490–499.

Jacob, P., Kahrilas, P. J., Logemann, J. A., Shah, V., & Ha, T. (1989). Upper esophageal sphincter opening and modulation during swallowing. *Gastroenterology, 97,* 1469–1478.

Johnson, R., McKenzie, S., Rosenquist, J., Lieberman, J., & Sievers, A. (1992). Dysphagia following stroke: Quantitative evaluation of pharyngeal transit times. *Archives of Physical Medicine and Rehabilitation, 73,* 419–423.

Kaatzke-McDonald, M., Post, E., & Davis, P. (1996). The effects of cold, touch, and chemical stimulation of the anterior faucial pillar on human swallowing. *Dysphagia, 11,* 198–206.

Kagaya, H., Baba, M., Saitoh, E., Okada, S., Yokoyama, M., & Muraoka, Y. (2011). Hyoid bone and larynx movements during electrical stimulation of motor points in laryngeal elevation muscles: A preliminary study. *Neuromodulation, 14,* 278–283.

Kagel, M., & Leopold, N. A. (1992). Dysphagia in Huntington's disease: A 16-year retrospective. *Dysphagia, 7,* 106–114.

Kahrilas, P., Logemann, J. A., Krugler, C., & Flanagan, E. (1991). Volitional augmentation of upper esophageal sphincter opening during swallowing. *American Journal of Physiology, 260,* G450–G456.

Khedr, E. M., Abo-Elfetoh, N., & Rothwell, J. C. (2009). Treatment of post-stroke dysphagia with repetitive transcranial magnetic stimulation. *Acta Neurologica Scandinavia, 119*, 155–161.

Kleim, K. A., Jones, T. A., & Schallert, T. (2003). Motor enrichment and the induction of plasticity before or after brain injury. *Neurochemical Research, 28*, 1757–1769.

Knauer, C. M., Castell, J. A., Dalton, C. B., Nowak, L., & Castell, D. O. (1990). Pharyngeal/upper esophageal sphincter pressure dynamics in humans. Effects of pharmacologic agents and thermal stimulation. *Digestive Diseases and Sciences, 35*, 774–780.

Koessler, W., Wanke, T., Winkler, G., Nader, A., Toifl, K., Kurz, H., & Zwick, H. (2001). 2 years' experience with inspiratory muscle training in patients with neuromuscular disorders. *Chest, 120*, 765–769.

Kumar, S., Wagner, C. W., Frayne, C., Zhu, L., Feng, W., & Schlaug, G. (2011) Noninvasive brain stimulation may improve stroke-related dysphagia: A pilot study. *Stroke, 42*, 1035–1040.

Lazarus, C. (2006). Tongue strength and exercise in healthy individuals and in head and neck cancer patients. *Seminars in Speech and Language: New Frontiers in Dysphagia Rehabilitation, 27*, 260–267.

Lazarus, C., Logemann, J. A., & Gibbons, P. (1993). Effects of maneuvers on swallowing function in a dysphagic oral cancer patient. *Head and Neck Surgery, 15*, 419–424.

Lazarus, C., Logemann, J. A., Song, C. W., Rademaker, A. W., & Kahrilas, P. J. (2002). Effects of voluntary maneuvers on tongue base function for swallowing. *Folia Phoniatrica et Logopaedica, 54*, 171–176.

Lazzara, G., Lazarus, C., & Logemann, J. A. (1986). Impact of thermal stimulation on the triggering of the swallow reflex. *Dysphagia, 1*, 73–77.

Leelamanit, V., Limsakul, C., & Geater, A. (2002). Synchronized electrical stimulation in treating pharyngeal dysphagia. *Laryngoscope, 112*, 2204–2210.

Logemann, J. A. (1983). *Evaluation and treatment of swallowing disorders*. San Diego, CA: College-Hill Press.

Logemann, J. A. (1997). Therapy for oropharyngeal swallowing disorders. In A. L. Perlman & K. Schulze-Delrieu (Eds.), *Deglutition and its disorders: Anatomy, physiology, clinical diagnosis, and management* (pp. 449–462). San Diego, CA: Singular.

Logemann, J. A., Kahrilas, P. J., Hurst, P., Davis, J., & Krugler, C. (1989). Effects of intraoral prosthetics on swallowing in patients with oral cancer. *Dysphagia, 4*, 118–120.

Logemann, J. A., Kahrilas, P. J., Kobara, M., & Vakil, B. (1989). The benefit of head rotation on pharyngoesophageal dysphagia. *Archives of Physical Medicine and Rehabilitation, 70*, 767–771.

Logemann, J. A., Pauloski, B. R., Colangelo, L., Lazarus, C., Fujiu, M., & Kahrilas, P. J. (1995). Effects of a sour bolus on oropharyngeal swallowing measures in patients with neurogenic dysphagia. *Journal of Speech and Hearing Research, 38*, 556–563.

Ludlow, C., Bielamowicz, S., Daniels Rosenberg, M., Abvalavanar, R., Rossini, K., Gillespie, . . . Carraro, U. (2000). Chronic intermittent stimulation of the thyroarytenoid muscle maintains dynamic control of glottal adduction. *Muscle and Nerve, 23*, 44–57.

Ludlow, C. L., Humbert, I., Saxon, J., Poletto, C., Sonies, B., & Crujido, L. (2007). Effects of surface electrical stimulation on hyolaryngeal movements in normal individuals at rest and during swallowing. *Dysphagia, 101*, 1657–1663.

Martin, B. (1994). Treatment of dysphagia in adults. In L. R. Cherney (Ed.), *Clinical management of dysphagia in adults and children* (Chap. 6). Frederick, MD: Aspen.

McBride, M. A., & Ergun, G. A. (1994). The endoscopic management of esophageal strictures. *Gastrointestinal Endoscopy Clinics of North America, 4*, 595–621.

McCabe, D., Ashford, J., Wheeler-Hegland, K., Frymark, T., Mullen, R., Musson, N., . . . Schooling, T. (2009). Evidence-based systematic review: Oropharyngeal dysphagia behavioral treatments. Part IV —impact of dysphagia treatment on individuals' postcancer treatments. *Journal Rehabilitation Research Development*, *46*, 205–214.

McCullough, G. H., Kamarunas, E., Mann, G. C., Schmidley, J. W., Robbins, J. A., & Crary, M. A. (2012). Effects of Mendelsohn maneuver on measures of swallowing duration post stroke. *Topics in Stroke Rehabilitation*, *19*, 234–243.

McHorney, C., Bricker, D., Kramer, A., Rosenbek, J., Robbins, J., Chignell, K. A., . . . Clarke, C., (2000). The SWAL-QOL outcomes tool for oropharyngeal dysphagia in adults: I. Conceptual foundation and item development. *Dysphagia*, *15*, 115–121.

McHorney, C., Bricker, D., Robbins, J., Kramer, A., Rosenbek, J., & Chignell, K. (2000). The SWAL-QOL outcomes tool for oropharyngeal dysphagia in adults: II. Item reduction and preliminary scaling. *Dysphagia*, *15*, 122–133.

McHorney, C., Martin-Harris, B., Robbins, J., & Rosenbek, J. (2006). Clinical validity of the SWAL-QOL and SWAL-CARE outcome tools with respect to bolus flow measures. *Dysphagia*, *21*, 141–148.

McHorney, C., Robbins, J., Lomax, K., Rosenbek, J., Chignell, K., Kramer, A., & Bricker, D. E. (2002). The SWAL-QOL and SWAL-CARE outcomes tool for oropharyngeal dysphagia in adults: III Documentation of reliability and validity. *Dysphagia*, *17*, 97–114.

McKenna, J. A., & Dedo, H. (1992). Cricopharyngeal myotomy. *Annals of Otology, Rhinology and Laryngology*, *101*, 216–221.

Mepani, R., Antonik, S., Massey, B., Kern, M., Logemann, J., Pauloski, B., . . . Shaker, R. (2009). Augmentation of deglutitive thyrohyoid muscle shortening by the Shaker exercise. *Dysphagia*, *24*, 26–31.

Meyer, G. W., & Castell, D. O. (1983). Anatomy and physiology of the esophageal body. In D. O. Castell & L. F. Johnson (Eds.), *Esophageal function in health and disease* (pp. 1–15). New York, NY: Elsevier Science.

Morris, H. L., Bardach, J., Jones, D., Christiansen, J. L., & Gray, S. D. (1995). Clinical results of pharyngeal flap surgery: The Iowa experience. *Plastic and Reconstructive Surgery*, *95*, 652–661.

Morris, S. E., & Klein, M. D. (1987). *Prefeeding skills: A comprehensive resource for feeding development.* Tuscon, AZ: Therapy Skill Builders.

Nudo, R. (2003). Adaptive plasticity in motor cortex: Implications for rehabilitation after brain injury. *Journal of Rehabilitative Medicine*, *41*(Suppl.), 7–10.

Nudo, R. (2005). Neural plasticity and functional recovery following cortical ischemic injury. *Conference Proceedings, IEEE Engineering in Medicine and Biology Society*, *4*, 4145–4148.

Nudo, R. (2007). Postinfarct cortical plasticity and behavioral recovery. *Stroke*, *38*, 840–845.

Nudo, R., & Friel, K. M. (1999). Cortical plasticity after stroke: Implications for rehabilitation. *Revue Neurologique* (Paris), *155*, 713–717.

Ogura, E., Matsuyama, M., Goto, T. K, Nakamura, Y., & Koyano, K. (2012). Brain activation during oral exercises used for dysphagia rehabilitation in healthy human subjects: A functional magnetic resonance imaging study. *Dysphagia*, *26*, 353–360.

Oh, J. C., Park, J. W., Cha, T. H., Woo, H. S., & Kim, D. K. (2012). Exercise using tongue-holding swallow does not improve swallowing function in normal subjects. *Journal of Speech and Hearing Research*, *38*, 110–123.

Palmer, P. M., McCulloch, T. M., Jaffe, D., & Neel, A. T. (2005). Effects of a sour bolus on the intramuscular electromyographic (EMG) activity of muscles in the submental region. *Dysphagia*, *20*, 210–217.

Pauloski, B. R., Logemann, J. A., Fox, J. C., & Colangelo, L. A. (1995). Biomechanical analysis of the pharyngeal swallow in postsurgical patients with anterior tongue and floor of mouth resection and distal flap reconstruction. *Journal of Speech and Hearing Research, 38,* 110–123.

Pelletier, C. A., & Lawless, H. T. (2003). Effect of citric acid and citric acid-sucrose mixtures on swallowing in neurogenic oropharyngeal dysphagia. *Dysphagia, 18,* 231–241.

Pitts, T., Bolser, D., Rosenbek, J., Troche, M., Okun, M. S., & Sapienza, C. (2009). Impact of expiratory muscle strength training on voluntary cough and swallow function in Parkinson disease. *Chest, 135,* 1301–1308.

Power, M., Fraser, C., Hobson, A., Rothwell, J. C., Mistry, S., Nicholson, D. A., . . . Hamdy, S. (2004). Changes in pharyngeal corticobulbar excitability and swallowing behavior after oral stimulation. *American Journal of Physiology-Gastrointestinal and Liver Physiology, 286,* G45–G50.

Riley, R. W., Powell, N. B., & Guilleminault, C. (1994). Obstructive sleep apnea and the hyoid: A revised surgical procedure. *Otolaryngology-Head and Neck Surgery, 111,* 717–721.

Robbins, J., Gangnon, R., Theis, S., Kays, S. A., & Hind, J. (2005). The effects of lingual exercise on swallowing in older adults. *Journal of the American Geriatric Society, 53,* 1483–1489.

Rosenbek, J. C., Robbins, J., Fishback, B., & Levine, R. (1991). Effects of thermal application in dysphagia after stroke. *Journal of Speech and Hearing Research, 34,* 1257–1267.

Rosenbek, J. C., Robbins, J. A., Roecker, E. B., Coyle, J. L., & Wood, J. L. (1996). A penetration-aspiration scale. *Dysphagia, 11,* 93–98.

Rosenthal, S., Sheppard, J. J., & Lotze, M. (1995). *Dysphagia in the child with developmental disabilities: Medical, clinical and family interventions.* San Diego, CA: Singular.

Sapienza, C., & Wheeler, K. (2006). Respiratory muscle strength training: Functional outcomes versus plasticity. *Seminars in Speech and Language, 27,* 236–244.

Schlaug, G., Renga, V., & Nair, D. (2008). Transcranial direct current stimulation in stroke recovery. *Archives of Neurology, 65,* 1571–1576.

Schmitz, J. P., Bitonti, D. A., & Lemke, R. R. (1996). Hyoid myotomy and suspension for obstructive sleep apnea syndrome. *Journal of Oral and Maxillofacial Surgery, 54,* 1339–1345.

Shaker, R., Easterling, K., Kern, M., Nitschke, T., Massey, D., Daniels, S., . . . Dikeman, K. (2002). Rehabilitation of swallowing by exercise in tube-fed patients with pharyngeal dysphagia secondary to abnormal UES opening. *Gastroenterology, 122,* 1314–1321.

Shaker, R., Kern, M., Bardan, E., Taylor, A., Stewart, E. T., Hoffmann, R. G., . . . Bonnevier, J. (1997). Augmentation of deglutitive upper esophageal sphincter opening in the elderly by exercise. *American Journal of Physiology, 272,* G1518–G1522.

Shaw, D. W., Cook, I. J., Jamieson, G. G., Gabb, M., Simula, M., & Dent, E. J. (1996). Influence of surgery on deglutitive upper oesophageal sphincter mechanics in Zenker's diverticulum. *Gut, 38,* 806–811.

Shelton, R., Lindquist, A., Arndt, W., Elbert, M., & Youngstrom, K. (1971). Effect of speech bulb reduction on movement of the posterior wall of the pharynx and posture of the tongue. *Cleft Palate Journal, 8,* 10–17.

Sher, A. E., Schechtman, K. B., & Piccirillo, J. F. (1996). The efficacy of surgical modifications of the upper airway in adults with obstructive sleep apnea syndrome. *Sleep, 19,* 156–177.

Silverman, E. P., Sapienza, C. M., Saleem, A., Carmichael, C., Davenport, P. W., Hoffman-Ruddy, B., & Okun, M. S. (2006). Tutorial on maximum inspiratory and expiratory mouth pressures in individuals with idiopathic Parkinson disease (IPD) and the preliminary results of an expiratory muscle strength training program. *NeuroRehabilitation, 21,* 71–79.

Sinclair, W. J. (1970). Initiation of reflex swallowing forms the naso- and oro-pharynx. *American Journal of Physiology, 218,* 956–959.

St. Guily, J. L., Moine, A., Perie, S., Bokowy, C., Angelard, B., & Chaussade, S. (1995). Role of pharyngeal propulsion as an indicator for upper esophageal sphincter myotomy. *Laryngoscope, 105,* 723–727.

St. Guily, J. L., Perie, S., Willig, T., Chaussade, S., Eymard, V., & Angelard, B. (1994). Swallowing disorders in muscular diseases: Functional assessment and indications of cricopharyngeal myotomy. *Ear, Nose and Throat Journal, 3,* 34–40.

Stathopoulos, E., & Duchan, J. F. (2006). History and principles of exercise-based therapy: How they inform our current treatment. *Seminars in Speech and Language: New Frontiers in Dysphagia Rehabilitation, 27,* 227–235.

Stepnick, D. W., & Hayden, R. E. (1994). Options for reconstruction of the pharyngoesophageal defect. *Otolaryngology Clinics of North America, 27,* 1151–1158.

Sullivan, P., Hind, J. A., & Roecker, E. B. (2001). Lingual exercise protocol for head and neck cancer: A case study [Abstract]. *Dysphagia, 16,* 154.

Troche, M. S., Okun, M. S., Rosenbek, J. C., Musson, N., & Fernandez, H. H. (2010). Aspiration and swallowing in Parkinson disease and rehabilitation with EMST: A randomized trial. *Neurology, 23,* 1912–1919.

Weiss, C. (1971). Success of an obturator reduction program. *Cleft Palate Journal, 6,* 291–297.

Wheeler, K. M., Chiara, T., & Sapienza, C. M. (2007). Surface electromyographic activity of the submental muscles during swallowing and during expiratory pressure threshold training tasks. *Dysphagia, 22,* 108–116.

Wheeler-Hagland, K. M., Rosenbek, J. C., & Sapienza, C. M. (2008). Submental sEMG and hyoid movement during Mendelsohn maneuver, effortful swallow, and expiratory muscle strength training. *Journal of Speech and Language Hearing Research, 51,* 1072–1087.

Wheeler, R., Logemann, J. A., & Rosen, M. (1980). Maxillary reshaping prostheses: Effectiveness in improving speech and swallowing in post-surgical oral cancer patients. *Journal of Prosthetic Dentistry, 43,* 313–319.

Wolff, K. D., Dienemann, D., & Hoffmeister, B. (1995). Intraoral defect coverage with muscle flaps. *Journal of Oral and Maxillofacial Surgery, 53,* 680–685.

Wong, R., & Johnson, L. F. (1983). Achalasia. In D. O. Castell & L. F. Johnson (Eds.), *Esophageal function in health and disease* (pp. 99–124). New York, NY: Elsevier Science.

Wong, L., & Weiss, C. (1972). A clinical assessment of obturator-wearing cleft palate patients. *Journal of Prosthetic Dentistry, 27,* 632–633.

Yip, H., Kendall, K. A., & Leonard, R. J. (2005). Cricopharyngeal myotomy normalizes the opening size of the upper esophageal sphincter in cricopharyngeal dysfunction. *Laryngoscope, 116,* 93–96.

Zide, B. M. (1990). Deformities of the lips and cheeks. In J. G. McCarthy (Ed.), *Plastic surgery* (Chap. 38). Philadelphia, PA: W. B. Saunders.

Index

Note: Page numbers in **bold** reference nontext material.